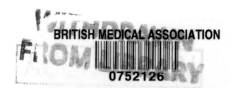

Evidence-Based
Pediatric Oncology

Evidence-Based Pediatric Oncology

Third Edition

Edited by

Ross Pinkerton, MB, BCh, BaO, MD

Executive Director, Division of Oncology
Royal Children's Hospital
Children's Health Queensland
Brisbane, QLD, Australia

Ananth Shankar, MD, FRCPCH

Consultant in Paediatric and Adolescent Oncology
University College London Hospitals NHS Foundation Trust
London, UK

Katherine K. Matthay, BA, MD

Mildred V. Strouss Professor of Translational Oncology
Director, Pediatric Hematology-Oncology
Department of Pediatrics
UCSF School of Medicine and
UCSF Benioff Children's Hospital
San Francisco, CA, USA

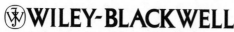
WILEY-BLACKWELL
A John Wiley & Sons, Ltd., Publication

BMJ|Books

Registered Office
John Wiley & Sons, Ltd, The Atrium, Southern Gate, Chichester, West Sussex, PO19 8SQ, UK

Editorial Offices
9600 Garsington Road, Oxford, OX4 2DQ, UK
The Atrium, Southern Gate, Chichester, West Sussex, PO19 8SQ, UK
111 River Street, Hoboken, NJ 07030-5774, USA

For details of our global editorial offices, for customer services and for information about how to apply for permission to reuse the copyright material in this book please see our website at www.wiley.com/wiley-blackwell

Library of Congress Cataloging-in-Publication Data

Evidence-based pediatric oncology / edited by Ross Pinkerton, Ananth Shankar, Katherine K. Matthay. – 3rd ed.
    p. ; cm.
  Includes bibliographical references and index.
  ISBN 978-0-470-65964-9 (hardback : alk. paper)
  I. Pinkerton, C. R. (C. Ross), 1950–   II. Shankar, A. G. (Ananth Gouri), 1962–   III. Matthay, Katherine.
  [DNLM: 1. Child–Case Reports.   2. Neoplasms–Case Reports.   3. Evidence-Based Medicine–Case Reports.   QZ 275]
  618.92′994–dc23
                                        2012044509

A catalogue record for this book is available from the British Library.

Wiley also publishes its books in a variety of electronic formats. Some content that appears in print may not be available in electronic books.

Cover image: High grade glioma imaged with ^{18}Fluorine PET MRI, photo reproduced courtesy of Professor AG Shankar
Cover design by Andy Meaden

Set in 9.5/12 pt Minion by SPi Publisher Services, Pondicherry, India
Printed and bound in Malaysia by Vivar Printing Sdn Bhd

1   2013

Contents

List of contributors, vii

Preface, ix

List of abbreviations, x

About the companion website, xv

Part 1: Solid tumors

1 Rhabdomyosarcoma, 3
Katherine K. Matthay
(Commentary by Meriel Jenney)

2 Osteosarcoma, 14
Katherine K. Matthay
(Commentary by Maria Michelagnoli)

3 Ewing sarcoma, 25
Katherine K. Matthay
(Commentary by Steven G. DuBois)

4 Wilms tumor, 34
Ananth Shankar
(Commentary by Kathy Pritchard-Jones)

5 Neuroblastoma, 47
Katherine K. Matthay
(Commentary by Katherine K. Matthay)

6 Hepatoblastoma, 58
Ross Pinkerton
(Commentary by Penelope Brock)

7 Malignant germ cell tumors, 65
Ross Pinkerton
(Commentary by Ross Pinkerton)

8 Medulloblastoma, 69
Ross Pinkerton
(Commentary by Eric Bouffet)

9 Glioma, 81
Ross Pinkerton
(Commentary by Joann L. Ater)

10 Non-Hodgkin lymphoma, 88
Ross Pinkerton
(Commentary by Ross Pinkerton)

11 Hodgkin lymphoma, 105
Ross Pinkerton
(Commentary by Cindy L. Schwartz)

Part 2: Leukemia

Section 1: Acute myeloid leukemia

12 Acute myeloid leukemia
commentary, 119
Robert J. Arceci

13 Remission induction in acute myeloid
leukemia, 126
Ananth Shankar

14 Acute myeloid leukemia
consolidation, 135
Ananth Shankar

15 Maintenance treatment in acute myeloid
leukemia, 137
Ananth Shankar

16 Autologous bone marrow transplantation
in acute myeloid leukemia, 141
Ananth Shankar

17 Acute myeloid leukemia:
miscellaneous, 144
Ananth Shankar

Section 2: Childhood lymphoblastic leukemia

18 Childhood lymphoblastic leukemia commentary, 146
   Vaskar Saha

19 Remission induction in childhood lymphoblastic leukemia, 154
   Ananth Shankar

20 Central nervous system-directed therapy in childhood lymphoblastic leukemia, 168
   Ananth Shankar

21 Maintenance treatment in childhood lymphoblastic leukemia, 180
   Ananth Shankar

22 Relapsed childhood lymphoblastic leukemia, 198
   Ananth Shankar

23 Postinduction therapy in adolescents and young adults with acute lymphoblastic leukemia, 204
   Ananth Shankar

Part 3: Supportive care in pediatric oncology

24 Colony-stimulating factors, 209
   Ananth Shankar
   (Commentary by Victoria Grandage)

25 Cardioprotection in pediatric oncology, 230
   Ananth Shankar
   (Commentary by Gill A. Levitt)

26 Infections in pediatric and adolescent oncology, 243
   Ananth Shankar and Sara Stoneham
   (Commentary by Julia E. Clark)

Index, 269

List of contributors

Robert J. Arceci

King Fahd Professor of Pediatric Oncology
Johns Hopkins University
Baltimore, MD, USA

Joann L. Ater

Professor, Department of Pediatrics Patient Care
Division of Pediatrics
The University of Texas
MD Anderson Cancer Center
Houston, TX, USA

Eric Bouffet

Garron Family Chair in Childhood Cancer Research
Director, Paediatric Neuro-Oncology Program
Professor of Paediatrics
Hospital for Sick Children
Toronto, ON, Canada

Penelope Brock

Consultant in Paediatric Oncology
Great Ormond Street Hospital
London, UK

Julia E. Clark

Consultant in Paediatric Infectious Diseases
Royal Children's Hospital
Children's Health Queensland
Brisbane, QLD, Australia

Steven G. DuBois

Associate Professor of Pediatrics
UCSF School of Medicine and
UCSF Benioff Children's Hospital
San Francisco, CA, USA

Victoria Grandage

Children and Young Peoples Cancer Service
University College London Hospitals NHS
Foundation Trust
London, UK

Meriel Jenney

Consultant Paediatric Oncologist
Children's Hospital for Wales
Cardiff, UK

Gill A. Levitt

Consultant in Paediatric Oncology and Late Effects
Great Ormond Street Hospital
London, UK

Katherine K. Matthay

Mildred V. Strouss Professor of Translational Oncology
Director, Pediatric Hematology-Oncology
Department of Pediatrics
UCSF School of Medicine and
UCSF Benioff Children's Hospital
San Francisco, CA, USA

Maria Michelagnoli

Children and Young People Cancer Service
University College London Hospitals NHS
Foundation Trust
London, UK

Ross Pinkerton

Executive Director, Division of Oncology
Royal Children's Hospital
Children's Health Queensland
Brisbane, QLD, Australia

Kathy Pritchard-Jones

Professor of Paediatric Oncology
ICH - Molecular Haematology and Cancer Biology
Department of Cancer
Faculty of Population Health Sciences
University College London
London, UK

Vaskar Saha

Professor of Paediatric Oncology
School of Cancer and Enabling Sciences
The University of Manchester
Manchester Academic Health Science Centre
The Christie NHS Foundation Trust
Manchester, UK

Cindy L. Schwartz

Alan G. Hassenfel Professor of Pediatrics
The Warren Alpert Medical School of Brown University
Director of Pediatric Hematology/Oncology
Department of Pediatrics
Hasbro Children's Hospital
Providence, RI, USA

Ananth Shankar

Consultant in Paediatric and Adolescent Oncology
University College London Hospitals NHS Foundation Trust
London, UK

Sara Stoneham

Paediatric and Adolescent Consultant Oncologist
University College London Hospitals NHS Foundation Trust
London, UK

Preface

The aim of this book is to summarize the information that is available from published randomized trials in childhood cancer. These data should not only provide a rational evidence base for the current practice but also demonstrate particular gaps in our knowledge and indicate which new studies should be a priority.

In recent years, the rate of improvement in outcomes for children's cancers has tended to reach a plateau and it has become increasingly important to design trials that ask explicit questions, are powered to be reliable, and will provide answers in a reasonable time. The high cure rates require large numbers of patients to demonstrate relatively small incremental improvement, in the case of therapeutic studies, or equivalence, where avoiding late effects through dose reduction is the goal.

Consequently, the pediatric oncology literature is littered with small single-arm "studies" and reports of what is essentially "best standard practice" which, whilst of interest, often fail to make progress.

Reluctance to run large randomized trials has resulted in the overuse of unproven strategies, sometimes with significant early and late morbidity, such as in the empirical application of very high-dose therapy with stem cell rescue in solid tumors other than neuroblastoma. It may also lead to the slow application of effective treatments.

Similarly, because of the small number of randomized trials in most childhood solid tumors, formal meta-analysis is often not possible. The Cochrane Childhood Cancer Group, set up in 2006 and based in Amsterdam, made a valiant attempt to address this issue (see www.thecochranelibrary.com for available reviews). Unfortunately, it has often been faced with a paucity of data or has had to rely on studies covering many decades during which time treatment has changed considerably and meta-analysis may, therefore, be less informative.

Much current practice is based on protocols that appear to produce the most favorable results in single-arm studies. Many are associated with significant early and late morbidity which subsequent randomized evaluation proves to have been unjustified. It is, therefore, of importance that all novel strategies are adequately evaluated before they become accepted as standard practice. It is hoped that the data in this book will provide ready access to background information for those involved in trial design and also be of value to those early in their oncology careers who should be aware of what studies have been done but find that most textbooks provide only minimal details of these trials.

This edition has focused on studies published since the completion of the second edition in 2007. The conclusions from the studies in the last two editions are outlined in specific sections. We have again been fortunate to have persuaded many well-known figures in children's cancer to add short commentaries to each section. These focus on the major conclusions from the studies presented and also on future research priorities.

Ross Pinkerton
2013

List of abbreviations

6-MP	6-mercaptopurine		ARAC	cytosine arabinoside
6-TG	6-thioguanine		ASCO	American Society of Clinical Oncology
			ASCT	autologous stem cell transplant
AA	anaplastic astrocytoma		ASN	asparagine
ABMT	autologous bone marrow transplantation		ASP	asparaginase
			AST	aspartate aminotransferase
ABVD	doxorubicin, bleomycin, vinblastine, dacarbazine		ATRA	all-trans-retinoic acid
			AVA	doxorubicin plus vincristine and actinomycin (VA)
ABVE	doxorubicin, bleomycin, vincristine, etoposide			
ABVE-PC	doxorubicin, bleomycin, vincristine, etoposide, prednisone, cyclophosphamide		B-ALL	B-cell acute lymphoblastic leukemia
			BCD	cisplatin or bleomycin, cyclophosphamide, actinomycin D
ACOMP	doxorubicin, cyclophosphamide, vincristine, methylprednisolone, prednisone		BEP	bleomycin, etoposide, cisplatin
			BFM	Berlin-Frankfurt-Münster
			BL	Burkitt lymphoma
ACOP	doxorubicin, cyclophosphamide, vincristine, prednisone		BLL	Burkitt-like lymphoma
			BM	bone marrow
ACT-D	actinomycin D		BMT	bone marrow transplant
AE	adverse events		BNHL	B-cell non-Hodgkin lymphoma
AFP	α-fetoprotein		BuMel	busulfan and melphalan
ALCL	anaplastic large cell lymphoma			
ALK	anaplastic lymphoma kinase		CAA	cancer-associated anemia
ALL	acute lymphoblastic leukemia		CAI	catheter-associated infection
allo-BMT	allogeneic bone marrow transplantation		CALGB	Cancer and Leukemia Group B
			cALL	common acute lymphoblastic leukemia
allo-SCT	allogeneic stem cell transplantation		CC	continuation chemotherapy
ALPN	allopurinol		CCF	congestive cardiac failure
ALT	alanine aminotransferase		CCR	continuous clinical remission
AML	acute myeloid leukemia		CCSG	Children's Cancer Study Group
ANC	absolute neutrophil count		CCSK	clear cell sarcoma of kidney
AOP	doxorubicin, vincristine, prednisone		CDI	chemotherapy dose intensity
AP	Adriamycin/cisplatin		CDR	clinical decision rules
APL	acute promyelocytic leukemia		CEM	melphalan, etoposide, carboplatin
APTT	activated partial thromboplastin time		CFRT	conventional fractionated radiotherapy

CHF	congestive heart failure	DNPS	*de novo* purine synthesis
CHOP	cyclophosphamide, doxorubicin, vincristine, prednisone	DNR	daunorubicin
		DT	disproportionate thrombocytopenia
CI	confidence interval, cumulative incidence		
CLDB	cladribine	ECHO	echocardiography
CML	chronic myeloid leukemia	ECOG	Eastern Co-operative Oncology Group
CNS	central nervous system	EF	extended field
COG	Children's Oncology Group	EFS	event-free survival
COJEC	cisplatin, vincristine, carboplatin, etoposide, cyclophosphamide	EOI	European Osteosarcoma Intergroup
		EORTC	European Organization for Research into Treatment of Cancer
COMP	cyclophosphamide, vincristine, methotrexate, prednisone	EPO	erythropoietin
COP	cyclophosphamide, vincristine, prednisolone	EpSSG	European Paediatric Soft Tissue Sarcoma Group
COPAD	cyclophosphamide, vincristine, prednisone, doxorubicin	ETPALL	early T precursor acute lymphoblastic leukemia
COPAdM	cyclophosphamide, vincristine, prednisolone, doxorubicin, and high-dose methotrexate with intrathecal methotrexate	EVAIA	vincristine, doxorubicin, dactinomycin, ifosfamide with the addition of etoposide
COPP	cyclophosphamide, vincristine, prednisone, procarbazine	FBN	febrile neutropenia
		FDG-PET	fluorodeoxyglucose positron emission tomography
CR	complete remission/response		
CRBSI	catheter-related bloodstream infection	FFS	failure-free survival
CRT	cranial irradiation	FH	favorable histology
CS	craniospinal	FLAG-Ida	fludarabine, cytarabine, GCSF, idarubicin
CsA	cyclosporine A		
CSF	cerebrospinal fluid; colony-stimulating factor	FUO	fever of unknown origin
CSRT	craniospinal radiotherapy	GBM	glioblastoma multiforme
CT	chemotherapy; computed tomography; continuing therapy	G-CSF	granulocyte colony-stimulating factor
		G-CSFR	granulocyte colony-stimulating factor receptor
CVC	central venous catheter		
CVPP	cyclophosphamide, vincristine, procarbazine, prednisone	GFR	glomerular filtration rate
		GM-CSF	granulocyte macrophage colony-stimulating factor
DA	daunorubicin and ARA-C	GO	gemtuzumab ozogamicin
DAT	daunomycin, cytarabine, thioguanine		
DD	divided dose	HAM	high-dose cytosine arabinoside and mitoxantrone
DEX	dexamethasone		
DFCI	Dana-Farber Cancer Institute	Hb	hemoglobin
DFS	disease-free survival	HB	hepatoblastoma
DI	delayed intensification	HCR	hematological remission
DIPG	diffuse intrinsic pontine glioma	Hct	hematocrit
DLBCL	diffuse large B-cell lymphoma	HD	Hodgkin disease
DLCL	diffuse large cell lymphoma	HDAT	high dose cytarabine, daunomycin, thioguanine
DMC	data monitoring committee		

HDCT	high-dose chemotherapy		LV	left ventricular
HD L-ASP	high-dose L-asparaginase		LVEF	left ventricular ejection fraction
HDMP	high-dose methylprednisolone			
HDMTX	high-dose methotrexate		MAP	methotrexate, doxorubicin, cisplatin
HIDAC	high-dose cytarabine and L-asparaginase		MDD	minimal detectable disease
			MDS	myelodysplastic syndrome
HL	Hodgkin lymphoma		M-EDTA	minocycline and edetic acid
HLA	human leukocyte antigen		MFS	metastasis-free survival
HPLC	high-performance liquid chromatography		MGCT	malignant germ cell tumor
			MLBCL	mediastinal large B-cell lymphoma
HR	hazard ratio, high-risk		MOPP	mustine, vincristine, procarbazine, prednisolone
HSCT	hematopoietic stem cell transplantation			
HVOD	hepatic veno-occlusive disease		MRC	Medical Research Council
HYFRT	hyperfractionated radiotherapy		MRD	minimal residual disease
HYSN	hydrocortisone		MRI	magnetic resonance imaging
			MRSA	methicillin-resistant *Staph. aureus*
IA	intra-arterial		MSK	musculoskeletal; Memorial Sloan-Kettering
IBI	invasive bacterial infection			
IC	intensive chemotherapy		MT	maintenance treatment
ID	intermediate dose		mTOR	mammalian target of rapamycin
IDA	idarubicin		MTP	muramyl tripeptide
IE	ifosfamide and etoposide		MTX	methotrexate
IF	involved field		MTXN	mitoxantrone
IFI	invasive fungal infection		MTX/VCR	methotrexate and vincristine
IGF-1R	insulin-like growth factor-1 receptor			
IL	interleukin		NBL	neuroblastoma
IM	intramuscular; interim maintenance		NCI	National Cancer Institute
INRC	International Neuroblastoma Response Criteria		NHL	non-Hodgkin lymphoma
			NOS	not otherwise specified
INSS	International Neuroblastoma Staging System		NWTSG	National Wilms Tumor Study Group
IR	incomplete response; intermediate risk		OPP	oncovin, procarbazine, prednisone
IRSG	Intergroup Rhabdomyosarcoma Study Group		OR	odds ratio
			OS	overall survival; osteosarcoma
IT	intrathecal			
ITP	idiopathic thrombocytopenic purpura		PBSC	peripheral blood stem cell
IV	intravenous		PBSCT	peripheral blood stem cell transplantation
IVA	ifosfamide, vincristine, actinomycin D			
			PCR	polymerase chain reaction
L-ASP	L-asparaginase		PCV	prednisolone, CCNU, vincristine
LCL	large cell lymphoma		PD	progressive disease
LD	low-dose		PDN	prednisolone
LDH	lactate dehydrogenase		PEG	polyethylene glycol
LFS	leukemia-free survival		PEG ASP	pegylated asparaginase
LMB	Lymphome Maligne B		PET	positron emission tomography
LR	low risk		PFS	progression-free survival
LRFN	low-risk febrile neutropenia		PNET	primitive neuroectodermal tumor

PO	*per os*	T-ALL	T-cell acute lymphoblastic leukemia
POG	Pediatric Oncology Group	TCR	T-cell receptor
PR	partial response	TG	thioguanine
PRS	postrecurrence/relapse survival	TIT	triple intrathecal
PTCL	peripheral T-cell lymphoma	TLP	traumatic lumbar puncture
PVB	cisplatin, vinblastine, bleomycin	TNHL	T-cell non-Hodgkin lymphoma
		TPO	thrombopoietin
RCC	renal cell carcinoma	TRM	treatment-related mortality
RCT	randomized controlled trial		
RECIST	Response Evaluation Criteria for Solid Tumors	UDS	undifferentiated sarcoma
		UH	unfavorable histology
RER	rapid early response		
RFS	relapse-free survival	VA	vincristine and actinomycin
rhEPO	recombinant human EPO	VAC	vincristine, actinomycin D, cyclophosphamide
RHR	relative hazard rate		
RI	remission induction	VACA	vincristine, doxorubicin, dactinomycin, cyclophosphamide
RMS	rhabdomyosarcoma		
RQ-PCR	real-time quantitative polymerase chain reaction	VAI	vincristine, dactinomycin, ifosfamide
		VAIA	vincristine, doxorubicin, dactinomycin, ifosfamide
RR	relative risk; risk ratio		
RT	radiotherapy/radiation therapy	VCR	vincristine
RTOG	Radiation Therapy Oncology Group	VDC	vincristine, doxorubicin, cyclophosphamide
SD	standard deviation	VEGF	vascular endothelial growth factor
SDI	single delayed intensification	VGPR	very good partial response
SE	standard error	VIDE	vincristine, ifosfamide, doxorubicin, etoposide
SER	slow early response		
SFOP	French Society for Paediatric Oncology	VIE	vincristine, ifosfamide, etoposide
SIOP	International Society of Paediatric Oncology	VM	vincristine and melphalan
		VTC	vincristine, topetecan, cyclophosphamide
SIR	standardized incidence ratio		
SMN	second malignant neoplasm		
SR	standard risk	WBC	white blood cell
STD	fractionated actinomycin D	WHO	World Health Organization
STS	soft tissue sarcomas	WT	Wilms tumor

About the companion website

Website: Evidence-Based Medicine Series

The Evidence-Based Medicine Series has a website at:

www.evidencebasedseries.com

Where you can find:

- Links to companion websites with additional resources and updates for books in the series

- Details of all new and forthcoming titles

- Links to more Evidence-Based products: including the Cochrane Library, Essential Evidence Plus, and EBM Guidelines.

How to access the companion sites with additional resources and updates:

- Go to the Evidence-Based Series site: **www.evidencebasedseries.com**

- Select your book from the list of titles shown on the site

- If your book has a website with supplementary material, it will show an icon Companion Website next to the title

- Click on the icon to access the website

PART 1
Solid tumors

CHAPTER 1

Rhabdomyosarcoma

Katherine K. Matthay
UCSF School of Medicine, San Francisco, CA, USA

Commentary by Meriel Jenney

Philosophy of treatment of rhabdomyosarcoma

Soft tissue sarcomas (STS) account for about 8% of all childhood malignancies. Rhabdomyosarcoma (RMS) is the single most common diagnosis (accounting for approximately 60% of all STS). It is, consequently, the tumor which is best defined, although there are important differences in behavior between RMS and some of the non-RMS STS (e.g. metastatic potential, chemosensitivity).

Historically, there have been important differences in the philosophy of treatment of RMS between the major international collaborative groups. Although there is now good communication, and a convergence toward standard criteria for staging and pathological classification, the experience of reviewing the literature can be confusing, particularly with respect to the previous lack of use of standard terminology for staging and treatment stratification.

One of the most important philosophical differences between the International Society of Paediatric Oncology (SIOP MMT) studies and those of the Intergroup Rhabdomyosarcoma Study Group (IRSG) (and, to some extent, those of the German [CWS] and Italian [ICG] Cooperative Groups) relates to the method and timing of local treatment. In particular, to the place of radiotherapy (RT) in guaranteeing local control for patients who appear to achieve complete remission (CR) with chemotherapy, with or without "significant" surgery. The SIOP strategy recognizes that some patients can be cured without the use of radiotherapy or so-called "significant" surgery," i.e. surgery resulting in considerable long-term morbidity. However, with this approach local relapse rates are generally higher in the SIOP studies than those experienced elsewhere, although the SIOP experience has also made it clear that a significant number of patients who relapse may be cured with alternative treatment (the so-called "salvage gap" between event-free and overall survival). In the context of such differences, *overall* survival rather than *disease-free* or *progression-free* survival becomes the most important criterion for comparing studies and measuring outcome

Treatment: the general approach

Rhabdomyosarcoma can occur almost anywhere in the body (although a number of well-recognized sites have been defined, e.g. bladder, prostate, parameningeal, limb, genitourinary, and head and neck). This leads to a complexity in its treatment and although the majority of clinical trials have explored chemotherapeutic options for the treatment of RMS, the impact of the site of disease should not be overlooked. Experience in all studies has confirmed that a surgical-pathological classification, which groups patients according to the extent of residual

---

Evidence-Based Pediatric Oncology, Third Edition. Edited by Ross Pinkerton, Ananth Shankar and Katherine K. Matthay.
© 2013 John Wiley & Sons, Ltd. Published 2013 by John Wiley & Sons, Ltd.

tumor after the initial surgical procedure, predicts outcome. The great majority of patients (approximately 75%) will have macroscopic residual disease (IRS clinical group III) at the primary site at the start of chemotherapy (this is equivalent to pT3b in the SIOP postsurgical staging system). The additional adverse prognostic influence of tumor site, size (longest dimension >5 cm), histological subtype (alveolar versus embryonal) and patient age (>10 years) adds to the complexities of treatment stratification. All current clinical trials utilize some combination of the best-known prognostic factors to stratify treatment intensity for patients with good or poor predicted outcomes and the impetus for this approach comes as much from wishing to avoid overtreatment of patients with a good prospect for cure as improving cure rates for patients with less favorable disease.

The importance of multiagent chemotherapy, as part of co-ordinated multimodality treatment, has been clearly demonstrated for RMS. Cure rates have improved from approximately 25% in the early 1970s, when combination chemotherapy was first implemented, to the current overall 5-year survival rates of more than 70% that are generally achieved. Nevertheless, it is interesting to see how relatively little the results of randomized controlled trials have actually contributed to decision making in the selection of chemotherapy and to the development of the design of the sequential studies which have shown this improvement in survival over those years.

Lessons from studies of rhabdomyosarcoma

The IRSG was formed in 1972 as a collaboration between the two former pediatric oncology groups in North America (Children's Cancer Group and Pediatric Oncology Group [POG]) with the intention of investigating the biology and treatment of RMS (and undifferentiated sarcoma) in the first two decades of life. This group, whose work and publications have been pre-eminent in the field, now forms the Soft Tissue Sarcoma Committee of the Children's Oncology Group (COG). Results of treatment have improved significantly over time. The percentage of patients alive at 5 years has increased from 55% on the IRS-I protocol [1] to over 70% on the IRS-III and IRS-IV protocols [2,3].

Combinations of vincristine, actinomycin D, and cyclophosphamide (VAC) have been the mainstay of chemotherapy in all IRS studies. Actinomycin-D was originally given in a fractionated schedule but subsequent experience, including a randomized study from Italy [4], showed no advantage in terms of outcome and has suggested that fractionation may increase toxicity; single-dose scheduling is now standard across all studies. There have never been any results in the IRSG studies that challenge the use of these drugs as first-line therapy and the results of all randomized studies which compare other drugs with, or against, VA or VAC have failed to show significant advantage.

One of the most significant differences between the IRSG and European studies has been in the choice of alkylating agent that provides the backbone of first-line chemotherapy. Ifosfamide was introduced into clinical practice earlier in Europe than in the United States and phase II data are available which support its efficacy in RMS. IRS-IV [2, 3] attempted to answer the question of comparative efficacy by randomizing VAC (using an intensified cyclophosphamide dose of $2.2\,g/m^2$) against vincristine/dactinomycin/ifosfamide (VAI), which incorporated ifosfamide at a dose of $9\,g/m^2$. A third arm in this randomization included ifosfamide in combination with etoposide (VIE; vincristine, ifosfamide, etoposide). No difference was identified between the higher-dose VAC and the ifosfamide-containing schedules, and VAC remains the combination of choice for future IRSG (now COG) studies. The rationale for this is explained by the lower dose of cyclophosphamide and its shorter duration of administration, together with concern about the nephrotoxicity of ifosfamide. Nevertheless, the European Paediatric Soft Tissue Sarcoma Group (EpSSG) has chosen to retain ifosfamide as its standard combination as the experience of significant renal toxicity at cumulative ifosfamide doses less than $60\,g/m^2$ is now very small and there are preliminary data suggesting that the gonadal toxicity of ifosfamide may be significantly less than that of cyclophosphamide [5].

Vincristine, actinomycin D, and cyclophosphamide remains the chemotherapy backbone for IRS studies, as there has been little evidence of benefit from other agents. IRS-III included cisplatin and etoposide in a three-way randomization between VAC, VAC with doxorubicin and cisplatin, and VAC with doxorubicin, cisplatin, and etoposide. No advantage was seen in selected group III and all group IV patients and there were concerns about additive toxicity. IRS-IV (and an earlier IRS-IV pilot) explored the value of melphalan in patients with metastatic RMS or undifferentiated sarcoma. Patients were randomized to receive three courses of vincristine and melphalan (VM) or four of ifosfamide and etoposide (IE) [6]. There was no significant difference in initial complete and partial remission rates. However, patients receiving VM had a lower 3-year event-free and overall survival. Patients receiving this combination had greater hematological toxicity and, therefore, a lower tolerance of subsequent therapy. In the latest published randomized study by the COG (D9803) [7] in patients with intermediate-risk RMS, VAC was compared to a regimen of VAC alternating with vincristine, topotecan, and cyclophosphamide. Again, no benefit was seen with use of these agents.

Alternative agents of particular interest include doxorubicin (Adriamycin), which has been evaluated in a number of IRSG studies. A total of 1431 patients with group III and IV disease were randomized to receive or not receive doxorubicin in addition to VAC during studies in IRS-I to IRS-III. The results did not indicate any significant advantage for those who received doxorubicin. Furthermore, also in IRS-III, patients with group II (microscopic residual) tumors were randomized between vincristine and actinomycin (VA) alone and VA with doxorubicin without any significant difference in survival. Recent European studies (MMT 95 and CWS-ICG 96) both included randomizations between their ifosfamide-based standard chemotherapy options and an intensified six-drug combination, which also included epirubicin (with carboplatin and etoposide). In the MMT 95 study [8], 457 previously untreated patients with incompletely resected embryonal rhabdomyosarcoma, undifferentiated sarcoma, and soft tissue primitive neuroectodermal tumor were randomized to receive IVA (ifosfamide, vincristine, actinomycin D) or a six-drug combination (IVA + carboplatin, epirubicin, etoposide) both delivered over 27 weeks. Overall survival for all patients was 81% (95% confidence interval [CI], 77–84%) at 3 years but there was no significant difference in outcome in either overall or event-free survival between the two arms. Toxicity was significantly greater (infection, myelosuppression,

mucositis) in patients in the six-drug arm. However, in this and the previous studies, the dose intensity of the anthracyclines used was low which may have influenced the evaluation.

So doxorubicin remains a drug of interest in soft tissue sarcomas. A SIOP "window" study in chemotherapy-naïve patients with metastatic RMS has provided good new phase II data for the efficacy of doxorubicin, with response rates greater than 65% [9]. This has justified further evaluation of the role of doxorubicin in the treatment of RMS and this is now under investigation in a randomized study being undertaken by the EpSSG. A more intensive scheduling of doxorubicin is being tested within this study.

Other agents that have shown activity in RMS include irinotecan (CPT11), which in combination with vincristine in a recent COG window study had excellent PR and CR rates [10]. There is also evidence of benefit in the phase I setting [11]. The scheduling of this agent in the phase II setting [12] has been evaluated in patients with RMS, undifferentiated sarcoma or ectomesenchymoma at first relapse or with disease progression. Although preclinical models suggested that a prolonged administration schedule of irinotecan would be more effective than a short (more convenient) schedule, this study demonstrated equivalent response rates (26% for prolonged schedule versus 36% for short) in patients receiving the two schedules. The current COG IRS-V study has now included this combination (using the short schedule) in the latest randomized study.

Vinorelbine is well tolerated and has been evaluated in combination with daily oral cyclophosphamide in previously heavily treated patients with relapsed RMS with encouraging results [13,14]. This combination is now under investigation in the current EpSSG study in which patients who achieve CR with conventional chemotherapy and local treatment are randomized to stop therapy or to continue to receive a further 6 months of "maintenance" therapy with these two agents.

Radiotherapy has been a standard component of therapy for the majority of patients in the IRSG studies from the outset. Randomized studies within IRS-I to IRS-III have established that RT is unnecessary for group I (completely resected) patients with embryonal histology. Analyses from the same studies suggest that RT does offer an improved failure-free survival

(FFS) in patients with completely resected alveolar RMS or with undifferentiated sarcoma. Studies from the European groups have attempted to relate the use of RT to response to initial chemotherapy. The most radical approach is being used by the SIOP group which has tried to withhold RT in patients with group III (pT3b) disease if CR is achieved with initial chemotherapy ± conservative second surgery. In the MMT 89 study, which included 503 patients, the systematic use of RT was avoided in patients who achieved complete local tumor control with chemotherapy with or without surgery, Five-year overall survival (OS) and event-free survival (EFS) rates were 71% and 57%, respectively. The differences between EFS and OS reflected local treatment strategy and successful retreatment for some patients after relapse (the salvage gap). The authors concluded that selective avoidance of local therapy is justified in some patients, though further work is required to identify prospectively those for whom this is most applicable [15].

So this approach is warranted for some patients, for example, those with tumors of the orbit, where outcomes from different international groups have previously been formally compared at a joint international workshop (there were no significant differences in overall survival between international groups using different strategies for radiotherapy, despite differences in event-free survival) [16]. However, the role of radiotherapy is clearly important for other subgroups of patients (for example, those with parameningeal, limb, and/ or alveolar disease) and there is a need to try to define risk groups as accurately as possible at the outset to avoid overtreatment, and also to reduce the risk of relapse and the need for salvage therapy.

Doses of RT have, somewhat pragmatically, been tailored to age, with reduced doses in younger children, although there is no defined threshold below which late effects can be avoided and yet tumor control is still achieved. The place for hyperfractionated RT was explored in IRS-IV when randomized against conventional fractionation [17]. Although there was a higher incidence of severe skin reaction and nausea and vomiting in patients receiving hyperfractionated RT, it was generally well tolerated. However, there was no advantage in failure-free survival, and conventional RT continues to be used as standard therapy.

Lessons from studies of nonrhabdomyosarcoma soft tissue sarcomas

Although this chapter refers to two studies that include patients with non-RMS STS [18, 19], the former is the only published study which was specifically designed to answer a randomized question about the value of chemotherapy in this difficult and heterogeneous group of patients. Unfortunately, the power of this study was limited and further work needs to be undertaken to better understand optimal therapy. Perhaps the most important immediate question is to ascertain whether the treatment of children with non-RMS STS, particularly with the diagnoses more frequently seen in adults, should be assessed any differently than for adults with the same condition. If not, combined studies, particularly of new agents, could be productive.

An important recent development in Europe has been the initiation of a new EpSSG study specifically for children with non-RMS STS and this will facilitate the systematic collection of data from the consistent treatment of children with these rare tumors. There is also now regular communication across the Atlantic with respect to the classification and treatment of non-RMS STS. Separate approaches are offered for synovial sarcoma for "adult" type non-RMS STS and for unique pediatric histiotypes, and links with adult trials will also be important. None of these studies yet includes a randomized element and the numbers of patients in some of these rare diagnostic groups, even when collected at European level, still make this a logistical and statistical challenge.

Conclusion

Although considerable progress has been made in improving overall survival in RMS, progress has been incremental and intuitive, based on careful treatment planning, the co-ordination of chemotherapy with surgery and RT, and better prognostic treatment stratification. Relatively little has been learned about improving treatment from randomized studies but previous conclusions about the role of doxorubicin are being revisited and further new agents (irinotecan, vinorelbine) are under evaluation. The challenge for the future requires the development of a greater ability to selectively reduce treatment for some groups of patients with a high chance of cure and to identify better forms of therapy for those with a very poor prognosis. Patients with metastatic disease, for example, continue to have a very poor survival rate. Wider international collaboration is the key to providing a patient base that will allow timely and valid randomized studies.

References

1 Maurer HM, Beltangady M, Gehan EA et al. The Intergroup Rhabdomyosarcoma Study-1. *A final report. Cancer* 1988;**61**;209–20.

2 Crist W, Gehan EA, Ragab AH et al. The Third Intergroup Rhabdomyosarcoma Study. *J Clin Oncol* 1995;**13**:610–30.

3 Baker KS, Anderson JR, Link MP et al. Benefit of intensified therapy for patients with local or regional embryonal rhabdomyosarcoma: results from the Intergroup Rhabdomyosarcoma Study-IV. *J Clin Oncol* 2000;**18**:2427–34.

4 Carli M, Pastore G, Perilongo G et al. Tumor response and toxicity after single high-dose versus standard five-day divided-dose dactinomycin in childhood rhabdomyosarcoma. *J Clin Oncol* 1988;**6**:654–8.

5 Ridola V, Fawaz O, Aubier F et al. Testicular function of survivors of childhood cancer: a comparative study between ifosfamide- and cyclophosphamide-based regimens. *Eur J Cancer* 2009;**45**:814–18.

6 Breitfeld PP, Lyden E, Raney RB et al. Ifosfamide and etoposide are superior to vincrisitne and melphalan for paediatric metastatic rhabdomyosarcoma when administered with irradiation and combination chemotherapy: a report from the Intergroup Rhabdomyosarcoma Study Group 23 225–33. *J Pediatr Hematol Oncol* 2001;**23**(4):225–33.

7 Arndt CAS, Stoner JA, Hawkins DS et al. Vincristine, actinomycin and cyclophosphamide compared with vincristine, actinomycin and cyclophosphamide alternating with vincristine, topetecan and cyclophosphamide for intermediate-risk rhabdomyosarcoma: Children's Oncology Group study D9803. *J Clin Oncol* 2009;**27**:5182–8.

8 Oberlin O, Rey A, Sanchez de Toledo JHM et al. A randomised comparison of intensified (6 drugs) versus standard (3-drug) chemotherapy for high-risk non-metastatic rhabdomyosarcoma and other chemosensitive childhood soft tissue sarcoma: long term results from the International Society of Paediatric Oncology (SIOP) MMT 95 study. *J Clin Oncol* 2012;**30**:2457–65.

9 Bergeron C, Thiesse P, Rey A et al. Revisiting the role of doxorubicin in the treatment of rhabdomyosarcoma: an up-front window study in newly diagnosed children with high-risk metastatic disease. *Eur J Cancer* 2008;**44**:427–31.

10 Pappo AS, Lyden E, Breitfeld P et al. Two consecutive phase II window trials of irinotecan alone or in combination with vincristine for the treatment of metastatic rhabdomyosarcoma: the Children's Oncology Group. *J Clin Oncol* 2007;**25**:362–9.

11 Bisogno G, Riccardi R, Ruggiero A et al. Phase II study of a protracted irinotecan schedule in children with refractory or recurrent soft tissue sarcoma. *Cancer* 2006;**106**:703–7.

12 Mascarenhas L, Lyden ER, Breitfield PP et al. Randomized phase 11 window trial of two schedules of irinotecan with vincristine in patients with first relapse or progression of rhabdomyosarcoma: a report from the Children's Oncology Group. *J Clin Oncol* 2010;**28**:4658–63.

13 Casanova M, Ferrari A, Spreafico F et al. Vinorelbine in previously treated advanced childhood sarcomas: evidence of activity in rhabdomyosarcoma. *Cancer* 2002;**94**:3263–8.

14 Kuttesch JF Jr, Krailo MD, Madden T, Johansen M, Bleyer A, Children's Oncology Group. Phase II evaluation of intravenous vinorelbine (Navelbine) in recurrent or refractory pediatric malignancies: a Children's Oncology Group study. *Pediatr Blood Cancer* 2009;**53**:590–3.

15 Stevens MC, Rey A, Bouvet N et al. Treatment of non-metastatic rhabdomyosarcoma in childhood and adolescence: third study of the International Society of Paediatric Oncology – SIOP Malignant Mesenchymal Tumor 89. *J Clin Oncol* 2005;**23**:2618–28.

16 Oberlin O, Rey A, Anderson J et al, for the International Society of Paediatric Oncology Sarcoma Committee, Intergroup Rhabdomyosarcoma Study Group, Italian Cooperative Soft Tissue Sarcoma Group, German Collaborative Soft Tissue Sarcoma Group. Treatment of orbital rhabdomyosarcoma: survival and late effects of treatment – results of an international workshop. *J Clin Oncol* 2001;**19**:197–204.

17 Donaldson S, Meza J, Breneman J et al. Results from the IRS-IV randomised trial of hyperfractionated radiotherapy in children with rhabdomyosarcoma – a report from the IRSG. *Int J Radiat Oncol Biol Phys* 2001;**51**:718–28.

18 Pratt CB, Pappo AS, Gieser P et al. Role of adjuvant chemotherapy in the treatment of surgically resected pediatric non-rhabdomyosarcomatous soft tissue sarcomas. Oncology Group Study. *J Clin Oncol* 1999;**17**:1219–26.

19 Pratt CB, Maurer HM, Gieser P et al. Treatment of unresectable or metastatic pediatric soft tissue sarcomas with surgery, irradiation and chemotherapy: a Pediatric Oncology Group Study. *Med Ped Oncol* 1998;**30**:201–9.

Summary of previous studies

The evidence base for treatment strategies is particularly strong in this tumor type due to the long history of large randomized trials designed and executed by the IRSG and currently the COG. Between 1988 and 2001, 11 IRSG studies were published. There were two studies from the POG and single randomized trials from the SIOP and Italian (AIEOP) groups respectively. Much useful information has been gained from the large SIOP trials but most of these have not been randomized.

IRS-I, published in 1988 [1] had four objectives. First, to evaluate the role of local radiotherapy in IRS group I patients who received vincristine, actinomycin D, and cyclophosphamide (VAC). Second, to determine whether the addition of cyclophosphamide to vincristine and actinomycin was of benefit in group II patients who received local irradiation. Third, to document the complete remission rate achieved by pulsed VAC with local irradiation in patients with group III and IV disease and fourth, to evaluate the role of adding doxorubicin to VAC in group III and IV patients.

Patients under the age of 21 years with rhabdomyosarcoma or undifferentiated sarcoma were eligible; 686 patients were eligible for inclusion. In group I patients, disease-free survival (DFS) at 5 years was 81%, overall survival 93% in those receiving no radiation compared with 79% and 81% respectively for those who were irradiated and, in particular, there was no significant difference with regard to either local or distant relapse.

In group II patients, the disease-free survival again showed no difference between patients who received or did not receive radiation therapy with identical overall survival of 72% and disease-free survival of 72% and 66%, respectively, for those who received or did not receive cyclophosphamide. In group III, which included 380 patients, the complete response rate achieved combining pulsed VAC with local radiotherapy was 67% while it was 72% for those who received pulsed VAC plus doxorubicin and irradiation. There was no difference in the 5-year DFS between

those who received doxorubicin and those who did not – 43% versus 39% (p=0.91) or 5-year overall survival of 52% each for both treatment arms. In group IV patients, a complete response rate of 50% was achieved overall and although there was a trend to benefit from doxorubicin in these patients with regard to a more rapid complete response rate and lower relapse rate, there was no significant difference in DFS or OS.

IRS-II, reported in 1993 [2], addressed three questions: (1) the value of cyclophosphamide in favorable site/pathology (extremity alveolar lesions excluded) group I patients, (2) the role of pulsed VAC compared to VA in favorable group II patients (extremity alveolar lesions excluded), and (3) the role of doxorubicin in group III and IV patients excluding special pelvic sites. There were 776 evaluable patients in total although 999 eligible patients were included in the analysis. This study demonstrated that VA given for 1 year was equivalent to 2 years of VAC in group I patients not receiving local irradiation therapy with an overall survival of 85%. In group II patients, cyclophosphamide does not add benefit to VA with DFS of 69% in those not receiving cyclophosphamide compared to 74% for those receiving cyclophosphamide. Finally, in group III and IV patients, doxorubicin did not appear to significantly improve outcome, with almost identical CR rates and OS in those achieving CR.

IRS-III [3] was designed to determine the role of doxorubicin in addition to VAC in group II patients, and, secondly, to determine whether the addition of either cisplatin or cisplatin plus etoposide to pulsed VAdrC –VAC in group III and IV patients improves survival outcome. There were in total 1062 eligible patients, For group II patients, 5-year progression-free survival (PFS) was 56% versus 77% in those receiving doxorubicin. For group III patients in the three regimens, PFS was 70%, 62%, and 56% respectively – no significant difference. For group IV patients, PFS was 27%, 27%, and 30% respectively. The more complex chemotherapy did not therefore appear to have any significant advantage. Again, it is notable that although not achieving statistical significance, with the addition of anthracycline in group II patients, there is a trend towards lower relapse rates.

IRS-IV [4,5] compared three induction and continuation regimens based on the VAC protocol with the substitution of ifosfamide for cyclophosphamide (VAI) or the replacement of actinomycin and cyclophosphamide with ifosfamide and etoposide (VIE). Patients with local or local regional disease were included but any patient felt to be at risk of renal problems was assigned VAC. Also excluded were the good-risk group I patients with testis, orbit or eyelid primaries who received only VA. A total of 894 patients was included. The 3-year failure-free survival for VAC, VAI, and VIE was 74%, 74%, and 76% respectively. It was, therefore, concluded that none of the novel regimens had any advantage over the standard VAC protocol but it is notable that compared to previous IRS trials, a higher dose of cyclophosphamide was used ($2.2\,g/m^2$).

In patients with metastatic disease there was a randomized comparison between two drug pairs [6]. This utilized the novel and somewhat controversial "window" design where untreated patients receive as yet unproven single or combination chemotherapy. In this study, the drug pairs comprised vincristine/melphalan or ifosfamide/etoposide in untreated metastatic rhabdomyosarcoma; 151 patients were randomized. Complete response rates did not differ at week 12: 13% versus 12%, partial response (PR) rate 61% versus 67% and progression of disease 13% versus 12%. There was, however, a significantly worse 3-year EFS with the VM combination: 19% versus 33% (p=0.04). This was felt to be potentially due to the influence of melphalan on hemopoietic stem cell function resulting in poor tolerance of subsequent chemotherapy and consequent dose reduction.

Another component of IRS-IV reported by Donaldson [7] compared the effectiveness and toxicity of hyperfractionated versus conventionally delivered radiation therapy in group III patients; 599 patients were entered, 490 were eventually randomized. Conventional radiation consisted of 50.4 Gy in 28 fractions compared with 59.4 Gy in 1.1 Gy doses twice per day with a 6-h interval between doses. There was no significant difference in outcome between the two groups but hyperfractionation was associated with a significantly higher instance of severe skin reaction, nausea and vomiting, and mucositis.

The very early SIOP study run between 1975 and 1983 and published in 1985 [8] was an historically important trial, which determined whether the use of chemotherapy and radiation therapy prior to surgery could minimize treatment sequelae. Patients initially received one course of VAC and those who had a greater than 25% reduction were advised to continue with chemotherapy alone whereas others received extensive surgery or local radiation therapy. Overall outcome between the two arms indicated that in chemosensitive patients, the use of radiation or extensive surgery had no significant benefit providing complete response was achieved with combination of chemotherapy. This trial, despite its limitations, prepared the ground for the subsequent philosophy of trying to avoid radiation and aggressive surgery, a strategy, which has been subsequently refined in later single-arm studies. These studies have enabled identification of subgroups in whom outcome was likely to be compromised by an insufficiently aggressive approach to local control but, in contrast, a population in whom cure could be achieved with chemotherapy alone or in some cases chemotherapy followed by multimodality salvage treatment.

An Italian AIOP trial published in 1988 [9] compared two methods of administration of actinomycin as part of the VAC regimen. This was a very small trial and indicated that the fractionation of actinomycin D in divided doses daily over 5 days was no more effective in achieving response than a single dose.

Finally, two trials run by the Pediatric Oncology Group have been published. In 1998 Pratt et al. reported POG8654 [10], which compared VAC with VAC with the addition of dacarbazine (DTIC) in patients with group III or IV disease. This failed to show any significant benefit but included a very mixed group of tumor types in addition to rhabdomyosarcoma.

The second report in 1999 [11] evaluated whether the administration of chemotherapy following surgical resection of nonrhabdomyosarcomatous soft tissue sarcomas improved local or systemic control. In view of the continued controversy around the role of adjuvant therapy in this group of patients, this was of particular interest. Children with group I disease received no radiotherapy but were randomly assigned to receive chemotherapy with VAdrC or observation, those with group II disease received age-adjusted postoperative radiation therapy and were then randomly assigned to receive or not receive chemotherapy, and those with group III disease underwent second-look surgery 6–12 weeks after completed radiation therapy and if complete remission was documented, these were also randomized to receive or not receive adjuvant chemotherapy. This study failed to show any significant benefit from the chemotherapy but, unfortunately, was compromised by the heterogeneous nature of the different histologies.

References

1 Maurer HM, Beltangady M, Gehan EA *et al*. The Intergroup Rhabdomyosarcoma Study-1. A final report. *Cancer* 1988; **61**;209–20.
2 Maurer HM, Gehan EA, Beltangady M *et al*. The Intergroup Rhabdomyosarcoma Study-II. *Cancer* 1993;**71**:1904–22.
3 Crist W, Gehan EA, Ragab AH *et al*. The Third Intergroup Rhabdomyosarcoma Study. *J Clin Oncol* 1995;**13**:610–30.
4 Baker KS, Anderson JR, Link MP *et al*. Benefit of intensified therapy for patients with local or regional embryonal rhabdomyosarcoma: results from the Intergroup Rhabdomyosarcoma Study-IV. *J Clin Oncol* 2000;**18**:2427–34.
5 Crist W, Anderson J, Meza J *et al*. Intergroup Rhabdomyosarcoma Study-IV: results for patients with non-metastatic disease. *J Clin Oncol* 2001;**19**:3091–102.
6 Breitfeld PP, Lyden E, Raney RB *et al*. Ifosfamide and etoposide are superior to vincristine and melphalan for paediatric metastatic rhabdomyosarcoma when administered with irradiation and combination chemotherapy: a report from the Intergroup Rhabdomyosarcoma Study Group 23 225–33. *J Pediatr Hematol Oncol* 2001;**23**(4):225–33.
7 Donaldson S, Meza J, Breneman J *et al*. Results from the IRS-IV randomised trial of hyperfractionated radiotherapy in children with rhabdomyosarcoma – a report from the IRSG. *Int J Radiat Oncol Biol Phys* 2001;**51**:718–28.
8 Flamant F, Rodary C, Voute PA, Otten J. Primary chemotherapy in the treatment of rhabdomyosarcoma in children. Trial of the International Society of Pediatric Oncology (SIOP) preliminary results. *Radiother Oncol* 1985;**3**:227–36.
9 Carli M, Pastore G, Perilongo G *et al*. Tumor response and toxicity after single high-dose versus standard five-day divided-dose dactinomycin in childhood rhabdomyosarcoma. *J Clin Oncol* 1988;**6**:654–8.
10 Pratt CB, Maurer HM, Gieser P *et al*. Treatment of unresectable or metastatic pediatric soft tissue sarcomas with surgery, irradiation and chemotherapy: a Pediatric Oncology Group Study. *Med Ped Oncol* 1998;**30**:201–9.
11 Pratt CB, Pappo AS, Gieser P *et al*. Role of adjuvant chemotherapy in the treatment of surgically resected pediatric non-rhabdomyosarcomatous soft tissue sarcomas. Oncology Group Study. *J Clin Oncol* 1999;**17**:1219–26.

New studies

Study 1

Arndt CAS, Stoner JA, Hawkins DS *et al.* Vincristine, actinomycin and cyclophosphamide compared with vincristine, actinomycin and cyclophosphamide alternating with vincristine, topetecan and cyclophosphamide for intermediate-risk rhabdomyosarcoma: Children's Oncology Group study D9803. *J Clin Oncol* 2009;**27**:5182–8.

Objectives

To compare the outcome of patients with intermediate-risk rhabdomyosarcoma treated with standard VAC chemotherapy to the outcome of those treated with VAC alternating with vincristine, topetecan, and cyclophosphamide (VTC).

Study design

Intermediate-risk RMS defined as stages 2 and 3 clinical group III embryonal rhabdomyosarcoma and all nonmetastatic alveolar, undifferentiated sarcomas (UDS), and ectomesenchymoma. Tissue submission for central review was required to confirm histology and study eligibility. Eligibility criteria for study inclusion were previously untreated patients younger than 50 years, beginning therapy within 42 days after initial biopsy, serum bilirubin of <1.5 mg/dL, and normal serum creatinine for age. Patients were assigned to a clinical group by each participating institution following surgery on the basis of clinicopathological determination of extent of disease and degree of surgical resection, according to criteria of the IRS postsurgical grouping classification. If primary excision of a tumor was the definitive operation, patients were classified after this procedure provided it was performed within 42 days of the initial procedure and prior to chemotherapy. Lymph node sampling was based on primary site of disease and required for paratesticular RMS in boys older than age 10 years and in those with extremity tumors and recommended for clinically positive nodes prior to study enrollment.

Patients were randomly assigned to either VAC or VAC/VTC. Patients with parameningeal primary tumors with intracranial extension were assigned to VAC and immediate radiation therapy (nonrandomized). The drug doses used in this study were age adjusted and for children ≥3 years of age, the doses were vincristine 1.5 mg/m^2, dactinomycin 0.045 mg/kg, topotecan 0.75 mg/ m^2×5 days, cyclophosphamide 2.2 g/m^2 (when this was combined with dactinomycin) and 250 mg/ m^2×5 days (when combined with topotecan). For younger children, the doses of vincristine, dactinomycin, and cyclophosphamide in the VAC combination were according to body weight.

Patients were evaluated at weeks 12, 24 and end of therapy. Patients who responded poorly to induction chemotherapy were recommended to proceed to preoperative radiotherapy followed by second-look surgery at week 24. Patients received response-adjusted radiation therapy according to stage group and histological subtype at diagnosis and disease status after the second-look surgery, if done, at week 12. Radiation dose ranged from 36 to 50.4 Gy depending on risk grouping. Dactinomycin and topetecan were withheld during radiation therapy.

Statistics

The primary comparison was between the two randomized regimens. Patients were stratified into five groups: embryonal RMS, stage 2 or 3, group III; embryonal RMS, group IV, younger than 10 years; alveolar RMS or UDS, stage 1 or group 1; alveolar RMS or UDS, stage 2 or 3, group II/III; and parameningeal extension stage 2 or 3.

Long-term FFS was expected to be 64% on the basis of IRS-III and IRS-IV. The study was designed with an 80% power (two-sided α of 0.05) to detect an overall increase in the 5-year FFS from 64% with VAC to 75% with VAC/VTC. A total of 158 failures were required, and projected to occur after follow-up of 518 patients. Kaplan–Meier and log-rank tests were used for FFS and OS. The Cox proportional hazards regression modeling was used to estimate hazard ratios and investigate whether the effect of VAC/VTC differed by risk stratum. Median follow-up was 4.3 years (0–8.2 years).

Results

Patients recruited between 1999 and 2005 included 702 patients; 85 were ineligible for analysis, 516 were randomly assigned to either VAC (n=264) or VAC/VTC (n=252). There was high concordance between central path review and institutional diagnosis: 96% for alveolar, 85% embryonal. The percentage of courses in which therapy was administered as recommended as protocol was 89% or greater for each regimen.

Estimated 4-year FFS rates were 73% for VAC and 68% for VAC/VTC (p=0.3). This was similar to that for IRS-IV, at 69%. Within subgroups, there is a slightly higher risk of failure among patients with stage 2–3 or group II–III alveolar who were treated with VAC/VTC compared to VAC alone (p=0.05), with differences within other strata not significant.

Toxicity

There was little difference between toxicities between arms although patients on VAC were more likely to develop febrile neutropenia. There were 17 second malignancies: six on VAC/VTC, nine on randomized VAC and two on nonrandomized VAC.

Conclusions

The study confirmed previous reports of a higher failure risk in higher stage groups and in patients with alveolar compared to embryonal disease. However, the study did not show any improvement in outcome (failure-free survival) for intermediate-risk RMS when topetecan was substituted for dactinomycin in half the cycles.

Study 2

Mascarenhas L, Lyden ER, Breitfield PP *et al.* Randomized phase 11 window trial of two schedules of irinotecan with vincristine in patients with first relapse or progression of rhabdomyosarcoma: a report from the Children's Oncology Group. *J Clin Oncol* 2010;**28**:4658–63.

Objectives

To compare response rates for two schedules of irinotecan combined with vincristine in patients with rhabdomyosarcoma at first relapse or disease progression.

Study design

Eligible patients had biopsy-proven RMS, undifferentiated sarcoma or ectomesenchymoma and were younger than 21 years of age with a first relapse or disease progression and had Eastern Co-operative Oncology Group (ECOG) performance status of 2 or less and life expectancy of at least 2 months. There were strict definitions for adequate organ function and cardiac function. Patients who had received more than one prior chemotherapy treatment regimen, those with prior exposure to anthracyclines, ischemic heart disease, myeloablative chemotherapy, disease impinging on or within the brain and spinal cord and those who were pregnant or lactating were excluded.

Patients with unfavorable prognosis (alveolar histology at initial diagnosis, stage 1 clinical group I embryonal histology diagnosis with distant recurrence, or stages 2, 3 or 4 and clinical group II, III or IV embryonal histology at initial diagnosis) were randomly assigned to one of two schedules of irinotecan combined with vincristine.
- Regimen 1A included irinotecan 20 mg/m^2 per day IV for 5 days at weeks 1, 2, 4, and 5 with vincristine 1.5 mg/m^2 IV on day 1 of weeks 1, 2, 4, and 5.
- Regimen 1B included irinotecan 50 mg/m^2 per day IV for 5 days at weeks 1 and 4 with vincristine as in regimen 1A.

Disease response was assessed using the NCI Response Evaluation Criteria for Solid Tumors (RECIST) at week 6. Those with responsive disease, either complete or partial, continued to receive 44 weeks of multiagent chemotherapy that incorporated the assigned irinotecan-vincristine regimen.

Statistics

The analysis compared response rate, toxicities, failure-free survival, and overall survival of patients on regimens 1A and 1B. The study was powered to detect a 25% improvement in the response rate to regimen 1A compared to 1B (α=0.1, 1–β=0.9, one-sided test favoring regimen 1A since the only difference of clinical importance was an improved response with the more prolonged but inconvenient schedule).

A sample size of 51 patients per arm (102 randomly assigned patients) was required to detect a significant improvement in the response rate. Fisher's exact test was used to compare the difference in proportions for baseline patient characteristics and treatment response between regimens. Estimation for survival was performed using the Kaplan–Meier method and compared using the log-rank test.

Results

COG-ARST0121 enrolled 139 patients between July 2002 and October 2006; 93 were enrolled and randomly assigned between the prolonged regimen and the short regimen. Patient characteristics including age, histology, primary site, size of largest lesion and whether the recurrence was local, regional nodal or distant were all similar for those treated in 1A and 1B. There was, however, a larger proportion of males on 1B (70% versus 40%). Recurrences were local in 25 patients, regional nodal in seven, distant metastatic in 36, combined local and regional nodal in five, combined local and distant metastatic in 10 and combined local, regional nodal, and distant metastatic in two.

Toxicity

Fifty percent of patients on regimen 1A and 66% on 1B experienced at least grade 3 toxicity in the first 6 weeks of therapy. There was no statistically significant difference in the instance of diarrhea (22% versus 13%) or anemia (39% versus 28%). Neutropenia was less common on regimen 1A (16% versus 34%) but there was no difference in the incidence of febrile neutropenia.

The week 6 response could be assessed in 89 (42 in regimen 1A and 47 in regimen 1B) of the 92 randomly assigned patients. Three patients were nonevaluable: one withdrew consent, one did not complete treatment, and one was not assessable due to metal artifact on the scan. Overall response (CR+PR) rate in this study was 31%.

There was no significant difference in response rates between regimen 1A, 26%, and regimen B, 36% (p=0.36). There were no complete responses on regimen 1B compared to four complete responses on regimen 1A. Response rate in patients with alveolar RMS were significantly higher compared to embryonal or other: 48% versus 5% on regimen 1A and 48% versus 20% on regimen 1B (p=0.01 and 0.08 respectively). Failure-free survival was similar between both regimens: the 1-year FFS rates on regimens A and B were 37% and 38% respectively, declining to 14% and 15% at 3 years.

Conclusions

The trial revealed no difference in response rate between the two schedules, disproving the preclinical prediction of superior activity with prolonged schedules. The authors speculated that perhaps the addition of vincristine, one of the most active agents on RMS, could have diluted any differential effect.

CHAPTER 2

Osteosarcoma

Katherine K. Matthay
UCSF School of Medicine, San Francisco, CA, USA

Commentary by Maria Michelagnoli

The current dilemma in osteosarcoma management surrounds the role of a novel biological agent, liposomal muramyl tripeptide phosphatidyl ethanolamine (L-MTP-PE, mifurmatide). L-MTP-PE is a synthetic analog of a component of the *Mycobacterium* sp. cell wall and it acts as an immune adjuvant macrophage stimulant. The natural history of osteosarcoma in the prechemotherapy era was usually death within 18 months from pulmonary metastases, despite primary tumor control with ablative surgery. Interest in L-MTP-PE was initially generated as preclinical data demonstrated responses in metastatic pulmonary osteosarcoma in animal models. A large phase III randomized trial was conducted by the Pediatric Oncology Group (POG)/Children's Oncology Group (COG) in the US to provide evidence of efficacy and the authors cite a reduction of the mortality rate hazard ratio by one-third, in localized nonmetastatic disease [1] . The interpretation of the published reports of the study has, however, caused controversy [1,2,3]. Therefore, although the results are interesting, it is disputed whether they are strong enough to endorse immediate incorporation of this agent into patient care.

The context is that prior to these publications, there has been no significant improvement in survival for patients with osteosarcoma during the last two decades. This is despite increasingly aggressive, complex variations in systemic perioperative cytotoxic regimens. In addition, there have been considerable advances in imaging systems, supportive care, complex limb salvage surgery (including custom-made growing prostheses) and multidisciplinary working which, perhaps surprisingly, have not translated into further improved life expectancy. Therefore, does adjuvant use of L-MTP-PE represent a breakthrough? Before we can address this question, there has to be an understanding of progress in osteosarcoma management to date.

Clarity regarding the "gold standard" of chemotherapy regimen eludes the oncology community, in terms of numbers of agents required for best induction, dose intensity, and role of salvage chemotherapy postoperatively. In the prechemotherapy era, long-term survival was less than 20% with surgery alone. From the 1980s the practice of perioperative multiagent chemotherapy improved survival to 50–60% (25–35% for patients with axial and metastatic presentations) but substantial further improvement has not been consistently demonstrated since.

The case for incorporation of chemotherapy into the treatment plan was initially questionable. The Mayo Clinic ran a study randomizing patients to a methotrexate-based regimen or surgery only and reported 5-year survival rates of 50%, for both arms [4]. This result exceeded the achievements reported historically from surgery alone. Retrospectively, the rationale is that there was a lack of appreciation of the prognostic implication of grading systems. It was subsequently recognized that a larger proportion of low-grade

Evidence-Based Pediatric Oncology, Third Edition. Edited by Ross Pinkerton, Ananth Shankar and Katherine K. Matthay.
© 2013 John Wiley & Sons, Ltd. Published 2013 by John Wiley & Sons, Ltd.

tumors were allocated to the "surgery only" arm, hence the surprisingly good outcome.

Separately, at the Memorial Sloan-Kettering Cancer Center in New York, Rosen published a series of studies, using increasingly complex adjuvant multiagent chemotherapy strategies, based on methotrexate. The "T10 regimen" was associated with apparent survival rates of 90% at 2 years. No other group has been able to mimic these results in multi-institutional settings. Two further randomized trials conducted in the US still had ethical approval for a control arm of observation alone. Both of these demonstrated the necessity for chemotherapy to improve survival prospects, with observation arms matching historical results of 17% long-term survival [5,6]. Increasingly, prognostic factors (patient and tumor characteristics) were recognized as being responsible for some of the variability in outcomes between early clinical trials, as a result of unequal representation in treatment arms of small series.

There is a consensus from phase II and III studies that the following agents have been shown to be efficacious in osteosarcoma: doxorubicin Adriamycin (A), ifosfamide (I), high-dose methotrexate (M) with leucovorin rescue, and cisplatin (P).

From the 1980s onwards, the trend towards longer and more complex regimens was challenged by some of the European groups. The European Organization for Research into Treatment of Cancer (EORTC) published a randomized control trial using a modified T10 regimen, with reduced-intensity methotrexate. Overall survival was disappointing at 40–50% in all arms [7]. The European Osteosarcoma Intergroup (EOI) then published a series of three trials [8,9,10] using a regimen backbone of Adriamycin/cisplatin (AP) and investigated the addition of methotrexate, use of the T10 regimen, and dose intensity. No survival advantage for the experimental arms was demonstrated over standard AP therapy. However, in retrospect, suboptimal dose intensity of cisplatin and doxorubicin when administered concurrently with methotrexate may have compromised efficacy [8]. The COSS studies similarly failed to demonstrate benefits of additional therapies to either an MA control arm or AP [11,12].

Despite AP not being shown to be inferior to other treatments for osteosarcoma in a randomized setting, parallel studies elsewhere in Europe and the US reported consistently superior results using regimens incorporating methotrexate and/or ifosfamide. Designing clean randomized controlled trials investigating the role of high-dose methotrexate has proved elusive as methotrexate administration interferes with the concurrent dose intensity of additional agents. The Rizzoli Institute has published evidence of the benefit of high-dose methotrexate ($12\,g/m^2$) over moderate doses [13], which conceivably explains the poor results of the modified T10 regimen of the EORTC study [7]. The role of ifosfamide is also unclear. Its role was explored in the COG/POG study [1,2,3] but a survival advantage was not proven. However, in the study design, cisplatin was omitted in the ifosfamide-containing arms during the neoadjuvant chemotherapy phase. As a result, the role of ifosfamide is uncertain because its contribution as a substitute or adjunct is unclear.

Whether or not a fourth drug has to be added to MAP is still unknown. A random effects meta-analysis of stringently selected, but heterogeneous, randomized clinical trials in osteosarcoma has just been published [14] which provides justification for a three-drug strategy over a two-drug strategy but event-free survival (EFS) and overall survival (OS) were not altered when comparing three-drug regimens with four-drug regimens. Pragmatically, MAP +/- ifosfamide has been adopted in most practices.

Dose intensity has been explored specifically [3,10,15]. Interestingly, the impact on long-term survival was not improved by increasing the known active agents to limits of toxicity. Similarly, increasing the intratumoral exposure to active agents by using the intra-arterial route rather than an intravenous one failed to show differences in outcome [16,17,18].

Established prognostic factors have been validated in successive trials to determine likely good outcomes, e.g. young age, nonmetastatic disease, limb rather than axial primaries, and a good response histologically to neoadjuvant chemotherapy. This latter issue, which is one of the few factors amenable to changes in management, has become the Holy Grail for outcome improvement. However, despite optimal doses of active agents, obtaining a good histology response does not always translate into survival. The role of salvage chemotherapy if the histology response is suboptimal is not yet proven. The largest international, collaborative, multi-institutional randomized clinical trial in osteosarcoma to date, EURAMOS 1, has just finished recruiting a sufficiently large cohort of patients to address this question. All patients registered received a standard induction regimen consisting of two cycles of AP and four cycles of high-dose methotrexate, before proceeding to surgical resection. Postoperative therapy was determined by histological response of the tumor. Good responders were randomized between MAP and MAP+pegylated interferon-α2b; poor responders were randomized to continue MAP or to receive MAP plus ifosfamide and etoposide.

Meanwhile, there has been a dearth of new agents showing any promise in osteosarcoma. We are clearly at the limits of dose intensity and efficacy with current perioperative multiagent strategies. The future hope is, therefore, dependent on better understanding of the biology of osteosarcoma and the potential identification of novel biological markers for small molecule therapy, which has transformed the management approach in other sarcomas, or the potential of other therapeutic approaches such as bisphosphonate therapy and/or immunotherapy. This brings us back to L-MTP-PE.

Intergroup study 0133 [1,2,3] was a prospective, four-arm, multicenter, two-by-two factorial design in patients with newly diagnosed osteosarcoma, exploring both addition of ifosfamide to a three-drug regimen as well as the incorporation of L-MTP-PE. Induction chemotherapy required upfront randomization to one of four arms: methotrexate/doxorubicin/cisplatin +/- ifosfamide +/- L-MTP-PE postoperatively; surgery to the primary tumor took place after two cycles. The inclusion of ifosfamide at a dose of $9 g/m^2$ had no impact on EFS or OS. However, there was a trend towards better EFS with the addition of L-MTP-PE, with overall survival improving from 70% to 78% ($p=0.03$; relative risk 0.71).

The preliminary publication in 2005 [3] unfortunately failed to demonstrate a significant role for L-MTP-PE, as the results were influenced by an apparent interaction between ifosfamide and the novel agent; consequently the statistical modeling of sample size required to demonstrate the hypothesis appeared inadequate. The later publication in 2008 [1] referencing longer outcome data appeared to show the intended benefit in OS, without the statistical evidence of an interaction. Sceptics remain concerned that there is insufficient evidence to show that the benefits of L-MTP-PE are not related to the incorporation of ifosfamide.

Data regarding the outcome for metastatic patients were separately reported in 2009 [2]. A trend towards improved EFS and OS was observed in those exposed to L-MTP-PE but the results were not statistically significant. However, the study was underpowered to detect a difference in survival between the study arms.

L-MTP-PE was demonstrated to be safe and well tolerated. The scheduling of administration may cause additional clinical problems, as an additional 18 weeks of treatment will be required. A significant proportion of patients are teenagers and young adults, who may resist prolongation of treatment. Compliance was a significant issue within the study format.

On the basis of this trial's dataset (reviewed and republished in 2008 [2] the European Medicines Evaluation Agency's (EMEA) committee on medicinal products for human use (CHMP) approved the use of L-MTP-PE for the treatment of nonmetastatic, resectable osteosarcoma in March 2009, allowing the drug to be marketed in Europe and making this the first agent to have a licensed indication in osteosarcoma specifically including pediatric patients. However, the EMEA's US counterpart, the FDA, has to date refused to grant a marketing approval, on the grounds of insufficient evidence of a survival advantage to justify the not inconsiderable cost implication of adding this product to the standard chemotherapy regimen. There is continued concern about the burden of this treatment to patients and healthcare systems, without further confirmatory trials.

Without international agreement of the gold standard of care (with regard to dose intensity, the number of agents to be used, including whether or not ifosfamide should be incorporated, and whether there is a role for change of postoperative therapy with relative failure of induction therapy and whether management should include L-MTP-PE or not), large-scale randomized clinical trials such as EURAMOS are not feasible, with a standard control arm. A universally accepted standard of care is further compromised by the enormous healthcare costs involved with current access to this novel agent, causing potential selection bias in suitable patient recruits. The hope remains that there will be a way forward, incorporating the option of further investigational studies of this promising agent, using the climate of international collaboration, to make faster progress than the experience of the last two decades.

References

1 Meyers PA, Schwartz CL, Krailo MD et al. Osteosarcoma: the addition of muramyl tripeptide to chemotherapy improves overall survival--a report from the Children's Oncology Group. *J Clin Oncol* 2008; **26**(4):633–8.

2 Chou AJ, Kleinerman ES, Krailo MD et al. Addition of muramyl tripeptide to chemotherapy for patients with newly diagnosed metastatic osteosarcoma. *Cancer* 2009;**115**:5339–48.

3 Meyers PA, Schwartz CL, Krailo M et al. Osteosarcoma: a randomised, prospective trial of the addition of ifosfamide and/or myramyl tripeptide to cisplatin, doxorubicin, and high-dose methotrexate. *J Clin Oncol* 2005;**23**(9):2004–11.

4 Edmonson JH, Green SJ, Ivins JC et al. A controlled pilot study of high-dose methotrexate as postsurgical adjuvant treatment for primary osteosarcoma. *J Clin Oncol* 1984;**2**:152–6.

5 Link MP, Goorin AM, Miser AW et al. The effect of adjuvant chemotherapy on relapse-free survival in patients with osteosarcoma of the extremity. *N Engl J Med* 1986;**314**:1600–6.

6 Eilber F, Giuliano A, Eckardt J, Patterson K, Moseley S, Goodnight J. Adjuvant chemotherapy for osteosarcoma. A randomised prospective trial. *J Clin Oncol* 1987;**5**:21–6.

7 Burgers JMV, van Glabbeke M, Busson A et al. Osteosarcoma of the limbs. Report of the EORTC-SIOP 03 trial 20781 investigating the value of adjuvant treatment with chemotherapy and/or prophylactic lung irradiation. *Cancer* 1988;**61**:1024–31.

8 Bramwell VHC, Burgers M, Sneath R et al. A comparison of two short intensive adjuvant chemotherapy regimens in operable osteosarcoma of limbs in children and young adults: the first study of the European Osteosarcoma Intergroup. *J Clin Oncol* 1992;**10**:1579–91.

9 Souhami RL, Craft AW, van der Eijken JW et al. Randomized trial of two regimens of chemotherapy in operable osteosarcoma: a study of the European Osteosarcoma Intergroup. *Lancet* 1997;**350**:911–17.

10 Gelderblom H, Jinks RC, Sydes M et al; European Osteosarcoma Intergroup. Survival after recurrent osteosarcoma: data from 3 European Osteosarcoma Intergroup (EOI) randomized controlled trials. *Eur J Cancer* 2011;**47**(6):895-902. Epub 2011 Jan 6.

11 Winkler K, Beron G, Katz R et al. Neoadjuvant chemotherapy for osteogenic sarcoma: results of co-operative German–Austrian study. *J Clin Oncol* 1984;**2**:617–24.

12 Winkler K, Beron G, Delling G et al. Neoadjuvant chemotherapy of osteosarcoma: results of a randomized cooperative trial (COSS-82) with salvage chemotherapy based on histological tumor response. *J Clin Oncol* 1988;**6**:329–37.

13 Bacci G, Picci P, Ruggieri P et al. Primary chemotherapy and delayed surgery (neoadjuvant chemotherapy) for osteosarcoma of the extremities. *Cancer* 1990;**65**:2539–53.

14 Anninga JK, Gelderblom H, Fiocco M et al. Chemotherapeutic adjuvant treatment for osteosarcoma: where do we stand? *Eur J Cancer.* 2011;**47**(16):2431–45.

15 Meyers P, Gorlick R, Heller G et al. Intensification of pre-operative chemotherapy for osteogenic sarcoma: results of the Memorial Sloan-Kettering (T12) protocol. *J Clin Oncol* 1998;**16**:2452–8.

16 Jaffe N, Robertson R, Ayala A et al. Comparison of intra-arterial cis-diamminedi-chloroplatinum II with high-dose methotrexate and citrovorum factor rescue in the treatment of primary osteosarcoma. *J Clin Oncol* 1985;**3**:1101–4.

17 Winkler K, Bielack S, Delling G et al. Effect of intraarterial versus intravenous cisplatin in addition to systemic doxorubicin, high dose methotrexate, and ifosfamide on histologic tumour response in osteosarcoma (study COSS-86). *Cancer* 1990;**66**:1703–10.

18 Bacci G, Ferrari S, Tienghi A et al. A comparison of methods of loco-regional chemotherapy combined with systemic chemotherapy as neo-adjuvant treatment of osteosarcoma of the extremity. *Eur J Surg Oncol* 2001;**27**:98–104.

Summary of previous studies

The earliest study in osteosarcoma (OS) was the German COSS-80, testing (1) whether the addition of either cisplatin or bleomycin, cyclophosphamide, actinomycin D (BCD) improves the efficacy of a doxorubicin/high-dose methotrexate (HDMTX) regimen and (2) whether interferon is of benefit when given to patients following initial chemotherapy [1]. There were 116 evaluable patients, out of 214 originally registered, with nonmetastatic OS. There was no significant difference in disease-free survival (DFS) with the addition of either cisplatin (73%) or BCD (77%) or between patients given interferon (77%) or no interferon (73%), although all groups had an improved overall survival compared to a prior COSS study. Another study compared in a small number of patients with nonmetastatic OS the efficacy of intra-arterial cisplatin with high-dose intra-arterial or intravenous methotrexate [2]. Following HDMTX, there were 4/15 responses: three complete responses (CR), one partial response (PR); with cisplatin there were 9/15 responses, seven CR and two PR: $p = 0.06$. There was said to be more rapid pain relief with the cisplatin regimen but the small size of the study and variability in approach made the results inconclusive.

Several studies then attempted to compare surgery alone to various chemotherapy regimens. A study by Edmonson *et al.* tested the role of adjuvant postoperative chemotherapy in 38 nonmetastatic patients using a regimen based on high-dose methotrexate and vincristine (MTX/VCR) compared to surgery alone [3]. There was no significant difference in progression-free survival (PFS) (40%) in the groups, though the overall survival was unexpectedly high at 52%. In response to the questions raised about the value of chemotherapy by the Edmonson study, the POG tested whether adjuvant chemotherapy after surgical resection/amputation improved survival for nonmetastatic OS [4]. Of 113 eligible patients, only 36 accepted the randomization to surgery alone or chemotherapy including cyclophosphamide, methotrexate, doxorubicin, and cisplatin. Even with these small numbers, there was a 2-year relapse-free survival (RFS) of 17%

for those not receiving chemotherapy, compared with 66% in those receiving chemotherapy: $p < 0.001$. Overall survival was in the region of 70% and did not differ between the two arms, possibly due to salvage chemotherapy. Thus the conclusion of this study was that chemotherapy improved RFS in OS.

Another study also addressed the randomized question of whether there was any benefit to chemotherapy using both neoadjuvant and adjuvant chemotherapy compared to surgery alone [5]. The preoperative treatment included intra-arterial doxorubicin and radiotherapy; after definitive surgery, adjuvant chemotherapy was composed of HDMTX, vincristine (VCR), doxorubicin and bleomycin, cyclophosphamide, and actinomycin D (BCD). Of the 59 patients, 32 received adjuvant chemotherapy and 27 observation alone. Overall, 55% were disease free at 2 years of those allocated to chemotherapy, compared with 20% who did not receive chemotherapy: $p < 0.01$. Eighty percent receiving chemotherapy were alive, compared with 48%: $p < 0.001$.

After these studies established the advantage of chemotherapy to treat micrometastatic disease, the EORTC tested whether adding lung radiotherapy alone or added to combination chemotherapy would improve RFS and decrease the risk of metastases [6]. Patients with nonmetastatic OS had amputation (n = 168) or local radiotherapy (n = 37), and were randomly assigned to receive chemotherapy alone (n = 65) with vincristine, methotrexate, doxorubicin, cyclophosphamide, or 20 Gy of bilateral lung radiotherapy (n = 73), or chemotherapy followed by bilateral lung radiotherapy (n = 67). Disease-free survival at 5 years was 40% for chemotherapy alone, 44% for lung irradiation alone and 45% for combination therapy. Lung function was impaired in 14% of those receiving irradiation. The conclusion was that there was no significant difference between these approaches but a control arm with no adjuvant therapy was not included in the study design, and there was some imbalance in the local control measures.

A subsequent study from the EORTC, Medical Research Council (MRC), and UK Children's Cancer

Study Group (CCSG) compared two different chemotherapy regimens in localized OS: doxorubicin/cisplatin in one arm and HMTX combined with reduced dose intensity doxorubicin and cisplatin in the other arm [7]. Regimen A consisted of doxorubicin and cisplatin given every 3 weeks for six courses; regimen B consisted of HDMTX 10 days prior to doxorubicin/cisplatin, which was given approximately every 4 weeks. At 5 years, 39% of group A and 53% of group B were free of metastases. The DFS was 57% for group A, 41% for group B, p=0.05. Overall survival was 64% and 50%, respectively, which was not statistically significant. The conclusion was that the lower dose intensity cisplatin/doxorubicin arm was probably inferior, despite the addition of HDMTX. It appeared that the addition of methotrexate, whilst reducing platinum-related toxicity, did not compensate for a reduction in efficacy due to reduced dose and dose intensity.

A variation on this was reported by Bacci *et al.* comparing cisplatin combined with a moderate-dose MTX regimen or with a HDMTX regimen [8]. Good histological response was seen in 41 of 66 evaluable patients receiving HDMTX (62%), compared to 25/60 receiving moderate-dose MTX (42%) (p < 0.04). The subsequent chemotherapy depended on initial treatment. Those with a good response were initially continued on methotrexate and cisplatin alone, but initially poor outcome led to a change in strategy, with the addition of doxorubicin. In patients with a fair response, doxorubicin was added and those with a poor response were switched to a doxorubicin/BCD combination. The overall 5-year DFS for the HDMTX arm was 58%, and 42% for the moderate-dose MTX arm (p=0.07). Overall, the response predicted outcome with 65% versus 40% versus 10% overall survival for good, fair, and poor responders, respectively (p=0.01). It was concluded that HDMTX was significantly better than moderate-dose MTX in achieving a good histological response but within the current study did not lead to a significant improvement in outcome.

Another study from the COSS group attempted to compare intra-arterial with intravenous cisplatin given preoperatively followed by initial standard chemotherapy, using doxorubicin and HDMTX [9]. Of the 109 randomized patients who were evaluable, the intra-arterial route led to a 68% good response rate and the intravenous (IV) route to a 69% good response rate without major differences in toxicity. It was

concluded that the intra-arterial route does not add to the efficacy of cisplatin when given in combination with other active agents. A later study of the European Osteosarcoma Group compared two chemotherapy regimens: one with intensive shorter 18-week treatment with cisplatin and doxorubicin and the other a longer 44-week, more complex regimen based on the Rosen T10 protocol, which additionally included HDMTX, vincristine, and BCD [10]. Overall survival was identical in both arms: 65% at 3 years and 55% at 5 years, and PFS at 5 years was 44% in both groups. Good histological response was seen in 29% of each group, and was strongly predictive of survival.

The COSS-82 trial randomized preoperative chemotherapy to try to reduce toxicity, by testing whether HDMTX with bleomycin, actinomycin D, and cyclophosphamide were better than HDMTX with cisplatin and doxorubicin [11]. Poor responders in the BCD arm were then changed to cisplatin/doxorubicin. Overall, the 4-year metastasis-free survival (MFS) for poor responders was 44%, compared to 77% for favorable responders (p < 0.001). Of 125 patients evaluable, the favorable pathological response defined as > 90% tumor cell destruction was seen in 15/57 patients (26%) with BCD compared to 35/58 patients (60%) with doxorubicin/cisplatin (p < 0.001). The 4-year MFS was 49% for BCD versus 68% for doxorubicin/cisplatin (p=0.1), but 5-year MFS was 45% versus 68% (p < 0.05).

Since improved histological response from preoperative chemotherapy appeared to predict outcome, a subsequent trial from the Memorial Sloan-Kettering Cancer Center tested an intensified preoperative chemotherapy against the prior T10 regimen with an endpoint of histological response and overall outcome [12]. Regimen I (T10) used HDMTX and BCD prior to surgery at 8 weeks, with doxorubicin afterwards for good responders and doxorubicin/cisplatin for standard responders. The intensified regimen II consisted of HDMTX and BCD, but also included two cycles of doxorubicin/cisplatin prior to surgery at 12 weeks, then used the same postoperative chemotherapy as regimen I. The intensified regimen did not change histological response. There was no difference in outcome between the two regimens. Event-free survival at 5 year was 73% for regimen I and 78% for regimen II.

Another study was done to try again to compare the value of adding intra-arterial local cisplatin to systemic chemotherapy, using the primary endpoint of histological response [13]. Initially, 49 patients received intra-arterial (IA) chemotherapy and 39 intravenous (IV). This was part of a HDMTX, cisplatin and doxorubicin combination and the study was stopped early because of a higher response rate in the IA arm (77% versus 46% good response).The second component was a four-drug regimen with the addition of ifosfamide but asking the same question regarding IA chemotherapy. Overall, the good response rate was higher than in the previous study (76% versus 62%, p=0.04). There was, however, no statistically significant difference between the two study arms: 80% (71–90%), 95% confidence interval versus 71% (61–82%) for IA versus IV, respectively. Similarly, no difference in 5-year EFS was seen in either study (first study 53% versus 61%, second study 62% versus 54% for IA versus IV, respectively). With more aggressive chemotherapy including ifosfamide, IA chemotherapy was not superior to cisplatin given IV.

A Pediatric Oncology Group study then tested whether neoadjuvant chemotherapy compared to postoperative adjuvant chemotherapy improved outcome [14]. Chemotherapy was HDMTX, doxorubicin/cisplatin, and BCD. Overall 5-year EFS for group A was 69%, group B, 61%. Toxicity and surgical complications were the same. No difference was seen whether chemotherapy was given preoperatively or postoperatively with regard to EFS or nature of surgery. A high overall amputation rate was observed in both arms of this study (approximately half the patients).

A study of the combined POG and CCG then tested whether adding ifosfamide to a chemotherapy regimen of HDMTX, doxorubicin, and cisplatin would improve EFS for OS, and whether adding the immunomodulator muramyl tripeptide (MTP) to chemotherapy would improve outcome, using a factorial design [15]. Both metastatic and nonmetastatic patients were enrolled but this analysis was restricted to nonmetastatic OS. Regimen A comprised cisplatin/doxorubicin in weeks 0, 5, 12, and 17. Doxorubicin alone was given at weeks 22 and 27. HDMTX was administered in weeks 3, 4, 8, 9, 15, 16, 20, 21, 25, 26, 30, and 31. Regimen B included ifosfamide 1.8 g/m$_2$, daily for 5 days, with mesna given in weeks 0, 5, 17, 27, and 35. Cisplatin was given four times, all during maintenance therapy postoperative weeks 12, 22, 32, and 38. Doxorubicin and methotrexate were given in the same dose and timing as in regimen A. The total doses of doxorubicin and HDMTX were the same in the two arms. Following surgery there was no difference in the grade of necrosis between the protocols: Huvos grade III and IV; regimen A 125/292, regimen B, 140/292. The 5-year EFS for regimen A was 64% and regimen B, 53%. In the arm where regimen B was combined with MTP, the EFS at 5 years was 72%, whereas for regimen A combined with MTP, 5-year EFS was 63%. The overall trend for difference between the four arms was significant (p=0.04). The addition of ifosfamide was of no significant benefit. There was a possible benefit from MTP specifically when combined with ifosfamide for nonmetastatic OS.

References

1 Winkler K, Beron G, Katz R et al. Neoadjuvant chemotherapy for osteogenic sarcoma: results of co-operative German–Austrian study. J Clin Oncol 1984;2:617–24.

2 Jaffe N, Robertson R, Ayala A et al. Comparison of intra-arterial cis-diamminedi-chloroplatinum II with high-dose methotrexate and citrovorum factor rescue in the treatment of primary osteosarcoma. J Clin Oncol 1985;3:1101–4.

3 Edmonson JH, Green SJ, Ivins JC et al. A controlled pilot study of high-dose methotrexate as postsurgical adjuvant treatment for primary osteosarcoma. J Clin Oncol 1984;2:152–6.

4 Link MP, Goorin AM, Miser AW et al. The effect of adjuvant chemotherapy on relapse-free survival in patients with osteosarcoma of the extremity. N Engl J Med 1986;314:1600–6.

5 Eilber F, Giuliano A, Eckardt J, Patterson K, Moseley S, Goodnight J. Adjuvant chemotherapy for osteosarcoma. A randomised prospective trial. J Clin Oncol 1987;5:21–6.

6 Burgers JMV, van Glabbeke M, Busson A et al. Osteosarcoma of the limbs. Report of the EORTC-SIOP 03 trial 20781 investigating the value of adjuvant treatment with chemotherapy and/or prophylactic lung irradiation. Cancer 1988;61:1024–31.

7 Bramwell VHC, Burgers M, Sneath R et al. A comparison of two short intensive adjuvant chemotherapy regimens in operable osteosarcoma of limbs in children and young adults: the first study of the European Osteosarcoma Intergroup. J Clin Oncol 1992;10:1579–91.

8 Bacci G, Picci P, Ruggieri P et al. Primary chemotherapy and delayed surgery (neoadjuvant chemotherapy) for osteosarcoma of the extremities. Cancer 1990;65:2539–53.

9 Winkler K, Bielack S, Delling G et al. Effect of intraarterial versus intravenous cisplatin in addition to systemic doxorubicin, high dose methotrexate, and ifosfamide on histologic tumour response in osteosarcoma (study COSS-86). Cancer 1990;66:1703–10.

10 Souhami RL, Craft AW, van der Eijken JW et al. Randomized trial of two regimens of chemotherapy in

operable osteosarcoma: a study of the European Osteosarcoma Intergroup. *Lancet* 1997;**350**:911–17.

11 Winkler K, Beron G, Delling G *et al.* Neoadjuvant chemotherapy of osteosarcoma: results of a randomized cooperative trial (COSS-82) with salvage chemotherapy based on histological tumor response. *J Clin Oncol* 1988;**6**:329–37.

12 Meyers P, Gorlick R, Heller G *et al.* Intensification of preoperative chemotherapy for osteogenic sarcoma: results of the Memorial Sloan-Kettering (T12) protocol. *J Clin Oncol* 1998;**16**:2452–8.

13 Bacci G, Ferrari S, Tienghi A *et al.* A comparison of methods of loco-regional chemotherapy combined with systemic chemotherapy as neo-adjuvant treatment of osteosarcoma of the extremity. *Eur J Surg Oncol* 2001;**27**:98–104.

14 Goorin AM, Schwartzentruber DJ, Devidas M *et al.*, for the Pediatric Oncology Group. Presurgical chemotherapy compared with immediate surgery and adjuvant chemotherapy for non-metastatic osteosarcoma: Pediatric Oncology Group Study POG-8651. *J Clin Oncol* 2003;**21**:4662–3.

15 Meyers PA, Schwartz CL, Krailo M *et al.* Osteosarcoma: a randomised, prospective trial of the addition of ifosfamide and/or myramyl tripeptide to cisplatin, doxorubicin, and high-dose methotrexate. *J Clin Oncol* 2005;**23**(9):2004–11.

New studies

Study 1

Meyers PA, Schwartz CL, Krailo MD *et al*. Osteosarcoma: The addition of muramyl tripeptide to chemotherapy improves overall survival—A report from the Children's Oncology Group. *J Clin Oncol* 2008; 26:633–638.

Objectives

To compare three-drug chemotherapy with cisplatin, doxorubicin, and methotrexate with four-drug chemotherapy with cisplatin, doxorubicin, methotrexate, and ifosfamide for the treatment of osteosarcoma. To determine whether the addition of muramyl tripeptide (MTP) to chemotherapy enhances event-free survival (EFS) and overall survival in newly diagnosed patients with osteosarcoma. This is a repeat analysis of the prior paper published in 2005 now examining survival in addition to EFS.

Study design

Six hundred and sixty-two patients with osteosarcoma without clinically detectable metastatic disease and whose disease was considered resectable received one of four prospectively randomized treatments. All patients received identical cumulative doses of cisplatin, doxorubicin, and methotrexate and underwent definitive surgical resection of primary tumor. Patients were randomly assigned to receive or not to receive ifosfamide and/or MTP in a 2×2 factorial design. The primary end points for analysis were EFS and overall survival. The plan was to assess relative risks associated with two different chemotherapies and biologic intervention as marginal analyses within the factorial design. Marginal analyses are valid only if there is no evidence of interaction. Patients assigned to regimen A (methotrexate, doxorubicin, cisplatin) would be compared with patients assigned to regimen B (A+ifosfamide) after stratification for MTP-PE assignment to assess effects of the regimens. A similar approach was to be used for assessing effects of MTP-PE. Interaction between assigned chemotherapy

and assigned biologic agent was assessed using the proportional hazards regression model. Briefly, the following terms were included in the regression model: c, chemotherapy, coded as 1 if the patient was assigned regimen B and 0 otherwise; m, biologic agent, coded as 1 if the patient was assigned to receive MTP-PE and 0 otherwise; and interaction, coded as the product of c and m, that is, 1 if the patient received both regimen B and MTP-PE and 0 otherwise. A p value associated with the test of hypothesis

Results

The median follow-up for 422/662 patients with no adverse events at analysis was 7.7 years. Overall, 264 (47.1%) of 559 assessable patients exhibited grade 3 or 4 necrosis. There was no statistically significant difference between treatment arms in the probability of favorable grade 3 or 4 necrosis. The EFS for all patients was 66% at 4 years and 64% at 6 years from entry; overall survival was 81% at 4 years and 74% at 6 years. There was no significant difference in EFS or in the risk of death for the two chemotherapy regimens, A versus B. However, when the impact of the MTP was examined, there was a significantly lower risk of death for the two regimens that included the MTP-PE. Regimen A without MTP was associated with a probability of survival of 78% and 71% at 4 and 6 years, respectively. The addition of MTP achieved a probability of survival of 82% and 75% at 4 and 6 years, respectively. Regimen B without MTP was associated with a probability of survival of 77% and 70% at 4 and 6 years, respectively. Treatment with four chemotherapy drugs including ifosfamide and the addition of MTP (regimen B with MTP) resulted in a probability of survival of 86% and 81% at 4 and 6 years, respectively. For overall survival, the proportional hazards regression analysis p value associated with the test of the hypothesis of no interaction between the chemotherapy intervention and the MTP intervention was 0.60, which does not meet a conventional level of significance. In the stratified analysis there was no evidence of an interaction. The two chemotherapy regimens carried the same risk of death ($p=0.83$). The relative risk of death for patients randomly assigned to receive MTP was 0.71 (95% CI, 0.52 to 0.96; $p=0.03$).

Conclusions

Conclusion

The addition of ifosfamide to cisplatin, doxorubicin, and methotrexate did not enhance EFS or overall survival for patients with osteosarcoma. The addition of MTP to chemotherapy resulted in a statistically significant improvement in overall survival and a trend toward better EFS.

Study 2

Chou AJ, Kleinerman ES, Krailo MD *et al.* Addition of muramyl tripeptide to chemotherapy for patients with newly diagnosed metastatic osteosarcoma. *Cancer* 2009;**115**:5339–48.

Objectives

To test whether the addition of liposomal muramyl tripeptide phosphatidylethanolamine (L-MTP-PE) to chemotherapy has been shown to improve overall survival in patients with metastatic osteosarcoma (OS). This paper was a more detailed analysis of the prior study published in 2005 looking only at patients with metastatic OS.

Study design

This was the second aim in a factorial design of an intergroup phase III study of OS. The trial randomized patients to a regimen of three-drug chemotherapy with cisplatin, doxorubicin, and high-dose methotrexate (regimen A) or to the same three drugs with the addition of ifosfamide (regimen B). The addition of L-MTP-PE to chemotherapy was evaluated in both arms in a randomized fashion. Although L-MTP-PE treatment did not begin until week 12 of protocol therapy, randomization of treatment assignment was done at entry. This resulted in four treatment arms: A or B for chemotherapy, both with and without MTP-PE. The EFS and overall survival functions were estimated by the method of Kaplan and Meier. Relative risks and associated confidence intervals were estimated using a relative hazards model with the characteristic of inter-

est as the only variable in the model. Interaction between assigned chemotherapy and assigned biological agent was assessed using the relative hazards regression. To explore the joint relationships between therapy assignment, patient characteristics, and outcome, factors considered significantly related to outcome as single characteristics were incorporated into a relative risk regression model along with the randomized therapeutic assignment. Backward stepwise regression was used to evaluate whether therapeutic assignment was significantly related to outcome after adjustment for those previously identified important risk factors.

Results

The 5-year EFS for the entire cohort of 91 patients was 34% (95% confidence interval [CI] 24–45%). When analyzed according to chemotherapy regimen, the 5-year EFS for each of the regimens was as follows: (1) regimen A without MTP-PE 29% (95% CI 11–51%); (2) regimen A with MTP-PE 41% (95% CI 21–60%); (3) regimen B without MTP-PE 23% (95% CI 8–43%); and 4) regimen B with MTP-PE 44% (95% CI 23–64%). There was no statistical difference among the regimens, and no evidence of interaction between the chemotherapy and the MTP-PE assignment. The relative risk for adverse analytic events associated with randomization to receive L-MTP-PE was 0.72 ($p=0.23$; 95% CI 0.42–1.2). The EFS at 5 years was 42% for those randomized to receive MTP-PE versus 26% for those who were not. The EFS at 5 years was 34% for those randomized to four-drug chemotherapy versus 35% for those randomized to three-drug chemotherapy. Similarly, there was no significant difference in overall survival by chemotherapy regimen or by addition of MTP-PE (log-rank 0.60). Five-year overall survival for the entire cohort of 91 patients was 47% (95% CI 35–58%). When analyzed according to chemotherapy regimen, the 5-year overall survival for each of the chemotherapy groups was as follows: (1) regimen A without MTP-PE 53% (95% CI 28–73%); (2) regimen A with MTP 50% (95% CI 26–69%); (3) regimen B without MTP-PE 30% (95% CI 13–50%); and (4) regimen B with MTP-PE 57% (95% CI 33–75%). The relative risk for death associated with randomization to receive L-MTP-PE was 0.72 ($p=0.27$; 95% CI 0.40–1.3). The survival at 5 years was 53% for those randomized to receive MTP-PE versus 40% for those who were not.

Conclusions

The authors conclude that although the advantages for EFS and OS are not significant, there is an apparent advantage and also a reduction in relative risk of death with MTP-PE that is concordant with the results for nonmetastatic OS.

Study 3

Gelderblom H, Jinks RC, Sydes M *et al.* Survival after recurrent osteosarcoma: data from 3 European Osteosarcoma Intergroup (EOI) randomized controlled trials. *Eur J Cancer* 2011;47:895–902.

Objectives

To determine the factors affecting postrecurrence survival in OS using data from three prior randomized clinical trials.

Study design

Between 1983 and 2002, the European Osteosarcoma Intergroup accrued 1067 patients to three randomized controlled trials of pre- and postoperative chemotherapy for patients with resectable nonmetastatic high-grade osteosarcoma of the extremity. Control treatment in all trials was doxorubicin 75 mg/m$_2$ and cisplatin 100 mg/m$_2$. The comparators were additional high-dose methotrexate (BO02), T10-based multidrug regimen (BO03), and granulocyte-colony stimulating factor (G-CSF) intensified-DC (BO06). Postrecurrence survival (PRS) was investigated on combined data with standard survival analysis methods.

Results

Median recurrence-free survival was 31 months; eight recurrences were reported more than 5 years after diagnosis. In 564 patients with a recurrence (median 13 months post randomization), there was no difference in postrelapse survival between treatment arms. Patients whose disease recurred within 2 years after randomization had worse prognosis than those recurring after 2 years. Patients with good initial histological response to preoperative chemotherapy had better overall survival after recurrence than poor responders. Local relapse was more often reported after limb-saving procedures (2% versus 8%; amputation versus limb saving), independent of primary tumor site. Site of first recurrence (local 20%, lung 62%, "other" 19%) affected survival, as patients recurring with nonlung distant metastases only or any combination of local relapse, lung metastases, and nonlung metastases (=group "other") had significantly worse overall survival (local 39%, lung 19%, "other" 9% at 5 years).

Conclusions

These data describing a large series of patients with recurrent extremity osteosarcoma confirm the relationship between early recurrence and poor survival. There was better PRS in patients after good histological response to preoperative chemotherapy, or with local-only recurrence.

CHAPTER 3

Ewing sarcoma

Katherine K. Matthay

UCSF School of Medicine, San Francisco, CA, USA

Commentary by Steven G. DuBois

Outcomes for patients with localized Ewing sarcoma have improved dramatically over the past three decades. This improvement is a direct result of the large co-operative group clinical trials summarized in the subsequent chapter. These studies have helped to define standard approaches to localized Ewing sarcoma that result in 5-year event-free survival (EFS) rates in excess of 70%.

In North America, INT-0091 established a new standard of care for patients with localized Ewing sarcoma consisting of vincristine/doxorubicin/cyclophosphamide alternating with ifosfamide/etoposide [1]. Successor North American studies have attempted to improve outcomes further by intensifying therapy using several different strategies. INT-0154 (Study 1, below) evaluated the strategy of dose intensification, mainly by augmenting individual doses of cyclophosphamide and ifosfamide [2]. Unfortunately, this strategy did not improve outcomes in patients with localized disease. The next strategy was evaluated in Children's Oncology Group (COG) protocol AEWS0031 which evaluated intensifying therapy by compressing the interval between chemotherapy cycles to 2 weeks instead of 3 weeks. While the final results of this trial have not yet been published, preliminary results presented at the American Society of Clinical Oncology 2008 Annual Meeting demonstrated a significant improvement in 3-year EFS with interval compressed chemotherapy. The current COG trial for patients with

localized Ewing sarcoma (AEWS1031) seeks to intensify therapy by adding another active chemotherapy combination to standard therapy. This ongoing trial utilizes the results of study 9457 (Study 5, below) that demonstrated significant activity of topotecan and cyclophosphamide in Ewing sarcoma [3]. Patients on AEW1031 are randomized to standard therapy or to an experimental arm that also includes blocks of topotecan and cyclophosphamide therapy.

In Europe, early co-operative group clinical trials also demonstrated the activity of regimens that include vincristine, doxorubicin, dactinomycin, and cyclophosphamide (VACA). More recent European trials have established other treatment regimens that result in similar outcomes to those reported in North American studies. The EICESS-92 trial (Study 2, below) yielded satisfactory results for patients with small primary tumors treated initially with vincristine, doxorubicin, dactinomycin, and ifosfamide (VAIA) followed by either ongoing VAIA or VACA [4]. For patients with large primary tumors, EICESS-92 suggests the addition of etoposide to VAIA. The Italian/Scandinavian protocol III (Study 3, below) also confirms that a regimen utilizing vincristine, doxorubicin, cyclophosphamide, ifosfamide, and etoposide produces good outcomes for patients with localized disease [5]. The results of the most recent European co-operative study, Euro-Ewing 99, have not yet been published. However, preliminary results presented at the 2011 SIOP annual meeting

Evidence-Based Pediatric Oncology, Third Edition. Edited by Ross Pinkerton, Ananth Shankar and Katherine K. Matthay.
© 2013 John Wiley & Sons, Ltd. Published 2013 by John Wiley & Sons, Ltd.

indicated excellent outcomes following vincristine/ifosfamide/doxorubicin/etoposide (VIDE) induction chemotherapy and either vincristine/ dactinomycin/cyclophosphamide (VAC) or vincristine/dactinomycin/ifosfamide (VAI) consolidation chemotherapy for patients with small localized tumors.

In stark contrast to improvements in outcomes for patients with localized Ewing sarcoma, patients with metastatic Ewing sarcoma continue to have poor outcomes that have not improved substantially in the past several decades. Strategies that have been evaluated in this population include addition of new chemotherapy regimens and dose intensification. INT-0091 and EICESS-92 both added ifosfamide and etoposide to doxorubicin-based chemotherapy and failed to improve outcomes for patients with metastatic disease. Studies 5–7 are nonrandomized but are included as background to current trials. North American study 9457 (Study 5, below) incorporated topotecan and cyclophosphamide as well as dose-intensified chemotherapy [3]. Despite significant activity of topotecan and cyclophosphamide, this trial did not improve outcomes for this population. A successor COG study (INT-0091, arm C; Study 4, below) also evaluated dose intensification in this population and likewise failed to improve outcomes [6]. Of note, the strategy of interval compression has not yet been evaluated in patients with metastatic Ewing sarcoma.

Another series of studies have investigated high-dose therapy for patients with poor-risk Ewing sarcoma, most notably newly diagnosed metastatic disease. The combination of busulfan and melphalan as myeloablative therapy has shown promise in nonrandomized studies conducted by the French national co-operative group and by the Euro-Ewing group (Studies 6 and 7, below) [7,8]. In both studies, only patients with responsive disease were eligible for high-dose therapy and a proportion of patients eligible for high-dose therapy did not undergo assigned therapy, raising the possibility of selection bias in these nonrandomized studies. The Euro-Ewing 99 trial includes an ongoing study evaluating high-dose therapy in a randomized manner for patients with poor-risk tumors, including those with isolated pulmonary metastatic disease. The eagerly awaited results of this randomized trial will provide clarity about the role of high-dose therapy for Ewing sarcoma.

Perhaps the most notable observation from the studies summarized below is the lack of biological agents that have moved from early-phase clinical trials into larger phase II and III clinical trials for these patients. A growing body of preclinical and clinical data supports a role for inhibition of the insulin-like growth factor-1 receptor (IGF-1R), mammalian target of rapamycin (mTOR), and vascular endothelial growth factor (VEGF) pathways in Ewing sarcoma. Despite this evidence, phase II and III clinical trials that incorporate these agents are in planning stages only for patients with poor-risk Ewing sarcoma, including newly diagnosed metastatic disease and relapsed disease. Given the late effects of intensive multiagent chemotherapy in patients with localized disease and the lack of substantial improvement in outcomes for patients with metastatic disease, both patient populations may benefit from the addition of biologically targeted therapies in upcoming clinical trials.

References

1 Grier HE, Krailo MD, Tarbell NJ et al. Addition of ifosfamide and etoposide to standard chemotherapy for Ewing's sarcoma and primitive neuroectodermal tumor of bone. N Engl J Med 2003;348(8):694–701.

2 Granowetter L, Womer R, Devidas M et al. Dose-intensified compared with standard chemotherapy for non-metastatic Ewing sarcoma family of tumors: a Children's Oncology Group study. J Clin Oncol 2009;27:2536–41.

3 Bernstein ML, Devidas M, Lafreniere D et al. Intensive therapy with growth factor support for patients with Ewing tumor metastatic at diagnosis: Pediatric Oncology Group/Children's Cancer Group phase II study 9457 – a report from the Children's Oncology Group. J Clin Oncol 2006;24:152–9.

4 Paulussen M, Craft AW, Lewis I et al. Results of the EICESS-92 study: two randomized trials of Ewing's sarcoma treatment – cyclophosphamide compared with ifosfamide in standard-risk patients and assessment of benefit of etoposide added to standard treatment in high-risk patients. J Clin Oncol 2008;26:4385–93.

5 Ferrari S, Sundby Hall K, Luksch R et al. Non-metastatic Ewing family tumors: high-dose chemotherapy with stem cell rescue in poor responder patients – results of the Italian Sarcoma Group/Scandinavian Sarcoma Group III protocol. Ann Oncol 2011;22:1221–7.

6 Miser JS, Goldsby RE, Chen Z et al. Treatment of metastatic Ewing sarcoma/primitive neuroectodermal tumor of bone: evaluation of increasing the dose intensity of chemotherapy – a report from the Children's Oncology Group. Ped Blood Cancer 2007;49:894–900.

7 Oberlin O, Rey A, Desfachelles AS et al. Impact of high-dose busulfan plus melphalan as consolidation in metastatic Ewing tumors: a study by the Societé Francaise des Cancers de L'Enfant. J Clin Oncol 2006;24:3997–4002.

8 Ladenstein R, Potschger U, Le Deley MC et al. Primary disseminated multifocal Ewing sarcoma: results of the Euro-Ewing 99 Trial. J Clin Oncol 2010;28:3284–91.

Summary of previous studies

The first co-operative group trial for Ewing sarcoma was the North American First Intergroup Study [1] which included patients with newly diagnosed localized Ewing sarcoma and randomized to VAC or VAC plus doxorubicin or VAC plus whole-lung radiation (15–18 Gy). A total of 342 eligible patients were randomized. Patients randomized to VACA had superior outcomes compared to patients randomized to VAC (60% versus 24% relapse-free survival at 5 years). Patients randomized to VAC plus whole-lung radiotherapy had intermediate outcomes (44% relapse-free survival at 5 years). This study demonstrated the importance of doxorubicin in the management of patients with Ewing sarcoma and also the potential impact of whole-lung radiotherapy.

The second intergroup study included only patients with newly diagnosed nonpelvic primary tumors of bone [2]. Patients were randomized to one of two chemotherapy regimens: a higher-dose regimen given every 3 weeks or a lower-dose regimen given on a more protracted, weekly schedule. All patients received vincristine, doxorubicin, cyclophosphamide, and dactinomycin, though patients on the protracted schedule received less intensive doxorubicin therapy. Patients randomized to the higher-dose regimen had superior 5-year EFS (73% versus 56%; p=0.03), highlighting the importance of dose intensity in the treatment of Ewing sarcoma.

INT-0091 was the third North American intergroup study and included patients with newly diagnosed localized and metastatic Ewing sarcoma of bone [3]. Patients were randomized to receive vincristine/doxorubicin/cyclophosphamide (VDC) every 3 weeks or VDC alternating every 3 weeks with ifosfamide/etoposide (IE). A total of 398 patients with localized disease were randomized. Patients with localized disease randomized to the VDC/IE arm had superior outcomes (69% versus 54% 5-year EFS). The addition of IE to VDC did not improve outcomes for the 120 patients with metastatic disease [4]. These results established VDC/IE

as a new North American standard for patients with localized Ewing sarcoma.

In Europe, a series of national co-operative group early studies all utilized VAC or VACA-type regimens in a nonrandomized manner. These trials all yielded 5-year EFS rates of approximately 50% [5,6,7,8]. As in North America, successor trials evaluated the addition of ifosfamide to VACA chemotherapy.

The CESS-86 trial adopted a risk-stratified approach to the use of ifosfamide [9]. In this trial, patients with small extremity tumors received VACA chemotherapy while patients with large tumors or axial tumors received ifosfamide instead of cyclosphosphamide (VAIA). A total of 301 patients were included in this nonrandomized trial. While there was no statistically significant difference in outcomes between the two treatment groups on univariate analysis, multivariate analysis controlling for differences in tumor size and tumor site demonstrated that the VAIA arm was superior to the VACA arm.

Two co-operative group trials have specifically addressed optimal radiotherapy techniques for patients with Ewing sarcoma. The Pediatric Oncology Group conducted study 8346 to evaluate the optimal radiation field for patients with Ewing sarcoma of the bone [10]. A total of 104 patients were randomized to receive either whole-bone radiotherapy or radiotherapy to the involved field plus a 2 cm margin. There was no difference in the rate of local failure between these two arms and therefore involved field radiotherapy became standard approach for subsequent patients.

The CESS-86 trial also included a randomization for patients receiving definitive or postoperative radiotherapy as their mode of local control [11]. These patients were randomized to receive conventional fractionation or hyperfractionation. Forty-four patients received definitive radiotherapy and 93 received postoperative radiotherapy. There were no statistically significant differences in disease-free survival, overall survival, or local control rate between conventional fractionation and hyperfractionation.

References

1 Nesbit ME Jr, Gehan EA, Burgert EO Jr et al. Multimodal therapy for the management of primary, non-metastatic Ewing's sarcoma of bone: a long-term follow-up of the First Intergroup study. *J Clin Oncol* 1990;**8**(10):1664–74.

2 Burgert EO Jr, Nesbit ME, Garnsey LA et al. Multimodal therapy for the management of non-pelvic, localized Ewing's sarcoma of bone: intergroup study IESS-II. *J Clin Oncol* 1990;**8**(9):1514–24.

3 Grier HE, Krailo MD, Tarbell NJ et al. Addition of ifosfamide and etoposide to standard chemotherapy for Ewing's sarcoma and primitive neuroectodermal tumor of bone. *N Engl J Med* 2003;**348**(8):694–701.

4 Miser JS, Krailo MD, Tarbell NJ et al. Treatment of metastatic Ewing's sarcoma or primitive neuroectodermal tumor of bone: evaluation of combination ifosfamide and etoposide – a Children's Cancer Group and Pediatric Oncology Group study. *J Clin Oncol* 2004;**22**(14):2873–6.

5 Craft AW, Cotterill SJ, Bullimore JA, Pearson D. Long-term results from the first UKCCSG Ewing's Tumour Study (ET-1). United Kingdom Children's Cancer Study Group (UKCCSG) and the Medical Research Council Bone Sarcoma Working Party. *Eur J Cancer* 1997;**33**(7):1061–9.

6 Jurgens H, Exner U, Gadner H et al. Multidisciplinary treatment of primary Ewing's sarcoma of bone. A 6-year experience of a European Cooperative Trial. *Cancer* 1988;**61**(1):23–32.

7 Oberlin O, Deley MC, Bui BN et al. Prognostic factors in localized Ewing's tumours and peripheral neuroectodermal tumours: the third study of the French Society of Paediatric Oncology (EW88 study). *Br J Cancer* 2001;**85**(11):1646–54.

8 Oberlin O, Patte C, Demeocq F et al. The response to initial chemotherapy as a prognostic factor in localized Ewing's sarcoma. *Eur J Cancer Clin Oncol* 1985;**21**(4):463–7.

9 Paulussen M, Ahrens S, Dunst J et al. Localized Ewing tumor of bone: final results of the cooperative Ewing's Sarcoma Study CESS 86. *J Clin Oncol* 2001;**19**(6):1818–29.

10 Donaldson SS, Torrey M, Link MP et al. A multidisciplinary study investigating radiotherapy in Ewing's sarcoma: end results of POG #8346. Pediatric Oncology Group. *Int J Radiat Oncol Biol Phys* 1998;**42**(1):125–35.

11 Dunst J, Jurgens H, Sauer R et al. Radiation therapy in Ewing's sarcoma: an update of the CESS 86 trial. *Int J Radiat Oncol Biol Phys* 1995;**32**(4):919–30.

New studies

Study 1

Granowetter L, Womer R, Devidas M *et al.* Dose-intensified compared with standard chemotherapy for non-metastatic Ewing sarcoma family of tumors: a Children's Oncology Group study. *J Clin Oncol* 2009;**27**: 2536–41.

This was an intergroup study that included the Pediatric Oncology Group and the Children's Cancer Group. Patients were enrolled from 1995 to 1998.

Objectives

The goal of this trial was to determine whether a dose-intensified chemotherapy regimen improves event-free survival in patients with localized Ewing sarcoma of bone or soft tissue.

Study design

This open-label phase III clinical trial randomized patients at study entry to one of two chemotherapy treatment regimens. Patients randomized to the standard arm received 17 courses of multiagent chemotherapy with doses of vincristine/doxorubicin/cyclophosphamide alternating every 3 weeks with ifosfamide/etoposide, analogous to the experimental arm of INT-0091 [1]. Patients in the experimental, dose-intensified arm received 11 courses of dose-intensified chemotherapy with vincristine/doxorubicin/cyclophosphamide alternating every 3 weeks with ifosfamide/etoposide. The doses of cyclophosphamide and ifosfamide given per course were higher in the experimental arm and additional weekly doses of vincristine were given such that the cumulative doses of these agents were similar between the standard and dose-intensified arms. Local control was recommended at week 12 in both arms. This study enrolled 478 eligible patients (231 standard regimen; 247 intensified arm).

Results

At 5 years, the EFS and overall survival (OS) rates for the study population were 71.1% and 78.6%, respectively. There were no statistically significant differences in EFS or OS between the two randomized treatment arms. Specifically, the 5-year EFS for patients in the standard arm was 72.1% compared to 70.1% for patients in the intensified arm. The intensified arm was associated with higher rates of hematological, renal, gastrointestinal, and infectious toxicities.

Conclusions

Intensification of therapy using intensified dosing of cyclophosphamide and ifosfamide did not improve outcomes for patients with localized Ewing sarcoma and was associated with increased toxicity. Of note, this was the first co-operative group trial for patients with Ewing sarcoma to include patients with extraskeletal Ewing sarcoma.

Study 2

Paulussen M, Craft AW, Lewis I *et al.* Results of the EICESS-92 study: two randomized trials of Ewing's sarcoma treatment – cyclophosphamide compared with ifosfamide in standard-risk patients and assessment of benefit of etoposide added to standard treatment in high-risk patients. *J Clin Oncol* 2008;**26**:4385–93.

This study was carried out by the European Intergroup Co-operative Ewing's Sarcoma Study group from 1992 to 1999.

Objectives

The goal of this study was to compare cyclophosphamide to ifosfamide as a component of therapy for patients with newly diagnosed standard-risk Ewing sarcoma. A second goal was to compare a chemotherapy regimen with and without etoposide for patients with newly diagnosed high-risk Ewing sarcoma.

Study design

In this open-label, randomized trial, patients with newly diagnosed Ewing sarcoma of bone were assigned a risk category at study entry. Patients were classified as standard risk if they had small (<100 mL tumor volume) localized tumors. Patients were classified as high risk if they had large (≥100 mL tumor volume) tumors and/or metastatic disease. Patients with standard-risk disease received four courses of multiagent chemotherapy consisting of vincristine, ifosfamide, dactinomycin, and doxorubicin (VAIA). Following local control, standard-risk patients were then randomized to receive an additional 10 courses of VAIA or 10 courses of vincrisitine, cyclophosphamide, dactinomycin, and doxorubicin (VACA). Patients with high-risk disease were randomized at study entry to receive 14 courses of VAIA or 14 courses of VAIA with the addition of etoposide (EVAIA). A total of 647 patients enrolled and were treated. Of these, 155 patients were classified as standard risk and 492 patients as high risk.

Results

Outcomes among standard-risk patients were comparable between VAIA and VACA randomized treatment arms, with estimated 3-year EFS rates of 74% and 73% respectively. Among high-risk patients, there was a trend in favor of the EVAIA treatment arm, with estimated 3-year EFS of 52% for patients randomized to EVAIA and 47% for high-risk patients randomized to VAIA. However, this difference was not statistically significant. Subgroup analysis demonstrated an EFS hazard ratio of 0.80 in favor of EVAIA for high-risk patients with localized tumors compared to an EFS hazard ratio of 0.96 for high-risk patients with metastatic disease.

Conclusions

Vincristine, ifosfamide, dactinomycin, and doxorubicin and VACA provide equivalent outcomes for patients with newly diagnosed localized Ewing sarcoma with small primary tumors. The addition of etoposide to VAIA may improve outcomes for patients with localized Ewing sarcoma and large primary tumors.

Study 3

Ferrari S, Sundby Hall K, Luksch R et al. Non-metastatic Ewing family tumors: high-dose chemotherapy with stem cell rescue in poor responder patients – results of the Italian Sarcoma Group/Scandinavian Sarcoma Group III protocol. *Ann Oncol* 2011;**22**:1221–7.

This study was carried out by the Italian Sarcoma Group and the Scandinavian Sarcoma Group from 1999 to 2006.

Objectives

The goal of this study was to evaluate a response-adapted approach incorporating high-dose therapy for patients with localized Ewing sarcoma and poor response to initial therapy.

Study design

Patients ≤40 years of age with newly diagnosed localized Ewing sarcoma of bone or soft tissue were eligible for this open-label response-adapted trial. All patients initially received four courses of multiagent chemotherapy followed by local control measures. Patients were then classified as good or poor responders. Good responders had no more than microscopic foci of viable tumor at time of resection (for patients undergoing surgical local control) or complete radiographic resolution of the soft tissue component (for patients not undergoing surgical local control). All other patients were classified as poor responders. Good responders received an additional nine courses of multiagent chemotherapy. Poor responders without disease progression received an additional four courses of multiagent chemotherapy followed by high-dose therapy with busulfan/melphalan conditioning. A total of 300 patients enrolled and were treated. Of these, 49% were good responders. The remaining patients either had disease progression and were removed from therapy or were classified as poor responders and assigned to receive high-dose therapy. Of those assigned to receive high-dose therapy, 18% [n = 28/156] did not receive assigned therapy due to disease progression, failed stem cell harvest, or refusal by patient/provider.

Results

The estimated 5-year EFS rate for the overall population was 69% (95% confidence interval [CI] 63–74%). For patients with good response to initial therapy, the estimated 5-year EFS rate was 75% (95% CI 70–80%). For patients with poor response to initial therapy, the estimated 5-year EFS rate was 63% (95% CI 55–70%) for all poor-response patients and 72% (95% CI 64–80%) for patients who received high-dose therapy.

Conclusions

A response-adapted treatment regimen that includes high-dose therapy after an initially poor response yields satisfactory outcomes in patients with newly diagnosed localized Ewing sarcoma.

Study 4

Miser JS, Goldsby RE, Chen Z *et al*. Treatment of metastatic Ewing sarcoma/primitive neuroectodermal tumor of bone: evaluation of increasing the dose intensity of chemotherapy – a report from the Children's Oncology Group. *Ped Blood Cancer* 2007;**49**: 894–900.

This was an intergroup study that included the Pediatric Oncology Group and the Children's Cancer Group. Patients enrolled from 1992 to 1994.

Objectives

The goal of this trial was to determine whether intensified dosing of cyclophosphamide and etoposide improves outcomes for patients with newly diagnosed metastatic Ewing sarcoma.

Study design

This open-label single-arm trial included patients with newly diagnosed Ewing sarcoma of the bone with metastatic disease at initial presentation. All patients received 18 courses of chemotherapy at 3-week intervals. Chemotherapy consisted of vincristine/doxorubicin/cyclophosphamide alternating every 3 weeks with ifosfamide/etoposide. The doses of cyclophosphamide, ifosfamide, and doxorubicin given per course were intensified beyond those administered in the experimental arm of INT-0091: 2200 mg/m^2/dose versus 1200 mg/m^2/dose for cyclophosphamide; 2800 mg/m^2/dose versus 1800 mg/m^2/dose for ifosfamide; and 90 mg/m^2/course versus 75 mg/m^2/course for doxorubicin. In addition, patients in this study received weekly doses of vincristine during vincristine/doxorubicin/cyclophosphamide cycles. Local control was recommended after 12 weeks of neoadjuvant chemotherapy. Sixty patients enrolled and received this dose-intensified therapy.

Results

At 6 years from study entry, the estimated EFS rate was 28% and estimated overall survival rate was 29%. The estimated overall survival rate with this dose-intensified regimen was similar to that observed for patients on INT-0091 treated on either the standard arm (vincristine/doxorubicin/cyclophosphamide only) or experimental arm (vincristine/doxorubicin/cyclophosphamide alternating every 3 weeks with ifosfamide/etoposide). Of 60 patients treated, six developed secondary leukemia.

Conclusions

Intensifying therapy using augmented doses of cyclophosphamide, ifosfamide, and doxorubicin does not improve outcomes for patients with newly diagnosed Ewing sarcoma of bone.

Study 5

Bernstein ML, Devidas M, Lafreniere D *et al*. Intensive therapy with growth factor support for patients with Ewing tumor metastatic at diagnosis: Pediatric Oncology Group/Children's Cancer Group phase II study 9457 – a report from the Children's Oncology Group. *J Clin Oncol* 2006;**24**:152–9.

This study was carried out by the Pediatric Oncology Group and Children's Cancer Group from 1999 to 2000.

Objectives

The goals of this study were: (1) to evaluate the activity of topotecan or topotecan/cyclophosphamide in patients with newly diagnosed metastatic Ewing sarcoma; (2) to determine the efficacy of dose-intensified therapy for this population; and (3) to determine whether amifostine ameliorates regimen-associated myelosuppression.

Study design

Patients <31 years of age with newly diagnosed metastatic Ewing sarcoma of bone or primitive neuroectodermal tumor (PNET) were eligible. This trial included two courses of window therapy studied in sequence. The first cohort of patients received two courses of topotecan monotherapy before moving on to dose-intensified multiagent chemotherapy with vincristine/doxorubicin/cyclophosphamide, alternating every 3 weeks with ifosfamide/etoposide. The second cohort of patients received two courses of topotecan and cyclophosphamide before moving on to the same dose-intensified multiagent chemotherapy regimen. In addition, those patients who provided consent were randomized 1:1 to receive or not receive open-label amifostine prior to doses of cyclophosphamide and ifosfamide. Local control took place after seven courses of neoadjuvant therapy; 110 eligible patients enrolled and were treated. Of these, 76 patients agreed to participate in the window study and 69 patients agreed to participate in the amifostine randomization.

Results

The response rate during the topotecan monotherapy window was 8%. The response rate during the topotecan/cyclophosphamide window was 57%. The duration of severe neutropenia and thrombocytopenia was similar between patients randomized to receive or not receive amifostine. The estimated EFS rate at 2 years from study entry was 24%. Receipt of window therapy or amifostine did not appear to affect outcome.

Conclusions

This study demonstrates the significant activity of the combination of topotecan and cyclophosphamide in patients with Ewing sarcoma. However, dose intensification did not improve outcomes in this metastatic population. Amifostine did not protect against myelosuppression associated with this regimen.

Study 6

Oberlin O, Rey A, Desfachelles AS *et al.* Impact of high-dose busulfan plus melphalan as consolidation in metastatic Ewing tumors: a study by the Societé Francaise des Cancers de L'Enfant. *J Clin Oncol* 2006;24: 3997–4002.

This study was carried out by the Societé Francaise des Cancers de L'Enfant from 1991 to 1997.

Objectives

The goal of this study was to determine outcomes for patients with metastatic Ewing sarcoma who receive myeloablative therapy with busulfan/melphalan following an initial good response to induction chemotherapy.

Study design

Patients with newly diagnosed Ewing sarcoma of bone with evidence of metastatic disease at initial presentation were eligible. All patients received uniform initial neoadjuvant chemotherapy consisting of five courses of doxorubicin with cyclophosphamide and two courses of ifosfamide with etoposide. Patients with a complete response or a very good partial response to induction chemotherapy were nonrandomly assigned to undergo myeloablative therapy with busulfan/melphalan conditioning. Local control occurred either before or after high-dose therapy depending upon details of the planned local control. Ninety-seven patients enrolled and were treated. Of these, 75 patients underwent high-dose therapy. The remaining 22 patients had either persistent or progressive disease after induction chemotherapy and were therefore not candidates for high-dose therapy.

Results

The estimated 5-year EFS rate for all 97 patients was 37% ± 10%. Among those patients who had a good response to induction chemotherapy and therefore received high-dose therapy, the estimated 5-year EFS rate was 47% ± 11%. Patients with bone marrow metastatic disease at initial presentation had an estimated 5-year EFS rate of 4 ± 4%.

Conclusions

Myeloablative therapy with busulfan and melphalan may improve outcomes for patients with newly diagnosed metastatic Ewing sarcoma who have a complete response or very good partial response to initial therapy.

Study 7

Ladenstein R, Potschger U, Le Deley MC *et al.* Primary disseminated multifocal Ewing sarcoma: results of the Euro-Ewing 99 Trial. *J Clin Oncol* 2010;28:3284–91.

This study was carried out by the Euro-Ewing group from 1999 to 2005.

Objectives

The goal of this study was to report the outcome of patients with newly diagnosed widely metastatic Ewing sarcoma treated with multiagent chemotherapy followed by myeloablative chemotherapy with busulfan and melphalan conditioning.

Study design

Patients <50 years of age with newly diagnosed Ewing sarcoma and metastatic disease other than isolated lung metastases were eligible for this single-arm open-label trial. Patients received six cycles of vincristine, ifosfamide, doxorubicin, and etoposide (VIDE) chemotherapy followed by local control to primary tumor and metastatic sites. Patients then went on to receive one course of vincristine, dactinomycin, and ifosfamide. Patients with disease that responded to initial therapy were eligible to receive myeloablative therapy, with busulfan/melphalan conditioning recommended. Two hundred and eighty-one patients enrolled and were treated. Of these, 44 had early progression precluding high-dose therapy and 68 did not receive high-dose therapy due to patient/provider choice or failed stem cell collection. The remaining 169 patients received high-dose therapy, 80% with busulfan/melphalan conditioning.

Results

The estimated 3-year EFS rate for the overall study population [n=281] was 27%. Among patients with complete response to induction therapy who went on to receive high-dose therapy, the estimated 3-year EFS rate was 57% (standard deviation 10%).

Conclusions

The use of high-dose therapy may be a promising strategy for patients with widely metastatic Ewing sarcoma and a complete response to initial therapy.

CHAPTER 4

Wilms tumor

Ananth Shankar

University College London Hospitals NHS Foundation Trust, London, UK

Commentary by Kathy Pritchard-Jones

This chapter summarizes the huge progress that has been made since the early 1970s in the treatment of Wilms tumor and other renal tumors of childhood. Looking critically at the first trial of what is now the Renal Tumours Study Group of the International Society of Paediatric Oncology [1], the fact that barely over half of all children with Wilms tumor were relapse free after nephrectomy and radiotherapy, with or without very modest duration, single-agent actinomycin D is a startling reminder of the need for multiagent therapy in children with Wilms tumor.

The first two trials of the North American National Wilms Tumor Study Group (NWTSG) that ran in the same decade showed that in patients whose tumors were amenable to immediate nephrectomy and whose treatment was carefully controlled, relapse-free survival rates of over 80% could be achieved. Ever since, the majority of children with Wilms tumor have been offered entry into randomized trials that have sought to reduce both the duration and intensity of their therapy without compromising relapse-free survival. These have been consistently successful, to the extent that for children treated in the 1990s, a decreasing proportion were treated with radiotherapy or doxorubicin whilst event-free and overall survival continued to improve. This emphasizes the importance of randomized trials rather than relying on historical comparisons that could lead to erroneous conclusions being drawn, particularly in relation to the need for

doxorubicin or the required dose of radiotherapy. This also implies that many children with Wilms tumor are still being overtreated by current standard regimens.

The trials conducted in the 1970s enrolled hundreds rather than thousands of patients yet we still rely today on the conclusions of the NWTS-1 trial that combination chemotherapy with vincristine plus actinomycin D is superior to either agent alone. This hypothesis was tested by randomizing a total of 166 patients with group II or III Wilms tumor and was not tested in children with group I tumors, who received either agent alone. All subsequent randomized trials of chemotherapy have used the vincristine and actinomycin-D (VA) combination as the standard arm in low-stage tumors and the question has never been readdressed, despite the severe hepatotoxicity of actinomycin D in 1–2% of patients. Why is this, when in the same era, the UK Medical Research Council conducted single-arm, prospective clinical studies that gave only vincristine monotherapy to children with stage I tumors, with similar disease-free outcomes?

Subsequently, studies conducted by the UK Children's Cancer Study Group adopted vincristine monotherapy as standard practice for stage I, nonanaplastic Wilms tumor [2]. Due to the high level of evidence quality for inclusion in this book, such single-arm trials are not included for critique here, despite offering an interesting perspective on what is sufficient treatment for children with localized, stage I Wilms tumors.

Evidence-Based Pediatric Oncology, Third Edition. Edited by Ross Pinkerton, Ananth Shankar and Katherine K. Matthay.
© 2013 John Wiley & Sons, Ltd. Published 2013 by John Wiley & Sons, Ltd.

A recent "decision tree" analysis concluded that, within the controlled environment of registration in a clinical trial, it was acceptable to reconsider a "surgery-only" approach for very low-risk, tiny tumors in children aged <2 years [3]. However, the vincristine-only treatment arm performed well in this analysis and might be reasonably reconsidered in settings where the toxicity or availability of actinomycin D is a concern [4].

Perhaps the most important message to be gleaned from the last 40 years of randomized trials in Wilms tumor is that the long-term results of all the randomizations show equivalent overall survival and question the benefit of using doxorubicin in localized disease [5]. There are increasing concerns about the long-term risks of cardiotoxicity. A recent prospective long-term follow-up study showed that one in eight survivors of childhood Wilms tumor had severe cardiac dysfunction 30 years after treatment if they had received both irradiation and doxorubicin [6].

The SIOP-WT 2001 trial has addressed the question of which patients can be safely treated without doxorubicin, but closed too recently for its full publication to be included in this edition [7]. The designers of this trial took the view that it is unlikely that there is a completely safe dose schedule for use of doxorubicin in the very young age group who are typically affected by Wilms tumor. Therefore, it was decided to test the safety of complete removal of doxorubicin rather than a dose reduction in the relevant regimens. The design of this trial had to take into consideration the two previous randomized trials (NWTS-3, SIOP-6) conducted in the 1980s, where both randomizations were closed early due to an excess of relapses in the "no doxorubicin" arms. However, in the SIOP-6 trial, there was no difference in event-free survival in the final analysis and other differences in postoperative treatment intensity may have accounted for the apparent early superiority of the doxorubicin arm. In the NWTS-3 trial, the advantage of doxorubicin was seen only in stage III patients randomized to a reduced dose (10.8 Gy) of flank radiotherapy. In both studies, the numbers of patients included in the doxorubicin randomizations were relatively small and there was no difference in overall survival on long-term follow-up. This justified a fresh look at the risk-benefits of doxorubicin in the treatment of children with Wilms tumor, provided that new information could be incorporated into the initial risk stratification process.

Two approaches to improving risk stratification have been developed in the 1990s. The NWTS-5 trial was the first and, so far, only clinical trial to test prospectively the prognostic value of a molecular biomarker, loss of heterozygosity for defined subregions of chromosomes 1p and 16q [8]. This impressive trial, enrolling over 2000 children with Wilms tumor, could not be included in this chapter as it was not a randomized trial design. However, this study has set the "best practice" standard for those who use immediate nephrectomy in the setting of quality-controlled review of pathology and surgical techniques, treatment, and outcomes.

The SIOP approach of neoadjuvant treatment of Wilms tumor provides the unique opportunity to look at the histological response *in vivo* of each child's tumor. Wilms tumors are subtyped according to the proportion of necrosis and the predominant cellular composition of the residual viable tumor. As described in this chapter for the German cohort of patients treated in the SIOP-93-01 trial, this has permitted the identification of a new high-risk category of Wilms tumor, "blastemal type," where a relatively high proportion of undifferentiated tumor cells survive preoperative chemotherapy [9]. This subtype has been excluded from the randomization in the design of the SIOP-WT 2001 trial and such patients continue to receive doxorubicin.

The UK investigators decided to address the question of which initial approach to the treatment of childhood renal tumors gave the optimum balance of tumor stage, to avoid the long-term risks of doxorubicin and radiotherapy whilst maintaining event-free and long-term survival [10]. This is the only trial that has ever attempted to randomize this surgical question, namely upfront nephrectomy versus preoperative chemotherapy with elective delayed nephrectomy, 7–8 weeks later. Given the long-standing, international controversies that have surrounded this question, it is not surprising that only 39% of eligible patients were randomized. The more favorable stage distribution and equivalent event-free survival led the UK investigators to subsequently adopt preoperative chemotherapy as their preferred initial treatment approach, joining the SIOP investigators for their WT 2001 randomized trial. The long-term outcomes of all children registered in the UKW-3 study have recently been published and show that 47% of all nonanaplastic Wilms tumors (i.e. stage I–V, including all metastatic and bilateral cases) received doxorubicin and 27% radiotherapy, with 90% 5-year overall survival [11]. This will form a useful baseline for future evaluation of the impact on population treatment and outcomes when a national study group changes its approach to first-line therapy for a relatively common childhood solid tumor.

It is doubtful that any further randomized trials of surgical approach to Wilms tumor will be performed. Furthermore, changes over time in the definition of "rupture" have done little to alleviate the ongoing controversy as to whether experienced surgeons can safely select children who are appropriate for immediate nephrectomy. The experience in the UKW-3 trial was that there was a higher rupture rate amongst the immediate nephrectomy cases, even though these tumors were, on average, smaller than those having preoperative chemotherapy.

The remaining challenge is how to make further refinements to risk-adapted use of current therapeutic agents on the background of an expected overall survival rate of ~90%. To improve survival, it is only a small minority of children with very high-risk tumor subtypes who need innovative therapies. However, all children with Wilms tumor could benefit if newer targeted and less toxic therapies could replace the antitumor activity of doxorubicin and radiotherapy. Trial design for safe and effective introduction of such agents is challenging, but should be achievable by the existing global co-operation between the international renal tumor groups. However, it requires greater knowledge than currently exists to understand the molecular pathways that drive resistance in Wilms tumor. The SIOP investigators are focused on molecular characterization of resistant blastema following chemotherapy. The Children's Oncology Group (COG) investigators have identified some molecular signatures of poor outcome in stage III nonanaplastic Wilms tumors, but the individual genetic pathways remain to be described [12]. Both groups define anaplastic Wilms tumor as high risk and despite its strong association with mutation of the *p53* gene, this has not yet been turned to therapeutic advantage. Finally, there is the possibility of using improving knowledge of genetic susceptibility to the toxic side-effects of chemotherapy to tailor effective treatment to a child's risk. The recent discovery of polymorphisms that indicate susceptibility to the cardiotoxic effects of doxorubicin could have clinical application in the not too distant future [13].

The final word should go to the evidence presented that addresses the needs of children with non-Wilms cancers of the kidney. They are individually extremely rare but collectively, they constitute almost 10% of all childhood renal tumors. Clear cell sarcoma of kidney (CCSK) (3%) and malignant rhabdoid tumor (2–3%) present at the same age as Wilms tumor whereas renal cell carcinoma (RCC) increases in incidence in adolescents, though can occur rarely in very young children. Whilst there is increasing knowledge of the molecular biology of childhood RCC and anecdotal evidence of activity of the same targeted tyrosine kinases as in adult RCC, the only randomized trial has been performed in CCSK. This was a subset analysis of the NWTS-4 trial which compared the duration of therapy and also the total dose of doxorubicin [14] for children with stage III and IV Wilms tumors and for those with CCSK. As there were only 40 patients with CCSK randomized, there was no statistically significant difference in event-free or overall survival. However, the event-free survival advantage to the longer duration arm that received the higher total dose of doxorubicin looks compelling and all current international protocols for the treatment of CCSK give these higher total doses of doxorubicin, albeit over a much shorter duration than in the NWTS-4 trial.

To conclude, there is still work to be done to optimize treatment for children with Wilms tumor. A subset of high-risk Wilms tumors along with the rarer non-Wilms tumors are in great need of therapeutic innovation. Only by global collaboration between co-operative groups and strong partnerships to exploit knowledge of biologically targeted therapies against common pathways in other childhood and adult cancers will progress be made in a timely fashion. These biology-driven approaches will not always follow randomized trial designs so the next edition of this chapter may need to broaden its inclusion criteria.

References

1 SIOP Renal Tumours Study Group: http://web.visu.uni-saarland.de/rtsg/

2 Pritchard-Jones K, Kelsey A, Vujanic G *et al*. Older age is an adverse prognostic factor in stage I, favorable histology Wilms tumor treated with vincristine monochemotherapy: a study by the United Kingdom Children's Cancer Study Group, Wilm's Tumor Working Group. *J Clin Oncol* 2003;**21**: 3269–75.

3 Frazier AL, Shamberger RC, Henderson TO, Diller L. Decision analysis to compare treatment strategies for Stage I/favorable histology Wilms tumor. *Pediatr Blood Cancer* 2010;**54**: 879–84.

4 Israels T, Chagaluka G, Pidini D *et al*. The efficacy and toxicity of SIOP preoperative chemotherapy in Malawian children with a Wilms tumour. *Pediatr Blood Cancer* 2012;**59**(4):636–41.

5 Green D. The treatment of stages I–IV favourable histology Wilms tumour . *J Clin Oncol* 2004;**22**:1366–72.

6 Van der Pal HJ, van Dalen EC, van Dalen EV *et al*. High risk of symptomatic cardiac events in childhood cancer survivors. *J Clin Oncol* 2012;**30**:1429–37.

7 Pritchard-Jones K, Graf N, Bergeron C *et al*. Doxorubicin can be safely omitted from the treatment of stage II/III, intermediate risk histology Wilms tumours: results of the SIOP WT 2001 randomized trial. *Pediatr Blood Cancer* 2011;**57**:741.

8 Grundy PE, Breslow NE, Li S, Perlman E *et al*. Loss of heterozygosity for chromosomes 1p and 16q is an adverse prognostic factor in favorable-histology Wilms tumor: a report from the National Wilms Tumor Study Group. *J Clin Oncol* 2005;**23**:7312–21.

9 Reinhard H, Semler O, Bürger D *et al*. Results of the SIOP 93-01/GPOH trial and study for the treatment of patients with unilateral non-metastatic Wilms tumor. *Klin Paediatr* 2004; **216**:132–40.

10 Mitchell C, Pritchard-Jones K, Shannon R *et al*. Immediate nephrectomy versus preoperative chemotherapy in the management of non-meta static Wilms tumour: results of a randomized trial (UKW3) by the UK Children's Cancer Study Group. *Eur J Cancer* 2006;**42**:2554–62.

11 Pritchard-Jones K, Moroz V, Vujanic G *et al*. Treatment and outcome of Wilms tumour patients: an analysis of all cases registered in the UKW3 trial. *Ann Oncol* 2012;**23**(9): 2457–63.

12 Huang CC, Gadd S, Breslow N *et al*. Predicting relapse in favorable histology Wilms tumor using gene expression analysis: a report from the Renal Tumor Committee of the Children's Oncology Group. *Clin Cancer Res* 2009;**15**: 1770–8.

13 Visscher H, Ross CJ, Rassekh SR *et al*. Pharmacogenomic prediction of anthracycline-induced cardiotoxicity in children. *J Clin Oncol* 2012;**30**:1422–8.

14 Seibel NL, Li S, Breslow NE *et al*. Effect of duration of treatment on treatment outcome for patients with clear-cell sarcoma of the kidney: a report from the National Wilms Tumor Study Group. *J Clin Oncol* 2004;**22**:468–73.

Summary of previous studies

The role of preoperative radiotherapy (RT) in the management of Wilms tumor (WT) was explored by two studies by Lemerle *et al.* [1, 2]. In the first study, based on imaging alone, patients were randomized to receive 20 Gy preoperative radiotherapy (arm A) or proceed straight away with primary nephrectomy (arm B). Following surgery, stage I patients in arm A received no further radiotherapy (they did receive chemotherapy). Arm B patients with stage I received 20 Gy postoperatively. Stage II patients received 30 Gy to the tumor bed while stage III patients with ruptured WT received 30 Gy whole-abdominal RT with additional booster doses where appropriate. A second randomization was to administer either a single dose of actinomycin D (ACT-D) postoperatively versus 3 weekly ACT-D for six courses. Stage distribution in arm A was stage I 31, II 33, and III 9 compared to 14, 28, and 22 respectively. In arm A, there were three tumor ruptures versus 20 in arm B. Relapse-free survival (RFS) and overall survival (OS) were 52% and 83% for arm A versus 44% and 71% for arm B. With regard to the ACT-D randomization, there was no difference in either RFS (54% versus 58%) or OS (82% versus 86%) between the two arms. It was concluded that while preoperative RT reduced the tumor rupture rate at surgery, this did not translate into improved RFS or OS because of the administration of postoperative RT.

The second study investigated whether preoperative chemotherapy (CT) was equivalent to preoperative RT in preventing surgical tumor ruptures in children with Wilms tumor. Eligible patients were randomized to receive either a combination of five doses of ACT-D plus 20 Gy local radiotherapy prior to nephrectomy (group R) or four doses of vincristine and two 3-day courses of ACT-D alone prior to nephrectomy (group C). Following nephrectomy, RT was given to both groups according to stage and preoperative treatment. Stage I patients received no postoperative RT while stages II and III received 15 Gy postoperative RT in group R and 30 Gy in group C. Although the stage distribution in group R (n=76) or C (n=88) was similar, a major change in pathological features, reflecting response, was higher in those who received preoperative RT

(53% versus 17%). There was no difference in OS between the groups. There was a trend in favor of group C patients with regard to overall recurrence-free survival. The authors concluded that preoperative chemotherapy was equivalent to preoperative radiotherapy in preventing tumor rupture. Additionally, they also noted that 43% of WT patients could be treated without RT when chemotherapy was given preoperatively.

The SIOP-6 trial and study reported by Tournade *et al.* [3] addressed the following issues on the management of WT: the duration of postoperative chemotherapy in patients with stage I disease, the role of local postoperative RT in stage II node-negative patients, and the role of doxorubicin in stage II node-positive and stage III patients. A 3-week preoperative chemotherapy regimen that consisted of vincristine and ACT-D was followed by surgery. Of a total of 1095 patients registered on the trial, only 509 were eventually randomized; 62% of patients were compliant with the trial-specific treatment. For stage I patients, the 2-year disease-free survival (DFS) was 92% in the short arm versus 88% in the long arm while the 5-year OS was 95% and 92% in the short and long treatment arms respectively. The number of abdominal recurrences (n=6) that developed in stage II, node-negative patients who did not receive postoperative RT caused the trial stopping rule to be activated. Subsequently, all node-negative patients received local RT. However, DFS rates were not significantly different in the two treatment arms (72% versus 78%). The doxorubicin randomization was prematurely stopped in node-positive stage II and stage III patients because of the early results of the North American national WT trial (NWTS-3) and other non-SIOP studies. Ultimate DFS was superior in those who received the doxorubicin-containing regimen (74% versus 49%; p < 0.03). It was concluded that a risk-adapted therapy to limit treatment-related sequelae was possible. A more intensive preoperative chemotherapy regimen is necessary to prevent abdominal recurrences for nonirradiated stage II N0 treated preoperatively and a three-drug protocol, including doxorubicin, is necessary for stages II N1 and III patients.

The Brazilian Wilms Tumor Study Group [4] conducted a randomized study that evaluated the toxicity and efficacy of fractionated ACT-D versus single-dose ACT-D. Patients were randomized to receive either a fractionated dose of 15 µg/kg of ACT-D over 5 days (arm A) or a single dose of 60 µg/kg (arm B). Chemotherapy courses were administered every 6 weeks. Of the 190 patients registered on the trial, only 156 were randomized. The 4-year RFS and OS rates were similar in both groups: 67% and 72% respectively in arm A and 67% and 75% respectively in arm B (p = 0.839 and 0.71 respectively). Additionally, patients in the single-dose arm had fewer hospital days compared to those who received fractionated doses. No significant difference in toxicity was observed between the two treatment groups of patients. It was concluded that while a single-dose schedule of ACT-D was as efficacious as and no more toxic than the fractionated dosing schedule of ACT-D, the single-dose schedule was more cost-effective.

During the late 1960s and early 1970s, the National Wilms Tumor Study Group trial 1(NWTS-1) [5] evaluated the following questions: the role of radiotherapy in group I patients; the efficacy of three chemotherapy regimens – vincristine alone, ACT-D alone or a combination of vincristine, and ACT-D in groups II and III patients as well as the role of preoperative vincristine in group IV patients. The radiation dose was adjusted for age and ranged from 18–24 Gy for children <18 months of age to 40 Gy in those >40 months. Out of the 606 patients registered in the trial, only 359 were randomized. For stage I patients <2 years of age, there was no difference in the DFS or OS between those who received RT or not (DFS 90% versus 88%, OS 97% versus 94% respectively). However, in children >2 years of age, the 2-year DFS in the RT group was significantly higher (77% versus 58%; p = 0.04) although this was not reflected in the OS (97% versus 91%). For group II and III patients, there appeared to be a significant survival advantage to the combination of vincristine plus ACT-D (VA); 2-year DFS for VA 81% versus 57% for ACT-D and 55% for vincristine alone. This was replicated in the OS of 86% for VA compared to 67% and 72% for ACT-D and vincristine respectively (p = 0.002). While the numbers were small (n = 13), stage IV patients who proceeded to immediate nephrectomy without preoperative vincristine appeared to have a better survival outcome (83% versus

29%; p = 0.02). The authors concluded that although stage I patients >2 years of age had a higher relapse rate without radiotherapy but as this did not translate to better OS, the late effects of RT did not justify the administration of RT to this group of good-risk patients. Additionally, they also concluded that for group II and III patients, the combination of vincristine and ACT-D was superior to either ACT-D or vincristine alone.

A report from the NWTS-2 trial evaluated the duration of treatment (6 months versus 15 months) in group I patients with WT and also assessed the value of the addition of doxorubicin to vincristine and ACT-D in patient groups II–IV [6]. Group I patients did not receive RT after nephrectomy and all received VA postoperatively at 6 weeks, 3 months, and 6 months. Group II–IV patients all received RT and the dose ranged from 18 Gy to 40 Gy depending on the age of the child. Group IV patients also received additional RT to metastatic sites. Patients were randomized to receive two (VA) or three drugs (doxorubicin plus VA, AVA) every 3 months for four doses. Of the 755 patients registered on the NWTS-2 trial, only 513 were randomized. For the 188 group I patients, there were no differences in survival outcome; 2-year RFS was 88%. RFS was also significantly better in group II–III patients with favorable histology (FH) who received doxorubicin. The 2-year RFS for group II–IV patients randomized to the three-drug AVA regimen was 77.1% versus 62.5% for the VA regimen (p < 0.0004). While the RFS was not significantly different between the two- and three-drug regimens in patients with unfavorable histology, the OS was superior for patients who received the three-drug regimen (p = 0.02). The authors concluded that a short treatment regimen is adequate for group I not receiving RT and the addition of doxorubicin improves survival outcome in all other risk groups, especially in those with favorable histology.

The NWTS-3 study explored the feasibility of further shortening the duration of treatment for stage I patients with FH WT, the role of doxorubicin and local radiotherapy in patients with stage II and III WT, and the addition of cyclophosphamide to the three-drug AVA regimen in patients with stage IV disease and unfavorable histology [7]. Stage II FH WT patients were randomized to receive or not receive 20 Gy local RT within 10 days of nephrectomy. Stage III FH WT patients were randomized between 10 and 20 Gy local RT. A total of 1465 patients were randomized. No significant difference was seen relating to the duration of treatment for stage I FH patients. The conclusions were less clear for the role of doxorubicin in the treatment of WT. When stages II and III were considered together, there was no difference in outcome. However, when stage III patients alone were considered, the relative risk of relapse for those who received VA compared to AVA was 1.6 (p=0.07), with fewer intra-abdominal relapses (4/134 versus 11/141) seen in those who received doxorubicin. More than half of the intra-abdominal relapses were seen in stage III patients who received reduced 10 Gy local RT without doxorubicin. RFS and OS were not different in stage II patients who received no RT versus 20 Gy RT or in stage III patients who received 10 Gy versus 20 Gy RT. For stage IV patients, the addition of cyclophosphamide to the three-drug AVA regimen did not improve survival outcome. A separate analysis for unfavorable histology showed that the outlook for patients with rhabdoid tumors was poor whether or not cyclophosphamide was added to the treatment regimen; only 25% were alive at 4 years in contrast to 75% of patients with clear cell sarcoma irrespective of the chemotherapy regimen. Four-year survival and RFS percentages for 279 patients with metastases at diagnosis or tumors of unfavorable histology were 73.0% and 68.1%.

The authors concluded that while the shorter duration treatment arm did not adversely affect survival outcome in stage I patients, after subset analysis corrected for certain aberrations they recommended that all stage I patients receive 6 months of treatment. While the efficacy of doxorubicin was not clearly demonstrated, the group favored the use of doxorubicin in stage III patients as it compensated for the lower dose of local RT. It was concluded that RT played no role in stage II patients. While the addition of cyclophosphamide to high-risk patients (stage IV and all stages in patients with unfavorable histology) did not improve survival outcome, it appeared to be of some benefit for patients with stage II–IV anaplastic WT. The apparently beneficial effect of cyclophosphamide in stages II–IV anaplastic tumors was carried forward to the next study (NWTS-4) to obtain clearer data.

The NWTS-4 trial evaluated the efficacy, toxicity, and cost-effectiveness of fractionated actinomycin D (STD) versus single-dose actinomycin D (PI) [8]. All patients <16 years of age with untreated stage I–IV FH WT, stage I anaplastic WT and stage I–IV CCSK

were included in the trial. After initial nephrectomy and lymph node biopsy, patients were randomized to receive a treatment that included vincristine and ACT-D either as a single dose or in divided doses. The initial ACT-D dose was 60 µg/kg but this was reduced to 45 µg/kg after concerns about hepatotoxicity. In summary, stage I patients received either 18 or 25 weeks of treatment with the frequency of ACT-D varying in addition to the schedule. For stage II patients, in addition to the schedule difference, the total number of doses differed: eight in one treatment arm and 21 in the other arm. In stage III patients and those with unfavorable histology, the number of doses of ACT-D varied between the treatment arms (10 versus six), as did the total number of doxorubicin doses (five versus nine), although the total dose was the same.

Although NTWSG-4 enrolled 3335 patients, ultimately, 536 low-risk patients were randomized to the STD arm versus 528 in the PI arm. The 2-year RFS for low-risk patients in the STD arm was 91.4% versus 91.3% in the intensive pulsed arm while for high-risk patients the 2 years RFS was 90% in the STD arm versus 87.3% in the PI arm. There was no difference in hematological toxicity between the two treatment arms. It was concluded that single-dose ACT-D was less toxic and equivalent in efficacy to the fractionated schedule for low-risk or high-risk WT or CCSK patients.

The NWTS-4 study group also evaluated the cost and efficacy of the various CT regimens used in the treatment of WT [9]. Previously untreated patients <16 years of age with stages II–IV FH WT as well as those with stage I–IV CCSK were included. There were two randomizations: randomization 1: between single-dose ACT-D (PI) versus divided dosing of ACT-D (STD); randomization 2: after completion of 6 months of CT to either stop or continue for an additional 9 months (6 versus 15 months). Of the 3230 patients registered, only 1756 were randomized. The 4-year RFS (stage II FH WT) randomized to the short arm (n=190) was 83.7% versus 88.2% in the long arm (n=187; p=0.11) while 4-year OS was 96.2% and 96.7% respectively (p=NS). Similarly, the 4-year RFS and OS for high-risk patients (stages III–IV; FH) randomized to the short arm (n=232) was 89.7% and 94.1% versus 88.8% and 94% respectively for patients who had the longer treatment (n=229). It was concluded that the shorter treatment program was very effective and was substantially more cost-effective and less toxic.

A subgroup analysis of the NWTS-4 study described by Green et al. [8] compared conventional standard therapy of vincristine, doxorubicin, and fractionated doses of actinomycin D (ST) against pulse intensive (PI) chemotherapy (vincristine, doxorubicin and single-dose actinomycin D) as well as the duration (short, 6 months, versus long, 9 months) of therapy in children with CCSK [10].While 86 children with CCSK were registered on the NWTS-4 study (male 59, female 27), only 53 underwent the first randomization. Twenty-seven patients were randomized to the ST arm and the remaining 26 to the PI arm. While the 8-year RFS rates for patients in the PI and ST arms were 71.8% and 69.6% respectively (p=0.81), the 8-year OS rates were 87.3% and 83.7% respectively (p=0.65). Only 40 patients took part in the second randomization (duration of treatment). The 5-year and 8-year RFS rates for patients randomized to the longer treatment arm was 87.8% at both time points versus 65.2% and 60.6% (p=0.08) respectively for patients in the short arm. Similarly, the 5-year and 8-year OS for patients in the longer treatment arm was 87.5% at both time points compared to 95.5% and 85.9% respectively for patients in the short arm (p=0.99). *It was concluded that while children with CCSK had a better RFS with longer treatment with vincristine, doxorubicin and actinomycin D, this did not translate into better overall survival.*

The SIOP-9 trial explored the optimal duration of preoperative chemotherapy (4 versus 8 weeks) in children with unilateral and nonmetastatic WT older than 6 months of age [11]. Eligible children aged >6 months to 16 years with untreated unilateral WT were only randomized if they had responded to the initial 4 weeks of chemotherapy with VA. Nephrectomy was carried out 1 week after completion of either 4 or 8 weeks VA chemotherapy. Subsequent treatment depended on the surgical stage. Out of the total of 852 children registered on the SIOP-9 trial, only 382 patients were randomized. There were no differences in the rupture rate at surgery (1% versus 3%), 2-year event-free survival (92% versus 87%) or in the site of failure between the two arms. In both treatment arms, 58% received stage I postoperative therapy. The authors concluded that there was no evidence of further downstaging by an additional 4 weeks of VA chemotherapy and that the 4-week schedule prenephrectomy chemotherapy should be considered the standard treatment.

A report by Green et al. included the combined results from the NWTS-3 and -4 trials of children with stages II–IV anaplastic WT who were treated with vincristine, actinomycin D, doxorubicin with cyclophosphamide (regimen J) or without cyclophosphamide (regimen DD-RT) [12]. Of the 72 randomized patients evaluated, 59 had diffuse anaplasia and the remaining 13 had focal anaplasia. Thirty-four patients received regimen DD-RT (AVA) and 38 were randomized to regimen J (AVA plus cyclophosphamide, AVAC). The 4-year RFS and OS rates were 35% (AVA) and 64.5% (AVAC) (p=0.03) and 38% and 61.4% (p=0.04) respectively. For children who had diffuse anaplasia, the RFS for regimen DD-RT was 27% versus 55% (p=0.02) for patients on regimen J. The authors concluded that children with focal anaplasia had an excellent prognosis when treated with vincristine, doxorubicin and actinomycin D. The addition of cyclophosphamide was of significant benefit in the treatment of children with stages II–IV diffuse anaplastic WT.

The SIOP-93 01 trial explored the reduction of postoperative chemotherapy in children with stage I intermediate risk and anaplastic histology WT to 4 weeks from the standard 18 weeks [13]. All patients had central review of pathology and had preoperative chemotherapy with weekly vincristine × 4 and one dose of ACT-D. After nephrectomy, patients were randomized to either stop (no further treatment; n=200) or receive two further courses of the same chemotherapy (STD; n=210). The 2-year EFS was 91.4% in the study arm versus 88.8% in the study arm and the 5-year OS was 97% and 95% for the standard and study arm patients respectively. Hematological toxicity was slightly greater in the longer duration treatment arm, especially anemia and thrombocytopenia. It was concluded that shortening the treatment duration did not compromise survival outcome but also reduced acute and late side-effects of treatment in patients with stage I intermediate and anaplastic histology WT.

References

1 Lemerle J, Voute PA, Tournade MF *et al.* Preoperative versus postoperative radiotherapy, single versus multiple courses of actinomycin D, in the treatment of Wilms tumor. Preliminary results of a controlled clinical trial conducted by the International Society of Paediatric Oncology (S.I.O.P.) *Cancer* 1976;**38**:647–54.

2 Lemerle J, Voute PA, Tournade MF *et al.* Effectiveness of preoperative chemotherapy in Wilms tumor: results of an International Society of Paediatric Oncology (SIOP) clinical trial. *J Clin Oncol* 1983;**1**:604–9.

3 Tournade MF, Com-Nougué C, Voûte PA *et al.* Results of the Sixth International Society of Pediatric Oncology Wilms Tumor Trial and Study: a risk-adapted therapeutic approach in Wilms tumor. *J Clin Oncol* 1993;**11**:1014–23.

4 De Camargo B, Franco EL. A randomized clinical trial of single-dose versus fractionated-dose dactinomycin in the treatment of Wilms tumor. Results after extended follow-up. Brazilian Wilms Tumor Study Group. *Cancer* 1994;**73**:3081–6.

5 D'Angio GJ, Evans AE, Breslow N *et al.* The treatment of Wilms tumor: results of the national Wilms tumor study. *Cancer* 1976;**38**:633–46.

6 D'Angio GJ, Evans A, Breslow N *et al.* The treatment of Wilms tumor: results of the Second National Wilms Tumor Study. *Cancer* 1981;**47**:2302–11.

7 D'Angio GJ, Breslow N, Beckwith JB *et al.* Treatment of Wilms tumor. Results of the Third National Wilms Tumor Study. *Cancer* 1989;**64**:349–60.

8 Green DM, Breslow NE, Beckwith JB *et al.* Comparison between single-dose and divided-dose administration of dactinomycin and doxorubicin for patients with Wilms tumor:

a report from the National Wilms Tumor Study Group. *J Clin Oncol* 1998;**16**:237–45.

9 Green DM, Breslow NE, Beckwith JB *et al.* Effect of duration of treatment on treatment outcome and cost of treatment for Wilms tumor: a report from the National Wilms Tumor Study Group. *J Clin Oncol* 1998;**16**:3744–51.

10 Seibel NL, Li S, Breslow NE *et al.* Effect of duration of treatment on treatment outcome for patients with clear-cell sarcoma of the kidney: a report from the National Wilms Tumor Study Group. *J Clin Oncol* 2004;**22**:468–73.

11 Tournade MF, Com-Nougué C, de Kraker J *et al.* Optimal duration of preoperative therapy in unilateral and nonmetastatic Wilms tumor in children older than 6 months: results of the Ninth International Society of Pediatric Oncology Wilms Tumor Trial and Study. *J Clin Oncol* 2001; **19**:488–500.

12 Green DM, Beckwith JB, Breslow NE *et al.* Treatment of children with stages II to IV anaplastic Wilms tumor: a report from the National Wilms Tumor Study Group. *J Clin Oncol* 1994;**12**:2126–31.

13 De Kraker J, Graf N, van Tinteren H *et al.* Reduction of postoperative chemotherapy in children with stage I intermediate-risk and anaplastic Wilms tumour (SIOP 93-01 trial): a randomised controlled trial. *Lancet* 2004;**364**:1229–35.

New studies

Study 1

Breslow NE, Ou SS, Beckwith JB *et al.* Doxorubicin for favorable histology, stage II–III Wilms tumor: results from the National Wilms Tumor Studies. *Cancer* 2004;**101**:1072–80.

Objectives

This report evaluated the efficacy of doxorubicin in children with stages II–III favorable histology Wilms tumor by reviewing the results of the National Wilms Tumour Studies 3 and 4.

Study design

Both NWTS-3 and 4 were multisite randomized trials for children <16 years of age with WT with or without anaplasia, clear cell sarcoma or rhabdoid tumor of kidney. Children with WT deemed inoperable without pretreatment were excluded. Details of eligibility criteria and staging treatment have been previously published (see references 7, 8 and 11 above). Patients with stage II FH WT in the NWTS-3 were randomized between no flank RT or 20 Gy RT and between treatment with doxorubicin (DOX) or without DOX in a factorial design. Patients with stage III/FH WT were randomized between 10 Gy RT or 20 Gy RT and between DOX or no DOX. In NWTS-4, the use of RT and DOX was determined by stage and histology. The analyses included patients whose treatment assignment was randomized and patients who were followed. The latter were eligible patients who were not randomized for various reasons but who were treated on protocol regimens and had the same requirements for data submission as randomized patients.

Between October 1979 and August 1986, 789 eligible patients with stage II–III FH WT were registered on the NWTS-3. Thirty-four patients were excluded (29 because of lack of baseline or pathology records and five because they had tumors in a solitary/fused kidney). Of the 1079 patients with stages II–III FH WT registered on NWTS-4 (August 1986 to September 1994), 54 were excluded because of lack of baseline details and a further 11 were excluded because they had tumors in a solitary/fused kidney.

Outcome endpoints were RFS, OS, and congestive heart failure (CHF).

Statistics

The time to event distributions and standard errors were estimated by actuarial methods. Differences among patient subgroups were evaluated by the log-rank test and estimates of relative risk (RR) were based on the Cox model.

Results
Treatment received

In NWTS-3, among patients with stage II WT, 41% received DOX and 42% received RT – most received high doses. Among patients with stage III WT, 64% received DOX and 98% received RT with equal representation for low (0.1–14.9 Gy) and high doses (>15 Gy).

In NWTS-4, 98% of patients with stage II WT received no RT and no DOX whereas among patients with stage III WT, 92% received low-dose RT and DOX.

Nonrandomized patients

Among the nonrandomized patients, 59% of patients who were treated with DOX received low-dose RT and 35% received high-dose RT whereas among patients who were not treated with DOX, the percentages who received low- and high-dose RT were 31% and 62% respectively.

The relative frequency of the two disease stages differed between the two studies, with equal numbers of patients with stage II (n=378) and III WT (n=377) on NWTS-3 but with more patients with stage II disease (n=580) than stage III WT (n=434) in NWTS-4. In addition, a greater proportion of patients in NWTS-4 with stage III disease received preoperative treatment

(19%) than in NWTS-3 (10%). Postrecurrence therapy also differed between NWTS-3 and NWTS-4.

Treatment outcome
Stage II WT patients had a lower risk of recurrence in NWTS-3 while in NWTS-4, the risk of recurrence was lower for patients with stage III disease.

Effects of DOX on disease recurrence and mortality
In total, 28 local recurrences occurred among 673 patients who received DOX compared to 12 in the 138 patients who did not receive DOX. For patients with stage II WT, the use of DOX did not reduce the risk of recurrent disease or decrease mortality. However, for patients with stage III/FH WT, DOX reduced the rate of recurrence by 50%, adjusted for study and RT dose. RR of any recurrent disease for stage II patients with DOX treatment was 1.02 (p=0.94) adjusted for study and RT dose whereas the RR for death was 1.39 (p=0.36). For stage III patients, the RR for local recurrence, general recurrence, and death was 0.43 (p=0.037), 0.56 (p=0.009) and 0.68 (p=0.173) respectively, adjusted for study and RT dose.

Congestive heart failure
Very few patients experienced CHF when included in the DOX efficacy analysis in combined NWTS-3 and -4. Only one patient who received DOX as initial treatment developed CHF (at 1.3 years and was alive at 19.1 years). Five patients who received DOX first for recurrent disease and thus were categorized as no DOX treatment in the first analysis developed CHF, of whom two subsequently died. Two other patients who also developed CHF were excluded because of preoperative therapy or lack of baseline records.

The risk of CHF was greatest for patients with left-sided WT (NWTS-3 and -4: nine CHF/1026 patients with left-sided tumor versus 2/959 in patients with right-sided WT).

Conclusions
It was concluded that despite a low risk of congestive heart failure with doxorubicin treatment, there was no conclusive evidence that front-line therapy with doxorubicin improved survival outcome.

Study 2
Reinhard H, Semler O, Bürger D et al. Results of the SIOP-93-01/GPOH trial and study for the treatment of patients with unilateral non-metastatic Wilms tumor. Klin Paediatr 2004;**216**:132–40.

Objectives
To determine whether a reduction in the postoperative chemotherapy duration for children with stage I WT with either anaplastic or intermediate-risk histology from the standard three courses to one course will adversely affect survival outcome.

Study design
The SIOP-93-01 trial/GPOH study was a multicenter randomized trial and included all newly diagnosed children with a renal tumor. Of the 1020 patients registered on the trial, 847 had a histologically confirmed WT, of whom 637 had a unilateral WT.

Outcome endpoint was event-free survival (EFS).

Randomization
Randomization was performed in 43.7% of all patients with stage I WT. There was no difference in EFS rates between both the treatment arms (90% versus 91%). In fact, the EFS rates were identical for stage I and stage II N0 (0.92) as well as for stage II N+ and stage III patients (0.82). The tumor volume after chemotherapy was a prognostic factor for intermediate-risk WT with the exception of epithelial and stromal predominant tumors.

Results
Five hundred and nineteen patients with unilateral nonmetastatic WT received postoperative chemotherapy. Histology distribution at surgery was as follows: low risk 3% (n=14), intermediate risk 90% (n=469) and high risk 7% (n=36). Stage distribution was stage I 61% (n=315), stage II 24% (n=126), stage III 7% (n=36), and stage II 5% (n=25). In 17 patients (3%) the tumor stage was unresolved. The median tumor volume shrank from 353 mL to 126 mL after preoperative chemotherapy. The 5-year EFS was 91% for all patients with unilateral WT without metastatic disease.

Conclusions
It was concluded that postoperative chemotherapy could be safely reduced to 4 weeks without worsening treatment outcome. The authors also concluded that

postoperative WT with a predominant blastemal component was to be regarded as high-risk tumor and that focal anaplasia which had a better prognosis than diffuse anaplasia had to be considered as intermediate-risk WT.

Please also refer to Chapter 25, Efficacy of anthracyclines in pediatric oncology, Study 5.

Study 3

Mitchell C, Pritchard-Jones K, Shannon R *et al.*, for the United Kingdom Cancer Study Group. Immediate nephrectomy versus preoperative chemotherapy in the management of non-metastatic Wilms tumour: results of a randomized trial (UKW3) by the UK Children's Cancer Study Group. *Eur J Cancer* 2006;**42**:2554–62.

Objectives

To determine if preoperative chemotherapy with vincristine and actinomycin D in children with nonmetastatic WT results in a more advantageous stage distribution and thus less treatment postoperatively for the whole group compared to those treated by immediate nephrectomy, whilst maintaining comparable EFS and OS.

Study design

The UKW-3 trial was open to all participating UK Children's Cancer Study Group (CCSG) centers in the UK and Ireland as well as in Oslo, Norway, and Adelaide in Australia, between October 1991 and March 2001. Eligible patients were aged between 6 months and 16 years with nonmetastatic WT that was deemed potentially operable by the local surgeon at diagnosis. Criteria for inoperability were tumor extension into the inferior vena cava or a very large fixed tumor. Other exclusion criteria were bilateral renal tumors, metastatic WT or patients in whom the diagnosis of WT was uncertain. Staging and histological subtyping were in accordance with the NWTS system. All histology was reviewed by an expert panel and confirmed as WT.

Randomization

Randomization was stratified by center with equal numbers of each treatment group in blocks of four. Eligible patients were randomly assigned to immediate nephrectomy (IN) or to biopsy, preoperative chemotherapy and delayed nephrectomy (DN) by a telephone call to the UK CCSG Data Centre at Leicester, UK. Out-of-hours randomization was by a single sealed envelope issued to each center.

Treatment

Patients randomized to preoperative chemotherapy received one injection a week for 6 weeks of vincristine and two doses of dactinomycin. Postoperative chemotherapy was dependent on pathological assessment of stage as well as the histological subtype of WT – favorable (FH) or unfavorable (UH) – and is detailed below.

Immediate nephrectomy

- FH stage 1 – vincristine alone × 10 weeks, stage II – vincristine plus dactinomycin × 26 weeks, stage III – vincristine, dactinomycin and doxorubicin plus 20 Gy hemi-abdomen RT, total duration of therapy 52 weeks, total doxorubicin dose 300 mg/m^2
- UH all stages – vincristine, dactinomycin and doxorubicin and 30 Gy to the hemi-abdomen for patients with stage III WT. Duration 1 year, total doxorubicin dose 360 mg/m^2

Delayed nephrectomy

- FH stage 1 – vincristine alone × 4 weeks, stage II – vincristine plus dactinomycin, stage III – vincristine, dactinomycin and doxorubicin plus 20 Gy hemi-abdomen RT
- UH all stages – vincristine, dactinomycin and doxorubicin and 30 Gy to the hemi-abdomen for patients with stage III WT

Statistics

The trial was designed to detect an increase in the proportion of stage I versus combined stages II and III from an anticipated 45% in the IN group to 60% in the DN group. It was determined that for a two-sided test of 5% and power of 80%, a trial size of 350 randomized patients equally between the two arms was needed. Sixty-three months after the start of the trial, the target size was reduced to 200 because of slow recruitment (agreed by the Data Monitoring and Safety Committee). As a result, the trial only had a 60% power to detect the level of improvement in staging anticipated at the beginning. Cumulative survival probabilities were calculated using the Kaplan–Meier method and the corresponding hazard ratios (HR) and 95% confidence interval (CI) estimated according to the Cox proportional hazard model. The potential influences of gender and age on the HRs were also investigated with the Cox model. The analyses compared all randomized patients irrespective of final histology between the treatment groups they were assigned. Median follow-up of randomized patients was 7 years and 2 months (range 48 days to 12 years and 1 month).

Results

Of the 842 patients with diagnosed renal tumors in the participating centers, 317 were ineligible for randomization according to the study entry criteria and a further 320 were not randomized for the following reasons: parental refusal (n=102), surgical preference (n=203) and not specified (n=15), giving a randomization rate of 205/525 (39%): 103 to IN and 102 to DN. Median age at diagnosis was 2 years and 10 months (range 6 months to 14 years).

Stage

Stage distribution in the IN and DN groups was stage I 54% versus 65%; stage II 15% versus 24%; and stage III 30% versus 10% respectively. The proportion of stage I patients in both treatment arms was greater than the 45% stage I after IN anticipated at trial design. The difference of 11% more stage I in favor of delayed surgery was not statistically significant (95% CI -3.1% to 24.1%; p=0.13). Nevertheless, with the shift of stage III to stage II tumors with preoperative chemotherapy, the corresponding and more sensitive test for trend was significant (p=0.008).

Tumor rupture

There were no peroperative tumor ruptures in the group who had DN versus 15 (15%) in the IN group. One patient in the IN group died of hepatic veno-occlusive disease (HVOD) secondary to a single dose of dactinomycin after surgery while one patient in the DN group developed HVOD after receiving the second dose of dactinomycin and died prior to surgery.

Relapses

Of the total of 40 relapses amongst the 205 randomized patients, 17 were in the IN group versus 23 in the DN group. Ten local relapses were in the DN group versus five in the IN group (p=NS). There were 10 distant relapses in each group. No relapses were seen in the track of the biopsy needle in the randomized patients.

Survival outcomes

Of the 42 events seen in the 205 randomized patients, 19 (13 deaths) occurred in the IN group versus 23 (11 deaths) in the DN group. The 5-year EFS was 79.6% (HR 1.25; 95% CI 0.68–2.30; p=0.52) for both treatment groups. Age and gender did not influence HR for EFS but reduced the differences between them with respect to OS

Conclusions

It was concluded that 6 weeks of preoperative chemotherapy with vincristine and dactinomycin in children with nonmetastatic WT resulted in a shift to more advantageous stage distribution and consequently to a reduction in therapy while maintaining excellent EFS and OS. Additionally, 20% of survivors were spared the late effects of doxorubicin treatment.

CHAPTER 5

Neuroblastoma

Katherine K. Matthay
UCSF School of Medicine, San Francisco, CA, USA

Commentary by Katherine K. Matthay

Long-term survival for high-risk neuroblastoma improved from approximately 10% before 1989 to greater than 30% by 2002 with the use of more intensive combination therapy and myeloablative therapy [1]. Intensification of induction was shown to be of benefit in the randomized trial by Pearson *et al.* [2] and this successful schedule was then incorporated into the ongoing SIOPEN high-risk trial, where a further randomized study showed that patients benefitted from using prophylactic granulocyte-colony stimulating factor (G-CSF) to support them through this induction [3]. Other studies tested the incorporation of topotecan, after the report in relapsed patients that topotecan with cyclophosphamide showed a significant response rate, and was superior to topotecan alone [4]. This regimen was then incorporated into a pilot study of induction, and shown to be feasible and to result in adequate peripheral blood stem cell (PBSC) harvests [5], and now is part of induction chemotherapy in an ongoing phase III Children's Oncology Group (COG) trial (ANBL0532) for high-risk neuroblastoma.

With the use of high-dose myeloablative chemotherapy, followed by therapy for minimal residual disease (MRD) with isotretinoin, the COG was able to show with long-term follow-up of their earlier randomized trial [6] that both modalities significantly improved survival for children with high-risk neuroblastoma [7], although due to the timing of the randomizations, the survival from diagnosis for the different groups could

not be accurately determined. Although the overall survival from time of second randomization was 59% for patients who were randomized to both bone marrow transplant (BMT) and isotretinoin, compared to 36% for those who received nonmyeloablative continuation therapy and no isotretinoin, the analysis of patients undergoing both randomizations excludes all those patients who progressed or had a poor response during induction and consolidation, and thus were not eligible for the second randomization, which may comprise up to 20% of patients initially enrolled on the study. Thus the 5-year overall survival (OS) from diagnosis for all 539 high-risk patients enrolled was only 36%. The stage III patients with high-risk features on this trial fared better, with 5-year OS of 59%; for the small number randomized to both BMT and isotretinoin, the OS was 100%. This analysis was limited by small numbers but raises the question of whether patients with stage III neuroblastoma lacking *MYCN* amplification should undergo myeloablative therapy or conventional chemotherapy [8].

The success of the trials showing that myeloablative therapy and treatment of MRD improved outcome led to the recent COG trial showing that the addition of immunotherapy with anti-GD2 monoclonal antibody and cytokines to isotretinoin significantly improved event-free survival (EFS) for patients with good response after autologous stem cell transplant (ASCT) [9]. In order to see if the increased toxicity of the therapy was due to the intensive cytokines, a randomized trial is

---

Evidence-Based Pediatric Oncology, Third Edition. Edited by Ross Pinkerton, Ananth Shankar and Katherine K. Matthay.
© 2013 John Wiley & Sons, Ltd. Published 2013 by John Wiley & Sons, Ltd.

ongoing in the European SIOPEN group, comparing isotretinoin with ch14.18 alone to isotretinoin with ch14.18 and low-dose interleukin (IL)-2.

Recently completed and ongoing randomized trials are in the process of analysis, but preliminary reports from the American Society of Clinical Oncology (ASCO) add two more important pieces of information to refine high-risk therapy. A report from Kreissman *et al.* for the COG showed that uniform intensive induction therapy and myeloablative chemotherapy with carboplatin, etoposide and melphalan for high-risk neuroblastoma resulted in similar EFS regardless of whether or not the PBSC were depleted of tumor cells by immunomagnetic purging [10]. This suggests that the relapse after transplant may be due to other sites of microscopic disease than just the hematopoietic system, and that further elimination of residual resistant tumor is necessary.

Another question is how to optimize the myeloablative portion of the therapy. In 2011, an ongoing SIOPEN study reported the preliminary analysis of their randomized trial utilizing the rapid cisplatin (C), vincristine (O), carboplatin (J), etoposide (E), and cyclophosphamide (C) (COJEC) induction followed by randomization to either a regimen of busulfan and melphalan (BuMel) or the COG regimen of melphalan, etoposide and carboplatin (CEM). The results reported at the ASCO 2011 meeting showed that the BuMel regimen was significantly superior to the CEM regimen, with a lower relapse rate and fewer severe toxicities, though toxic death rates were similar [11]. Three-year EFS for the BuMel regimen was 49%, compared to 33% for the CEM regimen, suggesting that in the context of the rapid COJEC induction, BuMel would be the preferred conditioning regimen. An ongoing randomized COG trial is testing a different myeloablative conditioning question: whether one or two tandem ASCT regimens would improve outcome, based on pilot data from a small single-arm trial [12].

For future approaches to overcoming resistance, pilot studies are testing the use of other targeted agents to improve response rate prior to myeloablative therapy with ^{131}I-MIBG combined with irinotecan (COG study ANBL09P1) [13, 14] or new therapies for microscopic residual disease, with immunocytokine therapy [15], new retinoids such as fenretinide [16, 17] or genetically targeted small molecule inhibitors, to mutated ALK (crizotinimb) [18], tumor vaccines, or Aurora kinase A inhibitors.

References

1 Moroz V, Machin D, Faldum A *et al.* Changes over three decades in outcome and the prognostic influence of age-at-diagnosis in young patients with neuroblastoma: a report from the International Neuroblastoma Risk Group Project. *Eur J Cancer* 2011;**47**(4):561–71.

2 Pearson AD, Pinkerton CR, Lewis IJ, Imeson J, Ellershaw C, Machin D. High-dose rapid and standard induction chemotherapy for patients aged over 1 year with stage 4 neuroblastoma: a randomised trial. *Lancet Oncol* 2008;**9**(3):247–56.

3 Ladenstein R, Valteau-Couanet D, Brock P *et al.* Randomized trial of prophylactic granulocyte colony-stimulating factor during rapid COJEC induction in pediatric patients with high-risk neuroblastoma: the European HR-NBL1/SIOPEN study. *J Clin Oncol* 2010;**28**(21):3516–24.

4 London WB, Frantz CN, Campbell LA *et al.* Phase II randomized comparison of topotecan plus cyclophosphamide versus topotecan alone in children with recurrent or refractory neuroblastoma: a Children's Oncology Group study. *J Clin Oncol* 2010;**28**(24):3808–15.

5 Park JR, Scott JR, Stewart CF *et al.* Pilot induction regimen incorporating pharmacokinetically guided topotecan for treatment of newly diagnosed high-risk neuroblastoma: a Children's Oncology Group study. *J Clin Oncol* 2011;**29**(33):4351–7.

6 Matthay KK, Villablanca JG, Seeger RC *et al.* Treatment of high-risk neuroblastoma with intensive chemotherapy, radiotherapy, autologous bone marrow transplantation, and 13-cis-retinoic acid. Children's Cancer Group. *N Engl J Med* 1999;**341**(16):1165–73.

7 Matthay KK, Reynolds CP, Seeger RC *et al.* Long-term results for children with high-risk neuroblastoma treated on a randomized trial of myeloablative therapy followed by 13-cis-retinoic acid: a Children's Oncology Group study. *J Clin Oncol* 2009;**27**(7):1007–13.

8 Park JR, Villablanca JG, London WB *et al.* Outcome of high-risk stage 3 neuroblastoma with myeloablative therapy and 13-cis-retinoic acid: a report from the Children's Oncology Group. *Pediatr Blood Cancer* 2009;**52**(1):44–50.

9 Yu AL, Gilman AL, Ozkaynak MF *et al.* Anti-GD2 antibody with GM-CSF, interleukin-2, and isotretinoin for neuroblastoma. *N Engl J Med* 2010;**363**(14):1324–34.

10 Kreissman SG, Villablanca JG, Seeger RC *et al.* A randomized phase 3 trial of myeloablative autologous peripheral blood stem cell (PBSC) transplant (ASCT) for high-risk neuroblastoma (HR-NB) employing immunomagnetic purged (P) versus unpurged (UP) PBSC: a Children's Oncology Group study. *J Clin Oncol* 2008;**26**:541.

11 Ladenstein RL, Poetschger U, Luksch R *et al.* Busulphan-melphalan as a myeloablative therapy (MAT) for high-risk neuroblastoma: results from the HR-NBL1/SIOPEN trial. *J Clin Oncol* 2011;**29**(suppl):abstr 2.

12 George RE, Li S, Medeiros-Nancarrow C *et al.* High-risk neuroblastoma treated with tandem autologous peripheral-blood stem cell-supported transplantation: long-term survival update. *J Clin Oncol* 2006;**24**(18):2891–6.

13 Matthay KK, Yanik G, Messina J *et al.* Phase II study on the effect of disease sites, age, and prior therapy on response to iodine-131-metaiodobenzylguanidine therapy in refractory neuroblastoma. *J Clin Oncol* 2007;**25**(9):1054–60.

14 DuBois SG, Chesler L, Groshen SG *et al.* Phase I study of vincristine, irinotecan, and 131I-MIBG for patients with relapsed or refractory neuroblastoma: a New Approach to Neuroblastoma Therapy (NANT) study. *J Clin Oncol* 2011;**29**(suppl): abstr 9513.

15 Shusterman S, London WB, Gillies SD *et al.* Antitumor activity of hu14.18-IL2 in patients with relapsed/refractory neuroblastoma: a Children's Oncology Group (COG) phase II study. *J Clin Oncol* 2010;**28**(33):4969–75.

16 Villablanca JG, London WB, Naranjo A *et al.* Phase II study of oral capsular 4-hydroxyphenylretinamide (4-HPR/fenretinide) in pediatric patients with refractory or recurrent neuroblastoma: a report from the Children's Oncology Group. *Clin Cancer Res* 2011;**17**(21):6858–66.

17 Cooper JP, Hwang K, Singh H *et al.* Fenretinide metabolism in humans and mice: utilizing pharmacological modulation of its metabolic pathway to increase systemic exposure. *Br J Pharmacol* 2011;**163**(6):1263–75.

18 George RE, Sanda T, Hanna M *et al.* Activating mutations in ALK provide a therapeutic target in neuroblastoma. *Nature* 2008;**455**(7215):975–8.

Summary of previous studies

All of the randomized trials from 1991 to 1995 for neuroblastoma (NBL) were focused on the patients with what we now consider high-risk NBL – patients older than 1 year with either regionally advanced or metastatic disease. The earliest trial by Castleberry *et al.* with the Pediatric Oncology Group (POG) was carried out between 1981 and 1989 and tested the role of local radiotherapy in patients >1 year of age with initially unresected stage C disease, i.e. those with complete or incomplete resection of primary nonmetastatic tumor, with positive intracavitary lymph nodes not adhered to primary tumor [1]. No biological studies were reported. All patients received chemotherapy with five courses of oral cyclophosphamide (day 1–7) and doxorubicin (day 8), given at 3-weekly intervals. Patients were randomized to receive local radiotherapy to the tumor plus regional lymph nodes (24 Gy for patients age 1–2 years and 30 Gy for those >2 years). Those with complete remission after second-look surgery received two further cycles of chemotherapy with alternating cyclophosphamide/ doxorubicin with cisplatin and VM-26. Patients on the radiotherapy arm had a significantly higher response rate, EFS, and OS.

The next three randomized trials were attempts to find improved induction chemotherapy for newly diagnosed patients. Castleberry *et al.* used a phase II investigational window to compare the response rate in newly diagnosed metastatic neuroblastoma to carboplatin versus iproplatin; ifosfamide and then epirubicin were given in a nonrandom fashion to separate sequential groups [2]. The major endpoint was the response to two courses of chemotherapy, after which patients proceeded to a randomization to two multiagent induction chemotherapy regimens. The partial response rate was 26/48 with carboplatin and 18/52 with iproplatin, with no significant difference in the overall objective response (partial response+minor response). In the sequential arm, the objective response rate was 70% with ifosfamide, 26% with epirubicin.

McWilliams *et al.* compared the response rate after five cycles of therapy in patients with metastatic neuroblastoma randomised at diagnosis to receive either cyclophosphamide (150 mg/m^2 po day 1–7) plus doxorubicin (35 mg/m^2) or cisplatin (90 mg/m^2) plus teniposide (100 mg/m^2) [3]. There was no significant difference in complete and partial response (including surgery), which was 59% versus 77% (p=0.077) respectively. There was also no difference in EFS at 5 years (6%). Coze *et al.* conducted a randomized trial with the French Society of Paediatric Oncology to test two different schedules of administration of cisplatin during induction therapy [4]. Initial chemotherapy comprised cyclophosphamide 1.5 g/m^2, doxorubicin 60 mg/m^2, vincristine 1.5 mg/ m$^2 \times 2$ (CADO), alternating with cisplatin 200 mg/m^2 divided over 5 days and etoposide 500 mg/m^2 (CVP) over 5 days. Patients were randomized to receive the cisplatin either as a continuous infusion over 5 days or as a 1-h bolus infusion, with the endpoint of reduction in creatinine clearance. The glomerular filtration rate (GFR) fell to below 90 mL/min/1.73 m^2 in 8% of those receiving continuous infusion cisplatin (n=43), compared to 18% with bolus infusion (n=48) (difference was not significant). The only significant difference between the two schedules was the degree of neutropenia after the first course of CVP, with 70% versus 43%, the higher incidence being in those who received continuous infusion (p=0.02), though there was no difference after the second course.

The next four studies all tested the role of myeloablative chemotherapy [5,6,7] and the treatment of MRD [5, 8] in outcome of high-risk neuroblastoma. Matthay *et al.* conducted a randomized trial from 1991 to 1996 to test whether myeloablative chemoradiotherapy with purged autologous BMT was superior to a nonmyeloablative continuation chemotherapy (CC), and whether a second randomization after BMT or CC to receive isotretinoin was superior to no further therapy [5]. The first randomization was carried out just prior to cycle 3 of chemotherapy at week 8 for all patients with nonprogressive disease. The second randomization followed BMT or week 34 of the end of CC. All patients were treated with the same induction chemotherapy and surgery, and then all without progressive disease went on to receive either chemoradiotherapy with carboplatin (1000 mg/m^2), etoposide (640 mg/m^2), melphalan (210 mg/m^2) and total body radiation (1000 cGy) or CC with three cycles at 28-day intervals of continuous infusion over 4 days of cisplatin (160 mg/m^2), doxorubicin (40 mg/m^2), and etoposide (500 mg/m^2) along with ifosfamide daily day 1–4 (2500 mg/m^2 daily) After CC or BMT therapy, isotretinoin was given orally 160 mg/m^2/day for 14 of 28 days for six cycles to randomized patients without biopsy-proven residual disease. The primary endpoint was EFS from time of randomization. There was a significant improvement in EFS for the patients randomized to BMT (34%) compared to CC (22%; p = 0.03). All consenting patients regardless of first randomization underwent the second randomization, and the EFS for those randomized to isotretinoin was 46%, compared to 29% for those randomized to no further therapy (p = 0.03). Overall survival was not significantly different, for either randomization.

Another study from the European Neuroblastoma Study Group (1983–85), reported by Pritchard *et al.* [6], actually preceded the CCG study temporally, and randomly tested myeloablative melphalan chemotherapy with autologous BMT to no further therapy. Patients who were in complete or good partial remission after 10 cycles of OPEC induction chemotherapy were randomized to either 180 mg/m^2 of high-dose melphalan followed by unpurged fresh autologous bone marrow or no further treatment. Of 167 patients registered, 90 achieved remission and 65 were randomized after 6–10 cycles of therapy. The difference in outcome was not significant, except when the analysis was restricted to stage 4 patients over 1 year at diagnosis (n = 48), for whom both outcome measures were significant for BMT: EFS (p = 0.01) and OS (p = 0.03).

A later comparison (1997–2002) of myeloablative therapy compared to a low-dose CC was reported by Berthold *et al.* with the German Society of Paediatric Oncology and Haematology [7]. Patients with stage 4 neuroblastoma over 1 year or with MYCN amplified tumors were treated with six cycles of a common induction chemotherapy, and then randomized

to receive myeloablative therapy with melphalan 180 mg/m^2, etoposide 40 mg/kg, carboplatin 500 mg/m^2 IV/1 h days -4 to -2, with stem cell infusion on day 0, or else maintenance therapy with four cycles of oral cyclophosphamide (150 mg/m^2/day days 1–8). Some patients received ch14.18 antibody or else isotretinoin after chemotherapy or transplant. The 3-year EFS of all 295 patients was 39% (95% confidence interval [CI] 33–45) and the 3-year OS was 58% (95% CI 52–64). There was a significant advantage for the group randomized to myeloablative therapy, with a 3-year EFS of 47%, compared to the maintenance chemotherapy group, with a 3-year EFS of 31% (p = 0.022). Kohler *et al.* tested a different schedule of isotretinoin in an ENSG study (1989–1997) done to establish whether 13-cis-retinoic acid used as continuation therapy after obtaining a good response to conventional chemotherapy could prolong disease-free survival in children with advanced neuroblastoma [8]. Children were treated in a double-blind, placebo-controlled study and given 0.75 mg/kg (≈22.5 mg/m^2) of isotretinoin (n = 88) or of placebo (n = 87) daily for 4 years. The 3-year EFS for isotretinoin was 37% versus 42% for those on placebo. Adjusting for prognostic factors, such as age, abdominal primary and bone marrow metastases, did not change the lack of difference between the two arms.

References

1 Castleberry RP, Kun LE, Shuster JJ et al. Radiotherapy improves the outlook for patients older than 1 year with Pediatric Oncology Group stage C neuroblastoma. *J Clin Oncol* 1991;**9**:789–95.

2 Castleberry RP, Cantor AB, Green AA et al. Phase II investigational window using carboplatin, iproplatin, ifosfamide, and epirubicin in children with untreated disseminated neuroblastoma: a Pediatric Oncology Group study [see comments]. *J Clin Oncol* 1994;**12**:1616–20.

3 McWilliams NB, Hayes FA, Green AA et al. Cyclophosphamide/doxorubicin versus cisplatin/teniposide in the treatment of children older than 12 months of age with disseminated neuroblastoma: a Pediatric Oncology Group randomized phase II study. *Med Pediatr Oncol* 1995;**24**:176–80.

4 Coze C, Hartmann O, Michon J et al. NB87 induction protocol for stage 4 neuroblastoma in children over 1 year of age: a report from the French Society of Pediatric Oncology. *J Clin Oncol* 1997;**15**:3433–40.

5 Matthay KK, Villablanca JG, Seeger RC et al. Treatment of high-risk neuroblastoma with intensive chemotherapy,

radiotherapy, autologous bone marrow transplantation, and 13-cis-retinoic acid. Children's Cancer Group. *N Engl J Med* 1999;**341**:1165–73.

6 Pritchard J, Cotterill SJ, Germond SM *et al.* High dose melphalan in the treatment of advanced neuroblastoma: results of a randomised trial (ENSG-1) by the European Neuroblastoma Study Group. *Pediatr Blood Cancer* 2005;**44**: 348–57.

7 Berthold F, Boos J, Burdach S *et al.* Myeloablative megatherapy with autologous stem-cell rescue versus oral maintenance chemotherapy as consolidation treatment in patients with high-risk neuroblastoma: a randomised controlled trial. *Lancet Oncol* 2005;**6**:649–58.

8 Kohler JA, Imeson J, Ellershaw C *et al.* A randomized trial of 13-cis retinoic acid in children with advanced neuroblastoma after high-dose therapy. *Br J Cancer* 2000;**83**:1124–7.

New studies

Study 1

Pearson AD, Pinkerton CR, Lewis IJ *et al*. High-dose rapid and standard induction chemotherapy for patients aged over 1 year with stage 4 neuroblastoma: a randomised trial. *Lancet Oncol* 2008;9:247–56.

Objectives

To assess whether an intensive chemotherapy protocol that had a 10-day interval between treatments would improve EFS in patients aged greater than or equal to1 year with high-risk neuroblastoma.

Study design

Children with newly diagnosed stage 4 neuroblastoma enrolled from 1990 to 1999 from 29 centers in Europe were randomly assigned to rapid treatment (cisplatin[C], vincristine [O], carboplatin [J], etoposide [E], and cyclophosphamide [C], known as COJEC) or standard treatment (vincristine [O], cisplatin [P], etoposide [E], and cyclophosphamide [C], i.e. OPEC, alternated with vincristine [O], carboplatin [J], etoposide [E], and cyclophosphamide [C], i.e. OJEC). Both regimens used the same total cumulative doses of each drug (except vincristine; $12\,mg/m^2$ rapid regimen versus $10.5\,mg/m^2$ standard regimen), but the dose intensity of the rapid regimen was 1.8 times higher than that of the standard regimen. The standard regimen was given every 21 days if patients showed hematological recovery, whereas the rapid regimen was given every 10 days irrespective of hematological recovery. Response to chemotherapy was assessed according to the conventional International Neuroblastoma Response Criteria (INRC). In responders, surgical excision of the primary tumor was attempted, followed by myeloablation (with $200\,mg/m^2$ of melphalan) and hematopoietic stem cell rescue. Primary endpoints were 3-year, 5-year, and 10-year EFS. Data were analyzed by intention to treat.

Results

One hundred and eleven patients in the standard group and 109 patients in the rapid group completed chemotherapy. Seventy-nine percent of patients in the standard group and 67% in the rapid group received at least 90% of the scheduled chemotherapy, and the relative dose intensity was 1.94 compared with the standard regimen. Three-year EFS was 24.2% for patients in the standard group and 31.0% for those in the rapid group (hazard ratio [HR] 0.86, 95% CI 0.66–1.14, p=0.30). Five-year EFS was 18.2% in the standard group and 30.2% in the rapid group, representing a difference of 12.0% (1.8 to 22.3), p=0.022. Ten-year EFS was 18.2% in the standard group and 27.1% in the rapid group, representing a difference of 8.9% (-1.2 to 19.0), p=0.085. Myeloablation was given a median of 55 days earlier in patients assigned rapid treatment than those assigned standard treatment. Infective complications (numbers of patients with febrile neutropenia and septicemia, and if given, time on antibiotic and antifungal treatment) and time in hospital were greater with rapid treatment. Occurrence of fungal infection was the same in both regimens.

Conclusions

Dose intensity can be increased with a rapid induction regimen in patients with high-risk neuroblastoma. There was no significant difference in OS between the rapid and standard regimens at 5 years and 10 years. However, an increasing difference in EFS after 3 years suggests that the efficacy of the rapid regimen is better than the standard regimen, despite the increased risk of infections.

Study 2

Matthay KK, Reynolds CP, Seeger RC *et al*. Long-term results for children with high-risk neuroblastoma treated on a randomized trial of myeloablative therapy followed by 13-cis-retinoic acid: a Children's Oncology Group study. *J Clin Oncol* 2009;27:1007–13.

Objectives

To assess the long-term outcome of patients enrolled on CCG-3891, a high-risk neuroblastoma study in which patients were randomly assigned to undergo autologous purged bone marrow transplantation

(ABMT) or to receive chemotherapy, and subsequent treatment with 13-cis-retinoic acid (cis-RA).

Study design

Patients received the same induction chemotherapy, with random assignment (n=379) to consolidation with myeloablative chemotherapy, total-body irradiation, and ABMT versus three cycles of intensive continuation chemotherapy. Patients who completed consolidation were randomly assigned to receive no further therapy or cis-RA for 6 months. All patients received initial therapy with cisplatin (60 mg/m^2), doxorubicin (30 mg/m^2 on day 2), etoposide (100 mg/m^2 on days 2 and 5), and cyclophosphamide (1000 mg/m^2 on days 3 and 4) for five cycles at 28-day intervals, plus surgery and radiotherapy for gross residual disease. For the transplantation group, the conditioning regimen consisted of carboplatin (1000 mg/m^2) and etoposide (640 mg/m^2) administered by continuous infusion over 96 h beginning 8 days before transplantation; melphalan (a bolus infusion of 140 mg/m^2 7 days before transplantation and a bolus infusion of 70 mg/m^2 6 days before transplantation); and total-body irradiation (333 cGy daily for the 3 days before transplantation), followed by an infusion of purged autologous bone marrow. The continuation chemotherapy group received three cycles of cisplatin (60 mg/m^2), etoposide (500 mg/m^2), and doxorubicin (40 mg/m^2), administered as a continuous infusion over 96 h and given simultaneously with a bolus injection of ifosfamide (2500 mg/m^2 on days 0–3) with mesna uroprotection, finally followed by granulocyte-colony stimulating factor. The first randomization was performed just before the third cycle of initial therapy, at week 8 of the protocol for patients without progressive disease. After transplantation or the end of continuation therapy, patients without disease progression were randomly assigned to receive six cycles of 13-cis-retinoic acid (160 mg/m^2/ day orally in two divided doses for 14 consecutive days in a 28-day cycle) or no further therapy.

The study design included two separate sequential random assignments in a quasi-factorial design. Patients with progressive disease (PD) before week 8 were ineligible for the first random assignment. Patients with PD or histologically confirmed disease at the completion of ABMT or CC were ineligible for the second random assignment. Patients ineligible for the first random assignment were nonrandomly assigned to CC (NRCC). If these patients remained progression free without documented tumor after CC, they were eligible for the second random assignment but were not included in the intention-to-treat analysis of the first random assignment. Treatment regimens were compared by intention-to-treat analyses, and the primary endpoint was EFS.

Results

The EFS for patients randomly assigned to ABMT was significantly higher than those randomly assigned to chemotherapy; the 5-year EFS was 30%±4% versus 19%±3%, respectively (p=0.04). The 5-year EFS (42%±5% versus 31%±5%) from the time of second random assignment was higher for cis-RA than for no further therapy, though it was not significant. Overall survival was significantly higher for each random assignment by a test of the log transformation of the survival estimates at 5 years (p=0.01). The 5-year OS from the second random assignment of patients who underwent both random assignments and who were assigned to ABMT/cis-RA was 59%±8%; for ABMT/no cis-RA, it was 41%±7%; for continuing chemotherapy/cis-RA, it was 38%±7%; and for chemotherapy/no cis-RA, it was 36%±7%.

Conclusion

Myeloablative therapy and autologous hematopoietic cell rescue result in significantly better 5-year EFS and OS than nonmyeloablative chemotherapy; cis-RA given after consolidation independently results in significantly improved OS.

Study 3

Park JR, Villablanca JG, London WB *et al.* Outcome of high-risk stage 3 neuroblastoma with myeloablative therapy and 13-cis-retinoic acid: a report from the Children's Oncology Group. *Pediatr Blood Cancer* 2009;**52**:44–50.

Objectives

To determine if intensive chemoradiotherapy with purged ABMT and/or 13-cis-retinoic acid (cis-RA) improved outcome for patients with high-risk neuroblastoma that was not metastatic to distant sites.

Study design

A retrospective cohort design was used to determine if myeloablative therapy for consolidation or cis-RA for

MRD would improve outcome. Seventy-two patients with International Neuroblastoma Staging System (INSS) stage III neuroblastoma were enrolled between 1991 and 1996 on the phase III CCG-3891 randomized trial (see Study 2 for specifics of treatment and analysis). Patients were analyzed on an intention-to-treat basis using a log-rank test.

Results

The 5-year EFS and OS rates for patients with stage III neuroblastoma were 55±6% and 59±6%, respectively (n=72). Patients randomized to ABMT (n=20) had 5-year EFS of 65±11% and OS of 65±11% compared to 41±11% (p=0.21) and 46±11% (p=0.23) for patients randomized to CC (n=23), respectively. Patients randomized to cis-RA (n=23) had 5-year EFS of 70±10% and OS of 78±9% compared to 63±12% (p=0.67) and 67±12% (p=0.55) for those receiving no further therapy (n=16), respectively. Patients randomized to both ABMT and cis-RA (n=6) had a 5-year EFS of 80±11% and OS of 100%.

Conclusions

Patients with high-risk stage III neuroblastoma have an overall poor prognosis despite aggressive chemoradiotherapy. Although there is an apparent improvement in outcome with ABMT and with 13-cis-RA, further studies are warranted to determine if myeloablative consolidation followed by 13-cis-RA maintenance therapy statistically significantly improves outcome for this group of high-risk but nonmetastatic patients.

Study 4

London WB, Frantz CN, Campbell LA *et al*. Phase II randomized comparison of topotecan plus cyclophosphamide versus topotecan alone in children with recurrent or refractory neuroblastoma: a Children's Oncology Group study. *J Clin Oncol* 2010;**28**:3808–15.

Objectives

To determine whether single-agent topotecan (TOPO) or combination topotecan and cyclophosphamide (TOPO/CTX) was superior in a phase II randomized trial in relapsed/refractory neuroblastoma. Because responders often underwent further therapies, novel statistical methods were required to compare the long-term outcome of the two treatments.

Study design

Children with refractory/recurrent neuroblastoma (only one prior aggressive chemotherapy regimen) were randomly assigned to daily 5-day topotecan (2 mg/m^2) or combination topotecan (0.75 mg/m^2) and cyclophosphamide (250 mg/m^2). A randomized two-stage group sequential design enrolled 119 eligible patients. Toxicity and response were estimated. Long-term outcome of protocol therapy was assessed using novel methods (causal inference), which allowed adjustment for the confounding effect of off-study therapies.

Results

Of 119 eligible patients, 71 previously underwent high-dose chemotherapy with ASCT as initial treatment, and 48 children had not. The median age at initial diagnosis was 3.6 years (range 0.5–18 years) and at enrollment was 5.6 years (range 1–19 years). The median time from initial diagnosis until enrollment was 18 months. Older age at diagnosis (p=0.0007) and single-copy *MYCN* (p=0.0002) were statistically significantly predictive of increased OS. Seven more responses were observed for TOPO/CTX (complete response [CR] plus partial response [PR], 18 [32%] of 57) than TOPO (CR+PR, 11 [19%] of 59; p=0.081); toxicity was similar. At 3 years, progression-free survival (PFS) and OS were 4%±2% and 15%±4%, respectively. While PFS was significantly better for TOPO/CTX (p=0.029), there was no difference in OS. Older age at diagnosis and lack of *MYCN* amplification predicted increased OS (p<0.05). Adjusting for randomized treatment effect and subsequent autologous stem cell transplantation, there was no difference between TOPO and TOPO/CTX in terms of the proportion alive at 2 years.

Conclusions

Topotecan + cyclophosphamide was superior to TOPO in terms of PFS, but there was no OS difference. After adjustment for subsequent therapies, no difference was detected in the proportion alive at 2 years. Causal inference methods for assessing long-term outcomes of phase II therapies after subsequent treatment can elucidate effects of initial therapies.

Study 5

Yu AL, Gilman AL, Ozkaynak MF *et al.* Anti-GD2 antibody with GM-CSF, interleukin-2, and isotretinoin for neuroblastoma. *N Engl J Med* 2010;**363**:1324–34.

Objectives

This study was done to determine whether adding ch14.18, a monoclonal antibody against the tumor-associated disialoganglioside GD2, GM-CSF, and interleukin-2 to standard isotretinoin therapy after intensive multimodal therapy would improve outcomes in high-risk neuroblastoma.

Study design

Patients with high-risk neuroblastoma who had a response to induction therapy and stem cell transplantation were randomly assigned, in a 1:1 ratio, to receive standard therapy (six cycles of isotretinoin) or immunotherapy (six cycles of isotretinoin and five concomitant cycles of ch14.18 in combination with alternating GM-CSF and interleukin-2). Eligibility requirements included high-risk neuroblastoma by COG criteria; age at diagnosis of under 31 years; completion of induction therapy, autologous stem cell transplantation, and radiotherapy; achievement of at least a partial response at the time of evaluation before autologous stem cell transplantation; autologous stem cell transplantation performed within 9 months after the initiation of induction therapy; enrollment between day 50 and day 100 after the final autologous stem cell transplantation; absence of progressive disease; and adequate organ function and a life expectancy of at least 2 months. Patients with biopsy-proven residual disease after autologous stem cell transplantation were eligible for enrollment but not for randomization and were non-randomly assigned to receive immunotherapy. They were excluded from the primary efficacy analysis.

Treatment consisted of either six cycles of isotretinoin alone at 160 mg/m^2/day for 14 of every 28 days (standard therapy) or six cycles of isotretinoin interspersed with five cycles of ch14.18 at a dose of 25 mg /m^2/day for 4 days, given in cycles 1, 3, 5 with GM-CSF 250 μg/m^2/day for 14 days starting 3 days prior to ch14.18, or with IL-2 during cycles 2 and 4, given continuous infusion, for 4 days during week 1 at a dose of 3×10^6 IU/m^2/day, as well as for 4 days during week 2 at a dose of 4.5×10^6 IU/m^2/day, concurrent with ch14.18 (immunotherapy).

The primary analysis was an intention-to-treat comparison of EFS in the two treatment groups. The study was designed to enroll 386 randomly assigned patients, for a statistical power of 80% with a two-sided log-rank test at a level of 0.05 (or a one-sided test at a level of 0.025) to detect an absolute difference of 15 percentage points between the two groups in the 3-year estimate of EFS (50% in the standard therapy group versus 65% in the immunotherapy group). A secondary analysis of overall survival in the intention-to-treat population, according to treatment group, was to be performed only if the two groups were found to differ significantly with regard to EFS. Comparability of the two treatment groups was tested in terms of their known prognostic factors and stratification factors at the time of study enrollment by using a chi-square test. P values of less than 0.05 were considered to indicate statistical significance.

Results

A total of 226 eligible patients were randomly assigned to a treatment group. In the immunotherapy group, a total of 52% of patients had pain of grade 3, 4, or 5, and 23% and 25% of patients had capillary leak syndrome and hypersensitivity reactions, respectively. With 61% of the number of expected events observed, the study met the criteria for early stopping owing to efficacy. The median duration of follow-up was 2.1 years for those who were alive and had not had a study event. Immunotherapy was superior to standard therapy with regard to rates of EFS (66±5% versus 46±5% at 2 years, p=0.01) and OS (86±4% versus 75±5% at 2 years, p=0.02 without adjustment for interim analyses).

The rate of EFS with immunotherapy was significantly greater in the subgroup of patients 1 year of age or older who had stage 4 disease (63±6% at 2 years) than for stage 4 patients in the standard therapy group (42±6% at 2 years, p=0.02). For the 25 patients nonrandomly assigned to immunotherapy for biopsy-proven residual disease, the EFS was 36±10% and OS was 76±9% (10 deaths due to progressive disease).

By univariate analysis of prognostic factors, stage 4 (versus 2, 3, 4s) and partial response (versus CR/VGPR) at time of transplant were significant adverse predictors of EFS; age, *MYCN* status, ploidy, histology, and number of ASCT infusions were not prognostic.

Conclusions

The addition of ch14.18, GM-CSF and IL-2 to isotretinoin therapy was associated with improved event-free and overall survival among children with high-risk neuroblastoma who had a response to initial chemotherapy and received immunotherapy within 100 days after autologous stem cell transplantation. These data suggest that more routine use of this immunotherapy regimen for such patients may be beneficial.

Study 6

Ladenstein R, Valteau-Couanet D, Brock P et al. Randomized trial of prophylactic granulocyte colony-stimulating factor during rapid COJEC induction in pediatric patients with high-risk neuroblastoma: the European HR-NBL1/SIOPEN study. *J Clin Oncol* 2010;**28**:3516–24.

Objectives

To determine in a randomized trial whether primary prophylactic (PP) versus symptom-triggered granulocyte colony-stimulating factor (GCSF; filgrastim) would reduce the incidence of febrile neutropenia during rapid COJEC induction.

Study design

From May 2002 to November 2005, 239 patients in 16 countries were randomly assigned to receive or not receive PPGCSF. There were 144 boys with a median age of 3.1 years (range 1–17 years), of whom 217 had INSS stage 4 and 22 had stage 2 or 3 *MYCN*-amplified disease. The prophylactic arm received a single daily dose of 5 μg/kg GCSF, starting after each of the eight COJEC chemotherapy cycles and stopping 24 h before the next cycle. Chemotherapy was administered every 10 days regardless of hematological recovery, provided that infection was controlled. Treating physicians were encouraged to use therapeutic GCSF in the control arm for severe or life-threatening infections together with antibiotics and antifungal therapy in children at particular risk (i.e. proven *Pseudomonas* or fungal infections, multiorgan dysfunction, or pneumonia). Secondary prophylaxis with GCSF (i.e. administration after one febrile neutropenic episode in subsequent cycles) was not recommended.

Randomization, on an intention-to-treat basis, was before day 2 of COJEC. Two-sided significance tests were used throughout (α 5%). The primary endpoint was reduction of febrile neutropenia during COJEC. The difference in the number of febrile episodes per course was primarily analyzed, following the pre-established analysis plan, using the modification of the two-sample *t* test described by Denne *et al*. Secondary endpoints included hospitalization days, documented infection rate, parenteral antibiotics days, number of packed red blood cell/platelet transfusions, chemotherapy delay, infection-related mortality, and signs of stem cell pool depletion using harvest days and numbers of CD34 cells. In addition, times to completion of COJEC, as a measure of chemotherapy dose intensity, and rate of remission at the end of induction and eligibility for myeloablative therapy randomization were studied.

Results

A total of 110 patients in the PPGCSF arm and 114 in the control arm completed the study. All 239 randomly assigned patients were included in the efficacy and safety analysis on an intention-to-treat basis; 232 were evaluable. In the control arm, an increasing number of patients received GCSF for clinical reasons with successive cycles: cycle 1, 5; cycle 2, 6; cycle 3, 10, cycle 4, 9; cycle 5, 12; cycle 6,12; cycle 7, 22; cycle 8, 37.

The patients randomized to the PPGCSF arm had significantly fewer median episodes of fever with neutropenia, median days with fever per cycle and during induction, median days of antibiotics, and median hospital days. The patients on PPGCSF also had less gastrointestinal toxicity and grade 4 neutropenia, and treatment delays. There was no significant difference in risk of grade 4 severe infection, fungal infection, or admission to intensive care. All four deaths were in patients randomized to the PPGCSF arm. The overall response rate was 72%, and importantly, there was no significant difference in bone marrow or skeletal or overall tumor response between the two groups, nor was there a difference in success of peripheral blood stem cell harvest.

Conclusions

Prophylactic GCSF during intensive timing induction therapy for high-risk neuroblastoma reduces the extent of myelosuppression, gastrointestinal toxicity, and hospitalization with fever and neutropenia, without apparent impact on response rate or toxic death rate.

CHAPTER 6

Hepatoblastoma

Ross Pinkerton
Royal Children's Hospital, Brisbane, QLD, Australia

Commentary by Penelope Brock

Liver tumors can be primary or secondary, benign or malignant. The most common primary liver cancer is hepatoblastoma (HB) and most tumors secrete α-fetoprotein (AFP). Hepatoblastoma makes up 1–3% of childhood cancers. Childhood cancers are rare and therefore hepatoblastoma is exceedingly rare, affecting about one in a million children. Despite its rarity, international collaboration and successive international clinical trials have made it one of the success stories of the last decades, improving the cure rate from 30% to the vast majority of children [1]. The two-thirds of children who have standard-risk or good prognostic disease are now curable, and over 80% are disease free at 3 years and beyond, with a combination of chemotherapy and surgery. In the remaining third with high-risk disease, clearance in the liver may require liver transplantation and clearance in the lungs requires dose-intensive chemotherapy but with these modalities, over 70% are disease free at 2 years and beyond.

Two randomized clinical trials in hepatoblastoma have been reported since 2006, one an Intergroup study from North America on advanced hepatoblastoma, P9645 [2], and the other an enlarged European SIOPEL study on standard-risk hepatoblastoma, SIOPEL-3 [3]. During this period, there have also been a few nonrandomized studies reported in high-risk hepatoblastoma from SIOPEL [4], as well as a very interesting new prognostic stratification for hepatoblastoma [5]. Due to the different staging systems used across the world,

comparison between these trials is difficult. The key difference is the surgically defined criteria used by North America in contrast to the image-defined criteria used by SIOPEL.

The first study, a North American Intergroup study from the Pediatric Oncology Group (POG) and the Children's Cancer Group (CCG), P9645, looked at intensifying platinum chemotherapy in advanced-stage hepatoblastoma and comparing it to the standard combination chemotherapy of cisplatin, 5-fluorouracil (5-FU), and vincristine (C5V) [2]. The issue was whether the potentially more toxic intensified platinum regimen was justified by improved outcome, which turned out not to be the case. There was an additional randomization to treat with or without amifostine, which was continued in all patients receiving C5V after cessation of the chemotherapy randomization.

One of the main criticisms of this trial is in the title itself: "Intensified platinum therapy is an ineffective strategy for improving outcome in paediatric patients with advanced hepatoblastoma." The hypothesis here, that dose intensification with an analog of cisplatin, carboplatin, can be considered equal to dose intensification with cisplatin, is flawed. Carboplatin has been shown to be less active than cisplatin in preclinical studies of hepatoblastoma [6]. The trial does not prove that dose intensification of cisplatin would be ineffective. In hepatoblastoma, one cannot assume that cisplatin and carboplatin are equally effective. In addition,

---

Evidence-Based Pediatric Oncology, Third Edition. Edited by Ross Pinkerton, Ananth Shankar and Katherine K. Matthay.
© 2013 John Wiley & Sons, Ltd. Published 2013 by John Wiley & Sons, Ltd.

carboplatin, like doxorubicin, causes myelosuppression and therefore cannot be dose intensified in the same way that cisplatin alone can. Carboplatin, however, has the advantage of being less nephro- and ototoxic. Although in malignant germ cell tumors carboplatin has successfully replaced cisplatin in combination chemotherapy in the UK, this Intergroup study has shown that it cannot replace cisplatin in the treatment of hepatoblastoma when used as a single agent.

Another controversial point raised in this trial is that advanced hepatoblastoma stage III, defined by surgical criteria, is used to measure treatment success. Treatment failure was declared when the tumor remained inoperable after chemotherapy. It is now accepted that when four sectors of the liver are involved at diagnosis (PRETEXT IV [7]), then liver transplantation should be considered as a curative treatment option. Even if excellent chemotherapy produces tumor shrinkage, the tumor may still remain inoperable. Liver transplantation has been successful in children with hepatoblastoma when there have been clear signs of chemotherapy response to treatment, i.e. falling AFP levels and reducing tumor size [8].

Metastatic disease is more comparable between the Intergroup and SIOPEL trials and is clearly defined by both the North American group as stage IV and in SIOPEL as "M" for metastatic. Unfortunately, the Intergroup studies do not present data for metastatic disease alone. These are the patients who carry the worst prognosis and who require the most intensive chemotherapy. In high-risk (defined as PRE Treatment EXT tent of disease – PRETEXT criteria and AFP <100 ng/mL [9]) hepatoblastoma, the SIOPEL group opted to dose intensify with cisplatin alternating with a combination of carboplatin and doxorubicin. Due to small numbers, this had to be a nonrandomized trial. Dose intensification with this multiagent chemotherapy regimen gave a 3-year overall event-free survival (EFS) of 65% [4] for the whole group while for patients with metastatic disease, the 3-year EFS was 56%. Although not published yet as a full article, the comparative analysis of the SIOPEL studies for metastatic disease was published in abstract form (SIOP 2011) which showed EFS for metastatic HB ranging from 28% at 5 years in SIOPEL-1 [10] to 74% at 2 years in SIOPEL-4. SIOPEL-4 used dose-intensified weekly cisplatin and standard doxorubicin [11]. This result

implies that dose intensifying the more active cisplatin agent together with doxorubicin is effective whereas dose intensifying the less effective carboplatin agent alongside cisplatin in HB is not.

In metastatic disease, two issues remain: first, the 25% of children who do not clear their disease in the lungs and second, the toxicity of the dose-intensive regimen. The use of doxorubicin in very young children carries a serious long-term risk of cardiotoxicity.

The second randomized study published in 2009 is from the SIOPEL group and shows that in standard-risk HB, as defined by the PRETEXT criteria PRETEXT I, II and III, doxorubicin can be safely removed from the chemotherapy regimen. As expected, toxicity was increased in the combination therapy group. It is exceptional in cancer that a single chemotherapy agent together with surgery is sufficient for cure. A previous example is a UK study showing a similar outcome in stage I Wilms tumor, which is curable with surgery and vincristine monotherapy.

The continuing challenge in standard-risk hepatoblastoma, and where current clinical trials are still focusing, is to reduce the toxicity of cisplatin. The Intergroup approach is to give less cisplatin to lower stage disease and both groups are interested in chemoprotectants. The Intergroup studied amifostine which unfortunately did not prove sufficiently useful [12] and SIOPEL are currently studying sodium thiosulfate. SIOPEL-6 is an open randomized trial particularly aimed at reducing the ototoxicity of cisplatin by introducing sodium thiosulfate as an otoprotectant.

In high-risk or poor prognostic disease, where all four surgical sectors of the liver are involved or there is metastatic disease or other high-risk factors, the challenge is to achieve clearance in both the lungs and the liver within the limits of treatment tolerance. Liver transplantation, particularly with living related donors, has already been shown to be successful. The important question to address for the future is how much chemotherapy do patients with advanced nonmetastatic stage III disease (defined by surgical and image-defined PRETEXT criteria) require?

In the future, ways need to be found to cure the remaining quarter of children with metastatic disease where residual lung metastases and lung progression are the limiting factors. Additional chemotherapy may be an option. Phase II studies have shown the efficacy of irinotecan in relapsed hepatoblastoma [13], presented orally at SIOP [14]. High-dose therapy has not been shown to be particularly beneficial. More targeted therapy may be possible in the future as activation of β-catenin is a hallmark of hepatoblastoma and when signaling pathways are elucidated, such as the c-Met pathway, then alternative treatment options may become available [15]. It may be that lung radiotherapy needs to be introduced into the treatment, as in Wilms tumor, to improve the cure rate for these children. Because hepatoblastoma has been so chemoresponsive, radiotherapy as a treatment modality has not been prioritized. However, hepatoblastoma, as most other embryological childhood tumors, is radiosensitive [16]. Additionally, there is possibly a very small group of patients in whom complete resection alone may be curative [17]. There is also an enormous challenge of rolling these treatment improvements out in a realistic way to benefit all children throughout the world and particularly in resource-challenged nations. This effort has been started in India. There is no doubt that cisplatin monotherapy is a safer option for children with standard-risk disease, reducing the risk of infection and the need for blood products [18].

References

1 Pritchard-Jones K, Stiller C. What can we learn from geographical comparisons of childhood cancer survival? *Br J Cancer* 2007;**96**(10):1493–7.

2 Malogolowkin MH, Katzenstein H, Krailo MD *et al*. Intensified platinum therapy is an ineffective strategy for improving outcome in pediatric patients with advanced hepatoblastoma. *J Clin Oncol* 2006;**24**(18):2879–84.

3 Perilongo G, Maibach R, Shafford E *et al*. Cisplatin versus cisplatin plus doxorubicin for standard-risk hepatoblastoma. *N Engl J Med* 2009;**361**(17):1662–70.

4 Zsíros J, Maibach R, Shafford E *et al*. Successful treatment of childhood high-risk hepatoblastoma with dose-intensive multiagent chemotherapy and surgery: final results of the SIOPEL-3HR study. *J Clin Oncol* 2010;**28**(15):2584–90.

5 Maibach R, Roebuck D, Brugieres L *et al*. Prognostic stratification for children with hepatoblastoma: the SIOPEL experience. *Eur J Cancer*. 2012;**48**(10):1543–9.

6 Fuchs J, Schmidt D, Pietsch T, Miller K, von Schweitz D. Successful transplantation of human hepatoblastoma into immunodeficient mice. *J Pediatr Surg* 1996;**31**:1241–6.

7 Roebuck DJ, Aronson D, Clapuyt P *et al*. PRETEXT: a revised staging system for primary malignant liver tumours of childhood developed by the SIOPEL group. *Pediatr Radiol* 2007;**37**(2):123–32.

8 Otte JB, Meyers RL. Liver transplantation. *J Pediatr Surg* 2006;**41**(3):607–8.

9 De Ioris M, Brugieres L, Zimmermann A *et al*. Hepatoblastoma with a low serum alpha-fetoprotein level at diagnosis: the SIOPEL group experience. *Eur J Cancer* 2008;**44**(4):545–50.

10 Perilongo G, Brown J, Shafford E *et al*. Hepatoblastoma presenting with lung metastases: treatment results of the first cooperative, prospective study of the International Society of Paediatric Oncology on childhood liver tumors. *Cancer* 2000;**89**(8):1845–53.

11 Casanova M, Brock P, Brugières L *et al*. Dose dense cisplatin improves survival in children presenting with metastatic hepatoblastoma: lessons from SIOPEL 1 to 4. *Pediatr Blood Cancer* 2011;**57**(5):724.

12 Katzenstein HM, Chang KW, Krailo M *et al*., for the Children's Oncology Group. Amifostine does not prevent platinum-induced hearing loss associated with the treatment of children with hepatoblastoma: a report of the Intergroup Hepatoblastoma Study P9645 as a part of the Children's Oncology Group. *Cancer* 2009;**115**(24):5828–35.

13 Bomgaars LR, Bernstein M, Krailo M *et al*. Phase II trial of irinotecan in children with refractory solid tumors: a Children's Oncology Group Study. *J Clin Oncol* 2007;**25**(29):4622–7.

14 Zsíros J, Childs M, Brugières L *et al*., on behalf of SIOPEL. Irinotecan single-drug treatment for children with refractory or recurrent hepatoblastoma – a phase II trial of the Childhood Liver Tumours Strategy Group (SIOPEL). *Pediatr Blood Cancer* 2009;**53**:745.

15 Purcell R, Childs M, Maibach R *et al*. HGF/c-Met related activation of β-catenin in hepatoblastoma. *J Exp Clin Cancer Res* 2011;**30**:96.

16 Habrand JL, Pritchard J. Role of radiotherapy in hepatoblastoma and hepatocellular carcinoma in children and adolescents: results of a survey conducted by the SIOP Liver Tumour Study Group. *Med Pediatr Oncol* 1991;**19**(3):208.

17 Malogolowkin MH, Katzenstein HM, Meyers RL *et al*. Complete surgical resection is curative for children with hepatoblastoma with pure fetal histology: a report from the Children's Oncology Group. *J Clin Oncol* 2011;**29**(24):3301–6.

18 Agarwala S, Ronghe MD, Aronson DC *et al*. Pilot of treatment guidelines for hepatoblastoma (HB) in resource challenged nations (RCN). *Pediatr Blood Cancer* 2009;**53**:745.

Summary of previous studies

Only one study in liver cancer was previously reported. This was from POG and CCG and performed between 1989 and 1992 and was designed to determine whether a combination of cisplatin/doxorubicin (regimen B) was more effective than cisplatin/vincristine/5-FU (regimen A) [1]. The latter was regarded as standard therapy in the USA at the time whereas cisplatin/doxorubicin was in use in European studies.

The issue was whether the potentially more toxic anthracycline-based combination was justified by improved outcome. Patients with stage I favorable histology (FH) were excluded and nonrandomly assigned to four courses of single-agent doxorubicin (regimen C). All other patients were randomized immediately after initial surgery and were stratified by stage. Favorable histology was defined as pure fetal histology with minimal mitoses. There were 182 patients with hepatoblastoma and 46 with hepatocellular carcinoma. Nine stage I patients with FH received regimen C. Of 173 randomized, 43 were stage I unfavorable, seven were stage II, 83 were stage III and 40 were stage IV. Overall 5-year EFS for regimen A was 57% and for regimen B 69% ($p=0.09$). Although there was no significant difference in EFS, the cumulative incidence of an adverse event at 4 years was significantly higher for patients in regimen A (39%) compared to regimen B (23%) ($p=0.02$). Predictably, regimen B had significantly more toxicity with longer hospital stay although infection rates were no different. It was concluded that while treatment outcome was not significantly different between the two regimens, the cisplatin/doxorubicin combination was more toxic.

The second publication reported a detailed subanalysis of patients with hepatocellular carcinoma treated in this trial [2]. Overall survival was much poorer, as would have been predicted, with EFS of 17%. There was no significant difference in outcome between patients on regimen A or regimen B but the numbers of patients in this cohort were relatively small.

References

1 Ortega JA, Douglass EC, Feusner JH *et al*. Randomised comparison of cisplatin/vincristine/fluorouracil and cisplatin/continuous infusion doxorubicin for treatment of pediatric hepatoblastoma: a report from the Children's Cancer Group and the Pediatric Oncology Group. *J Clin Oncol* 2000;**18**:2665–75.
2 Katzenstein H, Krailo M, Malogolowkin M *et al*. Fibrolamellar hepatocellular carcinoma in children and adolescents. *Cancer* 2003;**15**:2006–12.

New studies

Study 1

Malogolowkin MH, Katzenstein H, Krailo MD *et al.* Intensified platinum therapy is an ineffective strategy for improving outcome in paediatric patients with advanced hepatoblastoma. *J Clin Oncol* 2006;**24**:2879–84.

Objectives

To determine whether increasing platinum dose intensity by alternating carboplatin and cisplatin could improve outcome in patients with advanced hepatoblastoma.

Study design

This study was undertaken by the Paediatric Intergroup Hepatoblastoma Study Group (Study P9645) and took place between 1999 and 2002. It was designed as a factorial random assignment for patients with stage III and IV disease. Patients were under the age of 21 years and biopsy proven for previously untreated hepatoblastoma and the protocol required patients to have normal renal function. Surgical criteria for disease staging consisted of:

- stage I complete gross resection with clear margins
- stage II gross total resection with microscopic residual disease at the margins of the section
- stage III gross total resection with nodal involvement or tumor spill or incomplete resection with gross residual intrahepatic disease
- stage IV metastatic disease with either complete or incomplete resection of biopsy.

Central pathology review was required for all patients enrolled on the study. Patients with stage I or II disease were not considered for randomization, others were randomly assigned to receive C5V or CC with or without amifostine. Amifostine was used in a separate randomized trial evaluating the otoprotective effect of this compound. Each course of C5V consisted of cisplatin 100 mg/m^2 (or 3 mg/kg for patients <1 year of age) as a 4-h infusion on day 1 with vincristine 1.5 mg/m- and 5-FU 600 mg/m^2 IV both given on day 2. Regimen CC consisted of carboplatin 700 mg/m- given IV over 1 h

or 23 mg/kg for patients <10 kg or 18.5 mg/kg for patients <10 kg after two cycles followed by cisplatin 100 mg/m^2 on day 14, dosed as in the C5V regimen. Granulocyte-colony stimulating factor (G-CSF) was used after each CC cycle. Patients with a glomerular filtration rate (GFR) <100 mg/mL/min/1.73 m^2 were to have their carboplatin dose based on Calvert's formula to achieve an area under concentration curve of 6.

Patients were re-evaluated at the end of the initial chemotherapy phase of four cycles; those with unresectable disease at this time were considered as treatment failures. If there was residual disease after resection, patients received two more cycles of the same chemotherapy. Audiometry was performed before initiation of therapy and after cycle 4 and at completion of therapy. Response was evaluated based on AFP prior to each cycle of chemotherapy and imaging studies repeated after cycles 2, 4, and 6. Complete response (CR) was defined as no evidence of tumor on computed tomography (CT) or magnetic resonance imaging (MRI) and normal AFP for at least 4 weeks. Toxicities were graded according to the National Cancer Institute (NCI) guidelines.

Statistics

Patients were randomized after initial surgery and stratified according to stage. Stage I and II were treated with C5V with or without amifostine as part of a separate study. The dose intensity aspect of the trial was limited to those with stage III and IV disease. The study was planned to enrol patients for 5.5 years and follow the last patient for 3 years. Projected enrolment was 65 patients per year. The primary outcome comparison between the two treatment regimens was the risk for an adverse event. The equality of risk was to be assessed with a log-rank statistic stratified by stage of disease. This was projected to have 80% power to detect a 1.7-fold decrease in risk for adverse events for stage III or IV when using two-sided test 0.05. Interim monitoring was performed every 6 months after the 30th event was observed. The method of O'Brien and Fleming with a p-value of 0.005 for the stratified log-rank test was required to identify the study for possible termination of accrual.

Event-free survival was defined as the period from the date chemotherapy was started until the evidence of an event – progressive disease, death, diagnosis of a second malignant neoplasm or last contact, whichever occurred first. Survival was defined as the period from the date chemotherapy commenced until death or last contact. Statistical analysis was conducted on life-table estimates calculated by the method of Kaplan and Meier and the SD of the Kaplan–Meier estimate of the survivor function at selected points was calculated using Greenwood's formula. Risk for adverse event and death was compared across therapies and groups of patients using the log-rank statistic. Estimates for relative risks and 95% confidence intervals (CI) were calculated using the proportional hazards regression model with the relevant characteristic as the only variable and stratified as indicated. Outcome analysis was based on the assigned randomized treatment.

Results

One hundred and ninety-two eligible patients with stage III or IV disease were enrolled; 76 patients had experienced an adverse event at the time of the analysis, 72 had disease progression, four died on protocol therapy without evidence of disease progression. One patient had unexplained cardiopulmonary arrest, there was one postoperative complication and two had multiorgan failure, one of which was attributed to infection. A total of 109 patients were randomized, 56 to CC and 53 to C5V. As a result of semi-annual review by the Data and Safety Monitoring Committee of the COG, random assignment was discontinued after 3 years of enrolment because the projected improvement in long-term outcome associated with CC was statistically excluded as a possible outcome of the trial. The study was continued with patients assigned to receive C5V and randomly assigned to receive amifostine or not.

The 3-year EFS was 38% (90% CI 27–49%) for CC patients and 60% (90% CI 51–68%) for C5V (p=0.025). The increased risk for adverse event was evident after accounting for amifostine randomization and stage of disease. The 3-year survival was 56% (90% CI 44–68%) for CC patients versus 74% (90% CI 64–84%) for the C5V group (p=0.035).

Toxicity

There were significantly more transfusion requirements and thrombocytopenia associated with the patients randomized to CC. Although grade IV neutropenia was more common with C5V, ototoxicity was similar with both regimens with grade III or IV <8%.

Conclusions

Intensification of therapy by alternating platinum analogs and omitting 5-FU and vincristine increased the risk of adverse outcome in children with unresectable or metastatic hepatoblastoma.

Study 2

Perilongo G, Maibach R, Shafford E *et al*. Cisplatin versus cisplatin plus doxorubicin for standard-risk hepatoblastoma. *N Engl J Med* 2009;**361**:1662–70.

Objectives

To determine whether in children with standard-risk hepatoblastoma (defined as a tumor involving three or fewer sectors of the liver that is associated with an AFP level of >100 ng/mL), administration of preoperative cisplatin alone may be as effective as cisplatin plus doxorubicin.

Study design

This was an international co-operative prospective randomized trial run by the SIOPEL group (SIOP-3) between 1998 and 2006. Eligibility included age under 16 with previously untreated hepatoblastoma with standard-risk features, defined as a tumor entirely confined to the liver and involving not more than three hepatic sectors. During the trial the protocol was amended to exclude children presenting with an AFP <100 ng/L in view of the evidence of poor outcome for these patients. Tumor extension diagnosis was assessed by ultrasound, CT, and MRI and lung metastases identified by chest CT. Tumor extent was graded using the PRETEXT system developed by the SIOPEL group. Patients with PRETEXT I, II, or III hepatoblastoma and no evidence of extrahepatic disease were eligible for inclusion. In doubtful cases, participating centers could request a central review of imaging.

Diagnostic biopsy was mandatory in children under 6 months of age because of the wider range of differential diagnoses and the confounding AFP at this level. To avoid delay in starting therapy, all patients in whom the diagnosis of hepatoblastoma was confirmed received a single course of cisplatin while awaiting risk assessment. Within 15 days of diagnosis, patients were randomly assigned to cisplatin or cisplatin/doxorubicin. This was done centrally at the UK Children's Cancer Study Group (CCSG) study group data center and patients were assigned to one of the two study treatment groups by the minimization method.

The initial cisplatin cycle of 80 mg/m^2 was given as a continuous infusion over 24 h. The same doses of cisplatin were administered at 14-day intervals. For patients randomized to the cisplatin/doxorubicin regimen, cycles were given at 21-day intervals. Doxorubicin was given at a dose of 30 mg/m^2 as a continuous infusion over 24 h on days 2 and 3, i.e. total dose 30 mg/m^2. Tumor response was assessed after four cycles of cisplatin in the cisplatin group or after one cycle of cisplatin and three cycles of cisplatin plus doxorubicin in the cisplatin/doxorubicin group. If the tumor was considered to be resectable, surgery was attempted. Patients with complete resection were scheduled to receive two more cycles of either chemotherapy. If after the first four cycles there had been a response but the tumor was still unresectable, two more cycles of the same regimen were given but none after surgery. Thus each patient was scheduled to receive a maximum of six cycles of cisplatin in total. Dose adjustment was made for patients less than 10 kg (details not provided). The use of GCSF was not recommended. Hearing loss was evaluated according to the Brock criteria.

Statistics

This study design was based on a test of noninferiority of cisplatin compared to cisplatin/doxorubicin combination for the primary endpoint, i.e. the rate of complete resection. Cisplatin would be considered to be noninferior if the complete resection rate was not decreased by more than 10 percentage points from the 90% rate expected with the cisplatin/doxorubicin combination. Expected recruitment was 30–35 patients per year. Two-sided 95% CI was chosen for the final evaluation of the primary endpoint. Sample size was estimated at 250 patients to test noninferiority with a one-sided, two-sample difference in proportions test for the comparison of the rates of complete resection with an error rate fixed at 5% for incorrectly accepting noninferiority and a

power of 80%. The sample size yields a two-sided 95% CI with 60% power to exclude a 10% difference. Both a per-protocol and an intention-to-treat analysis were performed to avoid potential bias introduced by non-protocol chemotherapy administered before surgery. Kaplan–Meier survival estimates were compared with the log-rank test. The independent Data and Safety Monitoring Committee endorsed continuation of the trial at interim evaluations. A group-sequential approach involving a Lan-DeMets α-spending function with O'Brien–Fleming type boundaries was used to calculate the adjusted significance levels for five comparisons of the primary endpoints.

Results

A total of 92 institutions from 24 countries randomly assigned 267 patients. Of these, five were excluded because of diagnosis revised locally soon after initial diagnosis (nodular hyperplasia, hamartoma, benign nonspecified). A further seven were excluded due to lack of proper documentation. The intention-to-treat sample consisted of 255 patients, 126 on cisplatin alone and 129 on cisplatin/doxorubicin.

Response rate was 90% on cisplatin and 95% on cisplatin/doxorubicin and the rate of complete resection was 95% and 93% respectively. The intention-to-treat analysis showed the noninferiority of cisplatin by a margin of 10%. A per-protocol analysis was also carried out which confirmed no significant difference in either response or resection. A total of 34 randomly assigned patients had relapse or progression, 19 in the cisplatin group (15%) and 15 in the cisplatin/doxorubicin group (12%). Neither the risk of relapse nor risk of death differed between the two groups.

Toxicity

Hearing loss was evaluated according to the Brock criteria. Grade III and IV events were more frequent in the cisplatin/doxorubicin regimen than the cisplatin-only regimen: 74% versus 21%; this related to neutropenia and mucositis. There was no significant difference in ototoxicity or renal toxicity.

Conclusions

Compared with cisplatin/doxorubicin, cisplatin monotherapy achieved similar rates of complete resection and survival and therefore doxorubicin can be safely omitted from the treatment of standard-risk hepatoblastoma.

CHAPTER 7
Malignant germ cell tumors

Ross Pinkerton

Royal Children's Hospital, Brisbane, QLD, Australia

Commentary by Ross Pinkerton

The introduction of cisplatin-based treatment regimens in pediatric malignant germ cell tumors (MGCT) [1,2,3,4], based on effectiveness in adults with testicular tumors, had a dramatic effect on outcome, being clearly superior to previous regimens including vincristine, actinomycin D and cyclophosphamide (VAC). It is not clear whether regimens with higher doses of both cyclophosphamide or ifosfamide and doxorubicin would have achieved the same result but the late effects of such combinations made their use unattractive in a highly curable cancer. Subsequently, PVB (cisplatin, vinblastine, and bleomycin) or BEP (bleomycin, etoposide, and cisplatin) regimens became part of standard protocols, although many groups continued to add these drugs to VACA (vincristine, actinomycin D, doxorubicin, and cyclophosphamide) combinations, particularly in higher risk groups.

Few children's cancers illustrate better the difficulties in design and execution of randomized trials in rare cancers. The only randomized study in pediatric MGCT that has been completed is the CCG-8882/POG-9049 trial. This evaluated dose escalation across a wide range of prognostic subgroups and did not take account of the already excellent prognosis of those with gonadal and localized extragonadal tumors. The study introduced the high-dose cisplatin Einhorn regimen, which had been shown to have efficacy in relapsed or refractory testicular teratoma in adults. It was clear from earlier studies in metastatic neuroblastoma that this combination would have significant ototoxicity and renal toxicity, which one could argue would not be acceptable in children with already highly curable disease. The results of this study showed a small advantage for the high-dose regimen in terms of relapse-free survival (RFS) but not overall survival (OS). It is therefore difficult to conclude in what specific subgroups, if any, the significant toxicity of this treatment regimen is justified.

The United Kingdom Children's Cancer Study Group (UKCCSG) has taken the opposite approach and introduced carboplatin in the JEB regimen (carboplatin, etoposide, and bleomycin) to reduce cisplatin toxicity [5]. No alkylating agent or anthracycline was used. Although this regimen has never been evaluated in a randomized trial, the results have been encouraging but it appears important that a relatively higher dose of carboplatin (5–600 mg/m^2) is used. Poorer results have been reported by the French Paediatric Oncology Society (SFOP) group using lower doses than the glomerular filtration rate (GFR) formula-based dose method used in the UK protocol. For example, in the TGM 90 regimen, cisplatin, used at 100 mg/m^2 in TGM 85, was replaced by 400 mg/m^2 carboplatin. Complete remission (CR) rates were significantly lower with carboplatin (58%) compared to cisplatin (90%). Although most achieved CR with subsequent cisplatin, the overall survival for patients with localized disease was 78% with TGM 90 compared with 88% using TGM 85 [6].

Evidence-Based Pediatric Oncology, Third Edition. Edited by Ross Pinkerton, Ananth Shankar and Katherine K. Matthay.
© 2013 John Wiley & Sons, Ltd. Published 2013 by John Wiley & Sons, Ltd.

More recent nonrandomized studies have included investigation of the potential value of amifostine in children receiving high-dose BEP. The POG 9749 study failed to demonstrate any significant protective effect with such a strategy against ototoxicity.

An alternative dose intensification approach that was piloted by the COG (AGCT01P1) was the dose escalation of cyclophosphamide when added to standard-dose BEP in high-risk MGCT (stage III and IV extragonadal tumors). The dose range from 1.2 to 2.4 g/m² was acceptably tolerated but 1.8 g/m² is probably most appropriate in order to try and limit gonadal toxicity.

More recent single-arm studies by the UKCCSG, SFOP, and the German groups have focused on the refinement of treatment with patients stratified on the basis of clinical risk factors and compared outcome with historical series. The UKCCSG GC-3 study, for example, utilized the GFR-based JEB regimen and varied the number of courses on clinical stage and α-fetoprotein (AFP) levels.

Randomized trials in adults with good-risk testicular teratoma have shown that, compared with carboplatin, cisplatin-based chemotherapy provides a small but significant relapse-free advantage but some of these studies have also used a smaller dose of carboplatin than the UKCCSG [7, 8]. It would seem appropriate that the European and American groups consider a randomized trial to assess definitively the role of carboplatin and those studies should include adolescents in whom the divergence of treatment approach between pediatric and adult specialists may be most marked.

For the poorer risk groups, such as those with extragonadal primaries and high AFP level, the addition of IVAd (ifosfamide, vincristine, and doxorubicin) to PVB/JEB also warrants further evaluation.

High-dose chemotherapy with stem cell rescue has been used in relapse protocols following practice in adults where it has been associated with encouraging outcomes in platinum-refractory patients [9]. Randomized studies using this approach as first line in high-risk patients have failed to show significant benefit [10]. Whilst the number of children with relapsed MGCT is relatively small, second-line and third-line therapy could be the subject of combined

international studies. The COG, for example, recently completed a study to evaluate the use of a paclitaxel, ifosfamide, and carboplatin combination in recurrent or resistant MGCT.

References

1 Pinkerton CR, Pritchard J, Spitz L. High complete response rate in children with advanced germ cell tumours using cisplatin-containing combination chemotherapy. *J Clin Oncol* 1986;**4**:194–9.

2 Ablin AR, Krailo MD, Ramsay NK *et al*. Results of treatment of malignant germ cell tumours in 93 children: a report from the Children's Cancer Study Group. *J Clin Oncol* 1991; **9**:1782–92.

3 Schneider DT, Calaminus G, Reinhard H *et al*. Primary mediastinal germ cell tumors in children and adolescents: results of the German cooperative protocols MAKEI 83/86, 89 and 96. *J Clin Oncol* 2000;**18**:832–9.

4 Gobel U, Schneider DT, Calaminus G, Haas RJ, Schmidt P, Harms D. Germ-cell tumors in childhood and adolescence. GPOH MAKEI and the MAHO study groups. *Ann Oncol* 2000;**11**:263–71.

5 Mann JR, Raafat F, Robinson K *et al*. The United Kingdom Children's Cancer Study Group's second germ cell tumour study: carboplatin, etoposide and bleomycin are effective treatment for children with malignant extracranial germ cell tumours, with acceptable toxicity. *J Clin Oncol* 2000;**18**: 3809–18.

6 Baranzelli MC, Kramar A, Bouffet E *et al*. Prognostic factors in children with localized malignant nonseminomatous germ cell tumors. *J Clin Oncol* 1999;**17**:1212–18.

7 Bajorin DF, Sarosdy MF, Pfister DG *et al*. Randomized trial of etoposide and cisplatin versus etoposide and carboplatin in patients with good-risk germ cell tumors: a multiinstitutional study. *J Clin Oncol* 1993;**11**:598–606.

8 Horwich A, Sleijfer DT, Fossa SD *et al*. Randomized trial of bleomycin, etoposide, and cisplatin compared with bleomycin, etoposide, and carboplatin in good-prognosis metastatic nonseminomatous germ cell cancer: a multiinstitutional Medical Research Council/European Organization for Research and Treatment of Cancer trial. *J Clin Oncol* 1997;**15**:1844–52.

9 Einhorn LH, Williams SD, Chamness A, Brames MJ, Perkins SM, Abonour R. High-dose chemotherapy and stem- cell rescue for metastatic germ-cell tumors. *N Engl J Med* 2007; **357**:340–8.

10 Motzer RJ, Nichols CJ Margolin KA *et al*. Phase III randomized trial of conventional-dose chemotherapy with or without high-dose chemotherapy and autologous hematopoietic stem-cell rescue as first-line treatment for patients with poor-prognosis metastatic germ cell tumours. *J Clin Oncol* 2007;**25**:247–56.

Summary of previous studies

The only previous published randomized trial was carried out between 1990 and 1996 by the Pediatric Oncology Group and Children's Cancer Group (pediatric Intergroup study) [1]. The main objective of the study was to determine whether dose escalation of cisplatin in combination with etoposide and bleomycin improved event-free survival and survival in high-risk MGCT.

The study included patients with extracranial MGCT less than 21 years of age, no prior therapy other than surgical resection or biopsy, stage III or IV gonadal tumors, stages I–IV extragonadal tumors and relapsed stage III or IV MGCT from a previously resected stage I testicular tumor or recurrent immature or benign teratoma.

Those with testicular disease had radical inguinal orchiectomy and also resection of involved nodes if CT positive. For ovarian disease, there was unilateral oophorectomy for unilateral disease or bilateral oophorectomy if both ovaries were involved with preservation of fallopian tubes and uterus and debulking of all nodal or retroperitoneal disease and peritoneal disease. Surgical guidelines for the initial management of extragonadal MGCT depended on the primary tumor site.

Chemotherapy consisted of bleomycin day 1 and etoposide days 1–5, and cisplatin was randomized between $40\,mg/m^2$ daily $\times$ 5 versus $20\,mg/m^2$ daily $\times$ 5. Chemotherapy was given every 21 days.

Chemotherapy doses for infants younger than 12 months of age were calculated by body weight.

Patients were evaluated after four courses of chemotherapy. Those achieving CR (normal tumor markers and resolution of all imaging abnormalities) stopped chemotherapy, while the others (partial or less than partial response) underwent attempted resection. If there was pathological CR then no further treatment was given, otherwise two further courses.

Three hundred and seventeen patients were enrolled but only 299 were deemed eligible. Sites of disease were testis 60, ovarian 74, and extragonadal 165. Ten percent were stage I and II, 45% were stage III and 45% stage IV. Pathology was yolk sac tumor 65%, mixed 20%, germinoma 10%, and choriocarcinoma 3%. One

hundred and forty-nine were randomized to high-dose platinum and 150 to standard-dose platinum.

There was a significant event-free survival (EFS) advantage for those receiving high-dose platinum: 6-year EFS 89.6%±3.6% versus 80.5%±4.8% (p=0.028). There was no difference in overall survival (92% versus 86%). Patients randomized to high dose had reduced creatinine clearance in 7% versus 0% in children on the standard-dose BEP, low magnesium levels 13% versus 0% and objective hearing loss 14% versus 0%; 67% were reported to have required hearing aids in the high-dose arm. There were seven infection-related deaths, six in the high-dose arm.

It was concluded that there was an improvement in event-free survival, which was particularly noted in stage III and IV extragonadal tumors. Overall, there were four relapses in the high-dose arm versus 20 in the standard dose. However, excessive toxicity in the high-dose arm reduced benefit and also made this approach unacceptable in the context of a high cure rate.

Three subsequent publications reported the outcome in specific subgroups, namely mediastinal disease, retroperitoneal and abdominal, and sacrococcygeal [2,3,4]. These gave little further detail regarding the outcome but provided additional clinical information.

References

1 Cushing B, Giller R, Cullen J et al. Randomised comparison of combination chemotherapy with etoposide, bleomycin and either high-dose or standard dose cisplatin in children and adolescents with high-risk malignant germ cell tumours: a Paediatric Intergroup Study – Pediatric Oncology Group 3049 and Children's Cancer Group 8882. J Clin Oncol 2004;22:2691–700.

2 Billmire D, Vinocur C, Rescorla F et al. Malignant mediastinal germ cell tumours: an Intergroup study. J Pediatr Surg 2001;36:18–24.

3 Billmire D, Vinocur C, Rescorla F et al. Malignant retroperitoneal and abdominal germ cell tumours: an Intergroup study. J Pediatr Surg 2003;38:315–18.

4 Rescorla F, Billmire D, Stolar C et al. The effect of cisplatin dose and surgical resection in children with malignant germ cell tumours at the sacrococcygeal region: a pediatric intergroup trial (POG 9049/CCG8882). J Pediatr Surg 2001;36:12–17.

New studies

The authors have been unable to identify any new randomized trials in children with malignant germ cell tumors published since the previous edition of this book.

CHAPTER 8

Medulloblastoma

Ross Pinkerton

Royal Children's Hospital, Brisbane, QLD, Australia

Commentary by Eric Bouffet

Although this tumor was first identified in the late 1800s, the history of medulloblastoma started in 1930 with the landmark publications from Harvey Cushing and Percival Bailey [1,2]. During this time of heroic surgery, mortality was extremely high, greater than 30%, and radical removal was exceptional. Although Cushing noticed that patients with radical resection had a longer survival, most patients from his initial series succumbed rapidly, within a year or less. The longest survivor lived for 5 years after four posterior fossa surgeries and three radiation treatments. It took more than 20 years to make the next major advance in the management of medulloblastoma, which was the use of craniospinal radiation. Edith Paterson and the radiation oncology team at the Christie Hospital in Manchester reported in 1953 the results of a study that involved 12 medulloblastoma patients treated between 1932 and 1947 with postoperative whole central nervous system irradiation utilizing 250 kV x-rays. Five patients survived more than 5 years following this treatment, which confirmed Paterson's assumption that dissemination of this tumor within the central nervous system was present at diagnosis in all patients [3].

The subsequent evolution of medulloblastoma therapy is particularly complex and in the interpretation of results, one needs to take account of major changes that have occurred in radiology, anesthesia, neurosurgery, radiation, and medical oncology over the past four decades. In particular, imaging techniques have improved dramatically. Ventriculography, angiography, myelography, and even computed tomography (CT) have now all been supplanted by magnetic resonance imaging (MRI). In the first studies conducted by the International Society of Paediatric Oncology (SIOP) and the Radiation Therapy Oncology Group (RTOG), preoperative CT scan was the only mandatory imaging study required for staging [4, 5]. In subsequent studies, postoperative imaging and myelograms were requested but not always performed. Introduction of mandatory MRI scan of the brain and the spine only became standard in recent protocols. As far as cytological examination of the cerebrospinal fluid (CSF) is concerned, while North American protocols have included this test as a mandatory requirement for eligibility since the early 1990s, the SIOP group did not introduce this requirement until more recently. As a consequence, comparisons between studies over time are impossible as inconsistencies between staging procedures in published studies preclude any meaningful comparison. However, data from registries such as SEER demonstrate a significant improvement in survival, in particular during the period 1985–1995 [6,7]. This was a time of major advances in imaging techniques, with the introduction of the pre- and postoperative MRI scan as a standard tool to evaluate extent of disease and completeness of resection. This clearly suggests that allocation of treatment according to specific criteria (extent of resection and metastatic status) had a major impact on outcome.

Evidence-Based Pediatric Oncology, Third Edition. Edited by Ross Pinkerton, Ananth Shankar and Katherine K. Matthay.
© 2013 John Wiley & Sons, Ltd. Published 2013 by John Wiley & Sons, Ltd.

Early randomized studies

All these advances were made without the contribution of randomized trials and, in reality, the impact of randomized trials in the management of medulloblastoma has been marginal. The first SIOP and RTOG trials essentially contributed to the identification of high-risk groups, but neither trial concluded that the addition of chemotherapy was associated with a survival benefit [4,5]. The second SIOP study randomly assigned patients to receive either a 6-week module of postoperative chemotherapy followed by radiotherapy ("sandwich therapy") or immediate postoperative radiotherapy. In addition, patients defined as low risk were further randomized to receive either "standard" or "reduced' dose of craniospinal radiotherapy. The chemotherapy regimen consisted of procarbazine, methotrexate, and vincristine. The design of this study triggered divisions between European co-operative groups and as a consequence, accrual rate in this study was too low to provide meaningful conclusions. However, it is clear that an opportunity to reduce the dose of craniospinal radiation in low-risk patients was missed with this study, as the outcome of patients treated with reduced-dose craniospinal radiation following surgery was as good as those treated with a standard dose [8]. As a consequence, the SIOP group decided to maintain the 36 Gy dose of craniospinal radiation as standard of care for average-risk patients in the PNET-3 trial when North American institutions were increasingly using reduced dose for this specific group of patients [9,10].

In the late 1980s the North American Children's Cancer Group (CCG) also conducted a randomized study that triggered passionate debate. Following the promising results of a pilot study using "eight drugs in one day," i.e. vincristine, methylprednisolone, lomustine, hydroxyurea, procarbazine, cisplatin, cyclophosphamide, and cytarabine, the members of CCG decided to compare the old vincristine-lomustine combination with the new "eight in one" regimen that was showing spectacular activity in phase II studies [11]. To the surprise of CCG members, the vincristine-lomustine combination demonstrated significant survival benefit compared to the "eight in one" combination [12]. Several possible explanations were suggested to explain the inferiority of the "eight in one" arm. The treatment arms differed and in particular, in the "eight in one" arm, there was a delay in the administration of craniospinal

radiation and a difference in the vincristine dose intensity that could account for differences in survival, independently of the specific effect of the protocols of chemotherapy used. However, this study was extremely useful in identifying new prognostic factors, and in particular the superiority of the extent of resection over the classic T staging system that was taking into account the tumor size and tumor extent.

The late 1980s also show the limitations of the concept that randomization is a prerequisite to improving knowledge and patient survival. Following interesting pilot data from single institutions [13,14], the Pediatric Oncology Group initiated a randomized trial (POG 8631) in children older than 3 years in which two doses of craniospinal radiotherapy were compared, i.e. 36 Gy in 20 fractions and 23.4 Gy in 13 fractions, in good-risk patients defined by Chang stage, T1, T2, T3A with a subtotal of grossly complete resection (less than 1.5 cm^3 residual volume on the postoperative scan) and no evidence of dissemination. This study was prematurely closed because a planned interim statistical analysis revealed an increased rate of relapse, particularly neuraxis relapses, in patients receiving reduced-dose radiotherapy [15]. A follow-up analysis confirmed these results but showed that with time, the differences were less pronounced: the 8-year event-free survival (EFS) was 67% for patients treated with standard dose and 52% for those treated with reduced dose [16]. However, this trial did not include any chemotherapy and at the time the final results of this randomized trial were reported, a co-operative pilot study conducted by a limited number of North American institutions reported a 5-year event-free survival of 79% using reduced-dose craniospinal radiation with concurrent vincristine and subsequent cisplatin/lomustine and vincristine [10]. An attempt to compare standard-dose craniospinal radiation and reduced-dose radiation with concomitant vincristine followed by multiagent chemotherapy (vincristine, lomustine, and cisplatin) failed to accrue and the POG and CCG decided to adopt the reduced dose with chemotherapy as the standard for average-risk patients despite the negative results of POG 8631.

In Europe in the early 1990s, SIOP and the German HIT group initiated two randomized studies that provided important information regarding the role of chemotherapy in the treatment of medulloblastoma. In the SIOP study, patients aged 3–16 years old with histologically proven medulloblastoma and absence of leptomeningeal metastases on spinal MRI or myelogram (in the earlier phase of the study) were randomly assigned to receive either postoperative chemotherapy followed by craniospinal irradiation or craniospinal irradiation only. The chemotherapy regimen consisted of alternating cycles of vincristine/carboplatin/etoposide and etoposide/cyclophosphamide and the dose of craniospinal radiation was 36 Gy in 20 fractions. This was the first multicenter randomized study to demonstrate a significant advantage for sandwich chemotherapy combined with craniospinal radiation when compared with craniospinal radiation alone [9]. The HIT study was a randomized multicenter trial comparing postoperative neoadjuvant chemotherapy before radiation therapy and maintenance chemotherapy after immediate postoperative radiotherapy in patients with low- and high-risk medulloblastoma. In this protocol, the radiation dose to the craniospinal axis was 35.2 Gy in 22 fractions. The chemotherapy regimen was different in each arm. The group allocated to neoadjuvant chemotherapy received multiagent chemotherapy that included ifosfamide, etoposide, high-dose methotrexate, carboplatin, cytarabine, and cisplatin whereas patients in the maintenance chemotherapy arm received a combination of cisplatin, lomustine, and vincristine. This trial showed a survival advantage for M0 (no evidence of metastatic disease) and M1 (microscopic dissemination into the cerebrospinal fluid) patients treated with maintenance chemotherapy, again suggesting that delayed radiotherapy may have a negative impact on outcome [17,18].

Recent medulloblastoma trials

The confirmation that reduced-dose craniospinal radiation and adjuvant chemotherapy could become a standard treatment for average-risk patients (patients with total or near total resection and no evidence of metastatic disease) came from a large randomized study of two chemotherapy regimens. The COG9961 compared a combination of cisplatin, lomustine, and vincristine with a cisplatin, cyclophosphamide, and vincristine regimen. There was no difference in survival between the two arms. However, the excellent 81% 5-year event-free survival rate reported in this trial confirmed the possibility of using reduced-dose craniospinal radiation in the subset of patients with average-risk features [19]. Similar good survival rates were also reported by a co-operative group using sequential high-dose chemotherapy with autologous stem cell rescue following craniospinal radiation [20]. However, there is evidence that children still suffer significant learning and cognitive complications despite this reduced dose of radiation [21,22].

The results of these recent studies have raised the possibility that the dose of craniospinal radiation can be reduced even further in average-risk patients, and in 2004 the COG initiated a randomized study comparing standard-dose (23.4 Gy) versus reduced-dose (18 Gy) craniospinal radiotherapy and posterior fossa boost versus tumor bed boost radiotherapy in combination with chemotherapy in children 3–7 years of age with standard-risk medulloblastoma. The results of this recently closed study are awaited.

Interestingly, despite the important conclusions of the randomized PNET-3 trial, the SIOP group decided to adopt reduced-dose craniospinal radiation followed by multiagent chemotherapy as the standard treatment for patients with average-risk medulloblastoma. The design of the randomized PNET-4 trial was determined following the results of a pilot study conducted by the French group. In this study conducted between 1998 and 2001, patients with average-risk features were treated with twice-daily fraction for a total dose of 36 Gy to the neuraxis. The hypothesis was that hyperfractionation would allow an increase in biological dose to the tumor without increasing toxicity. This pilot study provided excellent survival data with promising neurocognitive outcomes that compared favorably with those described in patients treated with conventional radiation techniques [23]. The SIOP group designed a randomized study comparing postoperative radiotherapy, either as 23.4 Gy to the craniospinal axis or as hyperfractionated radiotherapy in patients with average-risk features. Both groups received weekly vincristine during radiation and maintenance chemotherapy with cisplatin, lomustine, and vincristine. Early results of this trial disclosed a survival rate similar to that observed in the North American study COG9961 [19]. However, there was no evidence of survival benefit associated with the use of hyperfractionated radiation [24]. The results of neurocognitive outcomes are still pending.

Future directions

Allocation of treatment in medulloblastoma patients has up to now been based on clinical and radiological staging. Recent transcriptional profiling studies from several research groups have suggested the existence of distinct molecular subgroups that differ in their demographics, transcriptomes, somatic genetic events, and clinical outcomes [25,26]. Co-operative groups are currently considering new protocols based on the molecular profiling of these tumors. However, this fragmentation into smaller subgroups will dramatically limit the possibility of conducting randomized studies. It is therefore likely that the design of future studies will essentially be nonrandomized and that progress in the management of medulloblastoma will be based on the results of single-arm studies.

References

1 Cushing H. Experiences with cerebellar medulloblastomas: critical review. *Acta Pathol Microbiol Scand* 1930;**1**:1–86.

2 Rutka JT, Hoffman HJ. Medulloblastoma: a historical perspective and overview. *J Neurooncol* 1996;**29**:1–7.

3 Paterson E, Farr RF. Cerebellar medulloblastoma: treatment by irradiation of the whole central nervous system. *Acta Radiol* 1953;**39**:323–36.

4 Tait DM, Thornton-Jones H, Bloom HJ et al. Adjuvant chemotherapy for medulloblastoma: the first multi-centre control trial of the International Society of Paediatric Oncology (SIOP I). *Eur J Cancer* 1990;**26**:464–9.

5 Evans AE, Jenkin RD, Sposto R et al. The treatment of medulloblastoma. Results of a prospective randomized trial of radiation therapy with and without CCNU, vincristine, and prednisone. *J Neurosurg* 1990;**72**:572–82.

6 McNeil DE, Cote TR, Clegg L et al. Incidence and trends in pediatric malignancies medulloblastoma/primitive neuroectodermal tumor: a SEER update. Surveillance Epidemiology and End Results. *Med Pediatr Oncol* 2002;**39**:190–4.

7 Smoll NR. Relative survival of childhood and adult medulloblastomas and primitive neuroectodermal tumors (PNETs). *Cancer* 2012;**118**:1313–22.

8 Bailey CC, Gnekow A, Wellek S et al. Prospective randomised trial of chemotherapy given before radiotherapy in childhood medulloblastoma. International Society of Paediatric Oncology (SIOP) and the (German) Society of Paediatric Oncology (GPO): SIOP II. *Med Pediatr Oncol* 1995;**25**:166–78.

9 Taylor RE, Bailey CC, Robinson K et al. Results of a randomized study of preradiation chemotherapy versus radiotherapy alone for nonmetastatic medulloblastoma: the International Society of Paediatric Oncology/United Kingdom Children's

Cancer Study Group PNET-3 Study. *J Clin Oncol* 2003;**21**:1581–91.

10 Packer RJ, Goldwein J, Nicholson HS et al. Treatment of children with medulloblastomas with reduced-dose craniospinal radiation therapy and adjuvant chemotherapy: a Children's Cancer Group study. *J Clin Oncol* 1999;**17**:2127–36.

11 Pendergrass TW, Milstein JM, Geyer JR et al. Eight drugs in one day chemotherapy for brain tumors: experience in 107 children and rationale for preradiation chemotherapy. *J Clin Oncol* 1987;**5**:1221–31.

12 Zeltzer PM, Boyett JM, Finlay JL et al. Metastasis stage, adjuvant treatment, and residual tumor are prognostic factors for medulloblastoma in children: conclusions from the Children's Cancer Group 921 randomized phase III study. *J Clin Oncol* 1999;**17**:832–45.

13 Tomita T, McLone DG. Medulloblastoma in childhood: results of radical resection and low-dose neuraxis radiation therapy. *J Neurosurg* 1986;**64**:238–42.

14 Halberg FE, Wara WM, Fippin LF et al. Low-dose craniospinal radiation therapy for medulloblastoma. *Int J Radiat Oncol Biol Phys* 1991;**20**:651–4.

15 Deutsch M, Thomas PR, Krischer J et al. Results of a prospective randomized trial comparing standard dose neuraxis irradiation (3,600 cGy/20) with reduced neuraxis irradiation (2,340 cGy/13) in patients with low-stage medulloblastoma. A combined Children's Cancer Group-Pediatric Oncology Group study. *Pediatr Neurosurg* 1996;**24**:167–76; discussion 176–7.

16 Thomas PR, Deutsch M, Kepner JL et al. Low-stage medulloblastoma: final analysis of trial comparing standard-dose with reduced-dose neuraxis irradiation. *J Clin Oncol* 2000;**18**:3004–11.

17 Kortmann RD, Kuhl J, Timmermann B et al. Postoperative neoadjuvant chemotherapy before radiotherapy as compared to immediate radiotherapy followed by maintenance chemotherapy in the treatment of medulloblastoma in childhood: results of the German prospective randomized trial HIT '91. *Int J Radiat Oncol Biol Phys* 2000;**46**:269–79.

18 Von Hoff K, Hinkes B, Gerber NU et al. Long-term outcome and clinical prognostic factors in children with medulloblastoma treated in the prospective randomised multicentre trial HIT'91. *Eur J Cancer* 2009;**45**:1209–17.

19 Packer RJ, Gajjar A, Vezina G et al. Phase III study of craniospinal radiation therapy followed by adjuvant chemotherapy for newly diagnosed average-risk medulloblastoma. *J Clin Oncol* 2006;**24**:4202–8.

20 Gajjar A, Chintagumpala M, Ashley D et al. Risk-adapted craniospinal radiotherapy followed by high-dose chemotherapy and stem-cell rescue in children with newly diagnosed medulloblastoma (St Jude Medulloblastoma-96): long-term results from a prospective, multicentre trial. *Lancet Oncol* 2006;**7**:813–20.

21 Mulhern RK, Palmer SL, Reddick WE et al. Risks of young age for selected neurocognitive deficits in medulloblastoma are associated with white matter loss. *J Clin Oncol* 2001;**19**:472–9.

22 Mulhern RK, Palmer SL, Merchant TE *et al.* Neurocognitive consequences of risk-adapted therapy for childhood medulloblastoma. *J Clin Oncol* 2005;**23**:5511–19.

23 Carrie C, Grill J, Figarella-Branger D *et al.* Online quality control, hyperfractionated radiotherapy alone and reduced boost volume for standard risk medulloblastoma: long-term results of MSFOP 98. *J Clin Oncol* 2009;**27**:1879–83.

24 Lannering B, Rutkowski S, Doz F *et al.* HIT-SIOP PNET4 – A Randomised multicentre study of hyperfractionated versus standard radiotherapy in children with standard risk medulloblastoma. *Pediatr Blood Cancer* 2010;**55**:806.

25 Northcott PA, Korshunov A, Witt H *et al.* Medulloblastoma comprises four distinct molecular variants. *J Clin Oncol* 2011;**29**:1408–14.

26 Taylor MD, Northcott PA, Korshunov A *et al.* Molecular subgroups of medulloblastoma: the current consensus. *Acta Neuropathol* 2012;**123**:465–72.

Summary of previous studies

The first reported comparison of two different adjuvant chemotherapy strategies in resected medulloblastoma was in 1980 [1]. In this study vincristine and cyclophosphamide were compared with vincristine combined with intrathecal (IT) methotrexate. Sixteen patients received cyclophosphamide and vincristine, 13 received vincristine and IT methotrexate. The local relapse rate with both combinations was 69%. It was concluded that neither regimen appeared to be particularly effective nor there was any difference between regimens. The very small study size limited the utility of this study.

A similar study published by the South West Oncology Study Group [2] in 1981 randomized children to receive radiation therapy alone or radiation followed by vincristine, hydrocortisone, and oral methotrexate given weekly for 4 weeks then monthly for a total of 1 year. Sixty-three patients were entered but only 34 were randomised – 16 to receive chemotherapy, of whom eight died, and 18 to receive no chemotherapy, of whom five died. It was concluded that there was no demonstrable advantage to adjuvant chemotherapy but the study was very small and underpowered.

Between 1975 and 1981 the Children's Cancer Study Group (CCSG) and RTOG evaluated the role of adding vincristine, prednisolone, and lomustine to standard surgery and radiation therapy [3]. Vincristine was given weekly for 8 weeks during radiation therapy and then eight 6-weekly cycles of vincristine, lomustine, and prednisolone were administered. One hundred and seventy-nine children were randomized – 88 to chemotherapy and radiotherapy and 91 to radiotherapy alone. Twelve patients switched treatment following randomization and 42 were electively treated without being randomized. The 5-year event-free survival was 52% for radiation treatment alone and 57% for those receiving chemotherapy. Overall, there was no significant difference. In the group with more advanced disease (M1–3 or T3–T4 disease), 19 received chemotherapy and radiotherapy and 11 radiotherapy alone. Event-free survival was 46% for

those receiving combination therapy compared to no survivors in the radiotherapy alone arm (p=0.006). Despite the large sample size, there were a number of methodological reservations regarding staging and adherence to allocated regimen limiting the value of the study.

Between 1986 and 1992 the CCG compared adjuvant prednisolone, CCNU, vincristine (PCV) with the novel eight in one regimen in high-risk patients defined as having M1–M4 or T3B–T4 disease [4]. Those with more than 1.5 mL of tumor residue following surgery were also eligible. Patients either received weekly vincristine for 8 weeks during radiation followed by eight cycles of PCV given every 6 weeks or alternatively two courses of eight in one chemotherapy prior to radiotherapy followed by eight cycles of eight in one given at 6-weekly intervals. A total of 212 patients were registered; nine were excluded due to inadequate data. Disease-free survival at 5 years was 63% ± 5% for PCV and 45% ± 5 for eight in one chemotherapy (p<0.006) The eight in one regimen was more toxic with regard to hematological complications, electrolyte, renal and ototoxicity. It was concluded that the eight in one regimen was both inferior and more toxic than standard PCV.

The first European collaborative SIOP study was published in 1990, although the study itself was carried out much earlier, between 1975 and 1979 [5]. This trial compared craniospinal irradiation alone with radiation given simultaneously with vincristine followed by a combination of vincristine and lomustine. Vincristine was given weekly during the 8 weeks of radiotherapy followed by a 4-week rest. Lomustine and vincristine were given as a 3-week cycle, every 6 weeks for a total of eight cycles. Patients with medulloblastoma or grade 3–4 ependymoma were eligible. A total of 286 patients with medulloblastoma were identified, of whom 141 were randomized to receive adjuvant chemotherapy and 145 radiotherapy alone. At 2 years, the EFS was 71% in the chemotherapy arm versus 53% in the radiotherapy alone arm (p<0.005). At subsequent follow-up there were more late relapses in the chemotherapy arm and as a result, there was no difference in the 10-year EFS rates (50% versus 46%; p=0.07). However, subgroup analysis suggested an advantage for chemotherapy. Of 94 patients with brainstem involvement, EFS was 55% for the chemotherapy arm versus 25% for the radiotherapy alone arm (p<0.005). Similarly, 91 patients with more advanced (T3–T4) disease who received chemotherapy had a better disease-free survival (40% versus 20%, p<0.002) and, finally, patients with incomplete resection (55% versus 36%, p<0.01). Although the trial did appear to demonstrate the value of adjuvant chemotherapy, the authors noted some reservations in this large multicenter international study including a number of problems with staging of patients.

The Pediatric Oncology Group conducted a similar study between 1979 and 1986, which was published in 1991 [6]. This addressed whether the addition of mustine, vincristine, procarbazine, prednisolone (MOPP) chemotherapy improved outcome when given after radiation therapy. Progression-free survival was the main outcome measure. Seventy-eight patients were eligible, seven refused randomisation. Five-year EFS was 68% for MOPP and 57% for radiation therapy alone (p=0.18). Only for children 5 years of age or older was there a statistically superior outcome with MOPP EFS: 77% versus 52% (p=0.05). For other groups, the trend was apparent but not statistically significant: subtotal excision 66% versus 56%, total excision 75% versus 58%. Stage T1–T2 64% versus 57%, T3 72% versus 61%. It was concluded that MOPP appeared to be advantageous in children over 5 years of age, particularly males, but the difference lost statistical significance beyond 7 years of follow-up.

Two studies have addressed the issue of radiation dose. The first is from the German GPO Group in conjunction with the International Society of Paediatric Oncology (SIOP) [7] which was carried out between 1984 and 1989. The study was designed first to evaluate the possible benefit of adding vincristine, procarbazine and high-dose methotrexate to radiotherapy and second, to evaluate the efficacy of reduced doses of radiation in low-risk patients. The patients were divided into two risk groups: the high-risk group included those with incomplete excision, brainstem involvement or metastases. The chemotherapy approach consisted of the "sandwich" approach with both pre- and postirradiation chemotherapy. A single course was given prior to radiation therapy and a further six cycles at 42-day intervals following irradiation. All poor-risk patients received standard radiation 35 Gy to the whole neuraxis with 20 Gy boost to the tumor. The low-risk group were further randomized to receive the same dose or 25 Gy with 30 Gy boost. A total of 446 patients were registered; 364 were analysed but 40 did not receive the treatment to which they were randomized. Overall EFS was 58% for those receiving sandwich chemotherapy and 60% for those receiving radiation therapy alone. There was no significant difference in any subgroup. For the 74 patients who received reduced-dose radiotherapy, the EFS was 55% compared to 68% (p=0.07) for the 79 patients who received the standard dose. When the groups were combined, for those receiving standard-dose radiotherapy (n=40) the EFS was 60% while in those who received reduced-dose irradiation (n=36), the EFS was 69%. In those receiving chemotherapy and standard-dose irradiation (n=38), EFS was 75% whereas in those receiving chemotherapy and reduced-dose irradiation (n=36), EFS was only 42%. Overall there appeared to be an adverse effect on survival associated with the insertion of chemotherapy prior to radiation where the radiation therapy dose was reduced. Again, the authors expressed some reservations about the quality of the data in this international collaborative trial. It was suggested that the dose of methotrexate might have been suboptimal but also that the delay in administration of radiation therapy might have an adverse effect on outcome.

A similar study carried out by the CCG and POG between 1986 and 1990 was reported in 1996 [8]. This addressed the issue of whether reduced-dose whole neuraxis radiation could safely be given to good-risk patients without adverse effects on recurrence rate and survival. In the control arm a total of 36 Gy was given in 20 fractions, 5 days per week, with posterior fossa boost of 18 Gy in 10 fractions. In the study arm doses were reduced to 23.4 Gy in 13 fractions to the whole neuraxis with a boost to the posterior fossa to achieve the same dose of 54 Gy as in the standard regimen. One hundred and twenty-six patients were randomized. Following randomization, 32 were deemed to have been ineligible. Outcome was analyzed both on the total group who were randomized (n=123) and all who were eligible (n=71). The good-risk low-stage subgroup comprised those with tumors T1–T2, more than 50% resection and <1.5 mL residue. Overall relapse rate for the whole population was 8% (n = 5/63) for standard dose versus 28% (n = 17/60) for reduced dose (p < 0.002). For eligible patients only, this was 6% (2/34) versus 32% (12/37) (p = 0.02). When any recurrences outside the posterior fossa were considered in the whole patient group, there were 7/60 relapses in the reduced-dose group versus 0/34 in the full-dose group (p < 0.004). It was concluded that in this good-risk group, dose reduction in the setting of radiation therapy alone leads to a higher failure rate.

The role of postoperative neoadjuvant chemotherapy given prior to radiotherapy was investigated by the German GPO group [9]. The study carried out between 1991 and 1997 was reported in 2000. The HIT '91 trial randomized patients to receive radiotherapy with vincristine followed by eight courses at 6-weekly intervals of lomustine, cisplatin, and vincristine or preradiation chemotherapy including ifosfamide, cisplatin, methotrexate, etoposide, and cytarabine. In the event of a partial or complete response, a further cycle was given prior to radiotherapy. In the event of stable disease or no response, radiation therapy was given and followed by lomustine, carboplatin, and vincristine. Radiation therapy comprised 35.2 Gy in 22 fractions for the whole neuraxis with a boost to 55.2 Gy to the primary site. One hundred and eighty-four patients were enrolled by 70 centers but only 137 were randomized; 72 received the neoadjuvant regimen and 65 received postradiation chemotherapy. Forty-seven patients were not randomized due to parental refusal. In those with M1 disease treated with preradiation chemotherapy, progression-free survival was 65% ± 5% at 3 years and with postradiation chemotherapy, 78% ± 6 (p < 0.03). It was concluded that although neoadjuvant chemotherapy is feasible, it did not appear to be of benefit and potentially had an adverse affect on outcome.

The most recent SIOP study run in conjunction with the UK CCSG PNET-3 study was reported in 2003 [10]. This was designed to determine whether chemotherapy given after surgery and before radiation therapy would improve outcome. The neoadjuvant regimen consisted of vincristine weekly for 10 weeks and four cycles of etoposide daily for 3 days, and carboplatin daily for 2 days alternating with cyclophosphamide. Following this, radiation therapy was given with a total dose 55 Gy to the posterior fossa. All patients (excluding those with leptomeningeal disease) were eligible, including those with M1 disease. Following staging, patients were randomly assigned to receive craniospinal radiation or prerradiation chemotherapy. Two hundred and seventeen patients were randomized; 27 were ineligible, 21 due to initial metastatic disease and six due to equivocal staging. Ninety patients received chemotherapy and radiotherapy, 89 patients received radiation therapy alone. Event-free survival was significantly better for those receiving combination therapy: EFS 78% (95% confidence interval [CI] 70–81) versus 65% (95% CI 55–75) at 3 years and 74% versus 59% at 5 years (p = 0.04). However, overall survival was not significantly different: 83% versus 76% at 3 years and 76% versus 65% at 5 years (p = 0.09). EFS was significantly better in those who took <50 days to complete the course of radiation therapy compared to those taking longer: EFS 78% versus 54% (p < 0.009). Ninety-nine patients had complete surgical resection at presentation and in these patients there was a significantly better EFS in those receiving combined therapy (p = 0.04). It was concluded that treatment with four courses with intensive chemotherapy is feasible prior to radiation therapy and advantageous, particularly in patients with surgical complete resection.

References

1 Gerosa M, DiStefano E, Carli M, Iraci G. Combined treatment of pediatric medulloblastoma. A review of an integrated program (two-arm chemotherapy trial) *Child's Brain* 1980;**6**:262–73.

2 Van Eys J, Chen T, Moore T, Cheek W, Sexauer C, Starling K. Adjuvant chemotherapy for medulloblastoma and ependymoma using IV vincristine, intrathecal methotrexate and intrathecal hydrocortisone. A Southwest Oncology Study Group study. *Cancer Treat Rep* 1981;**65**:681–4.

3 Evans AE, Jerkin DT, Spost R *et al*. Results of prospective randomised trial of radiation therapy with and without CCNU, vincristine and prednisone *J Neurosurg* 1990;**72**:572–82.

4 Zeltzer PM, Boyett JM, Findlay JL, Albright L, Rorke LB, Milstein JM. Metastasis stage, adjuvant treatment and residual tumor are prognostic factors for medulloblastoma in children; conclusions from the Children's Cancer Group 921 randomised phase III study. *J Clin Oncol* 1999;**17**:832–45.

5 Tait DM, Thornton Jones H, Bloom HJG, Lemerle V, Morris-Jones P. Adjuvant chemotherapy for medulloblastoma; the first multi-centre control trial of the International Society of Paediatric Oncology (SIOP-1). *Eur J Cancer* 1990;**26**:464–9.

6 Krischer JP, Ragab AH, Kun L *et al.* Nitrogen mustard, vincristine, procarbazine and prednisone as adjuvant chemotherapy in the treatment of medulloblastoma *J Neurosurg* 1991;**74**:905–9.

7 Bailey CC, Gneko A, Wellek S *et al.* Prospective randomised trial of chemotherapy given before radiotherapy in childhood medulloblastoma. International Society of Paediatric Oncology (SIOP) and the (German) Society of Paediatric Oncology (GPO): SIOP-II. *Med Pediatr Oncol* 1995;**25**:166–8.

8 Deutsch M, Thomas PRM, Krischer J *et al.* Results of a prospective randomised trial comparing standard dose neuraxis irradiation with reduced neuraxis irradiation in patients with low-stage medulloblastoma. *Pediatr Neurosurg* 1996;**24**:167–77.

9 Kartmann RD, Kuhl J, Timmermann B *et al.* Postoperative neoadjuvant chemotherapy before radiotherapy as compared to immediate radiotherapy followed by maintenance chemotherapy in the treatment of medulloblastoma in childhood; results of the German prospective randomised trial HIT 91. *Int J Radiat Oncol Biol Phys* 2000;**46**:269–79.

10 Taylor R, Bailey C, Robinson K *et al.*, International Society of Paediatric Oncology, United Kingdom Children's Cancer Study Group. Results of a randomised study of pre-radiation chemotherapy versus radiotherapy alone for non-metastatic medulloblastoma: the International Society for Paediatric Oncology/United Kingdom Children's Cancer Study Group PNET-3 Study. *J Clin Oncol* 2003;**21**:1581–91.

New studies

Study 1

Abd El-Aal HH, Mokhtar MM, Habib EE, El-Kashef AT, Fahmy ES. Medulloblastoma: conventional radiation therapy in comparison to chemo radiation therapy in the post-operative treatment of high-risk patients. *J Egyptian Natl Cancer Inst* 2005;**17**:301–7.

Objectives

To assess in high-risk medulloblastoma treated by surgery and radiation therapy whether adjuvant combination chemotherapy had additional value.

Study design

The study took place between 2001 and 2004 in a single center. Forty-eight prospectively presenting children were included. Eligibility criteria comprised minimum age of 3 years, maximum 18 years, no metastatic disease, Karnofsky performance >60 and diagnosis confirmed by biopsy or excision. High risk was defined on the basis of positive CSF cytology, T3 and T4 primary lesions, ependymal or glial differentiation, and <4 years of age.

Patients were randomized to receive postoperative craniospinal (CS) irradiation alone or combined postoperative chemotherapy and radiation therapy.

Outcome endpoints compared were response rates, disease-free (DFS) and overall survival (OS). Group I (radiation alone) included 21 patients, and group II (CS radiotherapy plus postoperative chemotherapy) had 27 patients. Radiation therapy consisted of 36 Gy to the whole neuraxis followed by boost of 20 Gy to the posterior fossa. Chemotherapy consisted of vincristine 1.4 mg/m^2 weekly during spinal radiation. Following CS irradiation, patients received four cycles of etoposide 100 mg/m^2 day 1–3 and cisplatin 75 mg/m^2 day 1. Chemotherapy was given every 21 days.

Statistics

Chi-square/Fisher exact tests compared independent proportions. Kaplan–Meier estimated overall disease-free survival rates and log-rank tests compared the groups. No details of required sample size or power prediction were provided. The method of randomization was not specified.

Results

Forty-three percent of tumours in group I were desmoplastic pathology and 33% in group II. In group I, a complete response occurred in 71% and in group II 59%. Progressive disease was not observed in any group I patient compared with 37% (n=9) in group II patients (p<0.004).

The OS for the whole study population was 57%. The 3-year OS for group I was 69% versus 49% in group II (p=0.09). Sixty-six percent of patients in group I remained disease free compared to only 24% in group II. The 3-year DFS was 61% and 49% for group I and II patients respectively.

Conclusions

It was concluded that in this setting, the use of adjuvant chemotherapy was of no benefit and in some cases treatment interruption during radiotherapy caused by myelosuppression adversely affected outcome.

Study 2

Packer RJ, Gajjar A, Vezina G *et al*. Phase III study of craniospinal radiation therapy followed by adjuvant chemotherapy for newly diagnosed average-risk medulloblastoma. *J Clin Oncol* 2006;**24**:4202–8.

Objectives

To evaluate two postradiotherapy chemotherapy regimens following reduced-dose craniospinal radiotherapy in children with average-risk medulloblastoma.

Study design

The study was carried out between 1996 and 2000 involving multiple sites. Eligibility criteria comprised patients between 3 and 21 years of age with no evidence of disseminated disease on MRI or cytology. Patients were to have <1.5 cm^2 of residual tumor on postoperative imaging performed within 21 days, preferably within 72 h, of surgery. No previous radiotherapy or chemotherapy other than corticosteroids was permitted and patients must have commenced treatment within 31 days of definitive surgery. Radiotherapy consisted of a dose of 23.4 Gy craniospinal radiation with posterior fossa boost of 32.4 Gy.

Following surgery, patients were randomized to receive cycles of regimen A or B. Regimen A consisted of lomustine 75 mg/m^2 orally day 0, cisplatin 75 mg/m^2 IV day 1 and vincristine 1.5 mg/m^2 days 1, 7, and 14. Regimen B consisted of cisplatin 75 mg/m^2 IV day 0, vincristine 1.5 mg/m^2 days 1, 7, and 14 and cyclophosphamide 1 g/m^2 over 1 h IV days 21 and 22. Patients were not to receive cisplatin if the creatinine clearance was <50% of baseline value and 50% dose reduction was mandated if there was a decrease in auditory acuity >30 decibels at 4000 Hz or >20 decibels at 500–3000 Hz. For grade 4 ototoxicity, cisplatin was withheld and not restarted unless follow-up audiograms returned to at least no more than grade 2 ototoxicity.

All preoperative and postoperative MRI imaging (97%) was centrally reviewed and 85% (358/421) of pathology was also reviewed centrally.

Statistics

Patients were stratified by age and brainstem involvement. The primary endpoint for analysis was time to treatment failure event (EFS) measured from the time of study enrollment. The original design required 240–300 randomly assigned patients to be enrolled over a 4-year period. With an assumed baseline EFS of 85% at 1 year and 70% long-term EFS and a minimum of 2 years follow-up, the power of the two-sided log-rank test was 79% for an improvement in long-term EFS from 70% to 85%. The rate of patient enrollment was higher than anticipated and for primary comparison, 379 patients were enrolled over 4 years and the analysis was performed with a minimum of 3 years follow-up. With the above assumptions, the study would have an 80% power to detect an increase in long-term EFS from 70% to 83% or a 13% improvement. All analyses followed intention-to-treat philosophy. Nonparametric EFS and survival curves were computed using the Kaplan–Meier method with

standard error (SE) via the Greenwood formula. Follow-up probabilities were estimated using the product limit estimate by censoring patients experiencing treatment failure events.

Results

Four hundred and twenty-one patients were enrolled in the study; 42 were excluded after central review. The remaining 379 patients included 66 who on central review had no clear evidence of excessive residual disease or metastases or where studies were of poor quality or incomplete submissions. Median follow-up was just over 5 years, with all patients having been observed for at least 3 years, 81% at least 4 years, and 57% at least 5 years. Five-year EFS and survival probabilities were 81% and 86% respectively. The 5-year EFS was 82% and 80% for regimens A and B respectively. Five-year overall survival was 87% and 85% respectively.

Toxicity

Virtually all patients experienced grade III or IV hematological toxicity at some time during therapy; grade IV hematological toxicities and infection occurred significantly more frequently in patients treated with regimen B. Electrolyte toxicity and poor performance scores occurred more frequently in patients treated on regimen A.

Conclusions

There was no observed difference in outcome between the two adjuvant chemotherapy regimens and overall there was encouraging EFS for children receiving reduced-dose craniospinal radiation plus chemotherapy.

Study 3

Von Hoff K, Hinkes B, Gerber NU *et al.* Long-term outcome and clinical prognostic factors in children with medulloblastoma treated in the prospective randomised multicentre trial HIT'91. *Eur J Cancer* 2009;**45**:1209–17.

This paper reports long-term follow-up of the HIT'91 study previously described to show benefit from maintenance chemotherapy. It analyses 280 patients aged 3–18 years included from 1991 to 1997 in a randomized trial comparing sandwich chemotherapy with postradiation maintenance chemotherapy. The median survival follow-up was 10 years. Overall, 187 patients had complete staging assessments and central histopathological review. Overall survival was higher after maintenance compared to sandwich treatment for those with M0 disease (overall survival 91% versus 62%, p<0.01) and also MI disease (70% versus 34%, p=0.02). For those with M2–3 disease, the 10-year overall survival was 42% and 45% respectively.

Conclusions

The authors concluded that the long-term survival outcome was improved with maintenance chemotherapy in patients with either localized (M0) or M1 medulloblastoma.

CHAPTER 9

Glioma

Ross Pinkerton
Royal Children's Hospital, Brisbane, QLD, Australia

Commentary by Joann L. Ater

Gliomas constitute over 50% of central nervous system tumors in children, and most are low grade. Several clinical trials address the treatment of low-grade glioma but none of the randomized studies is yet published. The high-grade glioma category of brain tumors includes anaplastic astrocytoma (AA), glioblastoma multiforme (GBM), high-grade mixed glioma, anaplastic oligodendroglioma and high-grade glioma not otherwise specified (NOS). They occur in any location in the central nervous system. Most studies that address treatment of high-grade glioma have focused primarily on either the supratentorial tumors or brainstem glioma. The supratentorial high-grade glioma group comprises only 10% of brain tumors treated in children under the age of 21 and children with intrinsic pontine glioma make up another 8–10% of pediatric brain tumors. There are only approximately 150 cases in each group diagnosed annually in the United States. The reports cited in this chapter are specifically related to either supratentorial and cerebellar high-grade gliomas or diffuse intrinsic pontine gliomas (DIPG).

With the limitations imposed by small numbers, randomized clinical trials can only be performed within co-operative groups such as the International Society of Pediatric Oncology (SIOP) and the Children's Oncology Group (COG). Indeed, all phase III studies included in this chapter are reports from these groups. However, over the last decade, COG has not initiated any randomized studies in pediatric high-grade glioma, choosing to focus on phase I and II trials based on preclinical laboratory and adult trial information. Regrettably, this is appropriate because the survival rates for diffuse intrinsic pontine glioma and high-grade glioma have changed little, if at all, over the last two decades, making retrospective comparisons more reliable.

Historically the prognosis of children with high-grade glioma has been poor. In fact, the prognosis appears to have decreased since the CCG-943 study that compared the addition of chemotherapy with lomustine and vincristine to radiation therapy alone. This study helped establish surgery, radiation, and chemotherapy as the standard approach for these tumors in children. However, in retrospect, some of the long-term survivors had atypical low-grade tumors rather than malignant glioma [1, 2]. Subsequent studies with even more intensive chemotherapy regimens added to surgery and radiation failed to increase survival and in some instances were associated with high rates of toxicity [3, 4]. In studies with central review, two clinical factors have consistently shown an association with outcome: histology and extent of tumor resection. In general, patients with glioblastoma multiforme have worse prognosis than those with a grade III glioma. Anaplastic oligodendrogliomas have

---

Evidence-Based Pediatric Oncology, Third Edition. Edited by Ross Pinkerton, Ananth Shankar and Katherine K. Matthay.
© 2013 John Wiley & Sons, Ltd. Published 2013 by John Wiley & Sons, Ltd.

a better outcome than other malignant gliomas [1, 3]. In addition, patients with tumors that are amenable to extensive resection have higher rates of long-term survival than those with less resectable tumors [5].

Surgery for diffuse intrinsic pontine glioma is not recommended. The fact that diffuse tumors can be identified noninvasively with magnetic resonance imaging (MRI) has diminished the role of biopsy in establishing diagnosis, except when atypical features are present [6]. Eighty-five percent to 90% of tumors that arise in the brainstem are diffuse intrinsic pontine anaplastic astrocytoma or glioblastoma multiforme, and 10–15% are focal low-grade astrocytomas. Recognition of the relatively favorable focal low-grade tumors is essential because of the relatively indolent course and distinctly different management. These tumors can be managed with surgery, observation, and radiation or chemotherapy at progression, with good outcome. Focal brainstem gliomas are now excluded from clinical trials on intrinsic brainstem tumors, such as the study reported by Mandell et al. for the Pediatric Oncology Group (POG-9239).

Radiation therapy

The role of radiation dose and schedule in pediatric high-grade glioma has been studied primarily in diffuse pontine glioma. There have been no randomized studies between surgery alone versus radiotherapy for high-grade gliomas in children. However, there is evidence based on a number of adult studies that radiotherapy is of benefit in at least relieving symptoms and prolonging survival [7].

In the 1980s and early 1990s, there was initial interest in whether higher doses and different schedules of radiation fractionation may be beneficial in treatment of brain tumors. This approach was utilized in the study by Mandell et al., which investigated the issue of higher dose hyperfractionated radiation for brainstem gliomas. Based on this study, standard radiation is still the recommended treatment for intrinsic pontine glioma because of the benefit derived from temporary clinical improvement in most patients and tumor response in about 30%. These trials of radiation in brainstem glioma are important because when carefully done, they demonstrated that hyperfractionation

provided no objective benefit in prolonging survival beyond the benefit achieved with standard radiation.

Chemotherapy

Over the last 5 years, several important phase II studies in high-grade glioma in children have been completed. In 2005, Stupp et al. reported a large randomized study of adult glioblastoma multiforme which showed significant improvement in survival with concomitant and adjuvant temozolomide with radiotherapy compared to radiotherapy alone [8]. This study was important in that it is the first randomized study in adult glioblastoma to show benefit of chemotherapy. The survival benefit was 2.5 months, which was significant statistically but represented only modest clinical improvement. Based on this study, several groups conducted pediatric trials with temozolomide given during radiotherapy and for 6 months after following the treatment reported by Stupp. In a COG study, the results with temozolomide for both high-grade gliomas and DIPG were similar to those obtained in the CCG-945 study with lomustine and vincristine following radiotherapy [9]. A French study of radiotherapy with temozolomide for DIPG also did not yield any significant improvement in outcome and was associated with higher toxicity compared to radiotherapy alone, with a 1-year overall survival (OS) of 50% [10]. Perhaps combinations with temozolomide will yield improved results. Early results with lomustine and temozolomide showed improved event-free survival (EFS) with the addition of lomustine, but no difference in overall survival [11].

Recently, bevacizumab alone or with irinotecan has been studied in pediatric high-grade gliomas based on promising results in adult glioblastoma, resulting in US Food and Drug Administration approval of this drug for treatment for malignant glioma [12]. However, so far the results in children have been disappointing. A phase II study of bevacizumab plus irinotecan in recurrent malignant glioma and DIPG showed no sustainable responses [13].

In an effort to improve efficacy of chemotherapy in childhood high-grade gliomas, investigators have began exploring the applicability of molecular targeted treatment strategies. However, while there is good evidence from the extensive research that has been done in defining molecular pathways of tumorigenesis in adult high-grade gliomas, there is relatively little information about pediatric gliomas. With the data that are accumulating, it appears that pediatric gliomas may be biologically distinct from adult primary malignant gliomas in that they infrequently exhibit deletions or mutations of the *PTEN* gene or amplification of *EGFR* [14]. In addition, pediatric malignant gliomas rarely arise from apparent low-grade precursors and rarely have mutations in the *IDH1* or *IDH2* genes [15]. Studies that have examined several molecular targeted treatment strategies in conjunction with radiotherapy known to target adult glioma tumorigenesis have yielded unsatisfactory results in children. For example, studies of the *PDGFR* inhibitor imatinib, the *EGFR* inhibitor gefitinib, and the farnysltransferase inhibitor tipofarnib have yielded disappointing results [16, 17, 18].

It appears that currently in childhood high-grade glioma, there is no new treatment that seems promising enough to commit to a large phase III study that will take many years. Thus, most groups such as COG are continuing to pursue phase I and II studies. In the future, with more individualized therapies directed at specific tumor markers, immunotherapy, antiangiogenic therapy, etc., we will need to devise more creative ways to measure response and efficacy of therapy. In addition, targeted therapy should be based, when possible, on sound laboratory studies in pediatric tumors.

Conclusions

The treatment of pediatric high-grade glioma continues to be a dilemma. The number of reported trials in childhood glioma is limited and their results are of insufficient power to provide unequivocal evidence-based outcomes for clear diagnostic, prognostic, and therapeutic directions. Two of the reasons for this conundrum are that there are too few well-conducted trials and current trials are based on adult preliminary studies, when the biology of childhood gliomas may be different. More well-co-ordinated trials incorporating biological correlations are needed. Despite the trials conducted to date, there is a compelling urgency to engage in clinical trials that will answer the questions that remain, many of which are generated by the very trials that were designed to settle some of these issues.

References

1 Hales RK, Shokek O, Burger PC *et al.* Prognostic factors in pediatric high-grade astrocytoma: the importance of accurate pathological diagnosis. *J Neurooncol* 2010;**99**:65–71.

2 Pollack IF, Boyett JM, Yates AJ *et al.* The influence of central review on outcome associations in childhood malignant gliomas: results from the CCG-945 experience. *Neurooncology* 2003;**5**:197–207.

3 Finlay JL, Boyett JM, Yates AJ *et al.* Randomized phase III trial in childhood high-grade astrocytoma comparing vincristine, lomustine, and prednisone with the eight-in-1-day regimen. *J Clin Oncol* 1993;**13**:112–23.

4 MacDonald TJ, Arenson EB, Ater J *et al.* Phase II study of high-dose chemotherapy before radiation in children with newly diagnosed high-grade astrocytoma: final analysis of Children's Cancer Group Study 9933. *Cancer* 2005;**104**:2862–71.

5 Wisoff JH, Boyett JM, Berger MS *et al.* Current neurosurgical management and the impact of extent of resection in the treatment of malignant gliomas of childhood. A report of the Children's Cancer Group trial CCG-945. *J Neurosurg* 1998;**89**:52–9.

6 Albright AL, Packer RJ, Zimmerman R *et al.* Magnetic resonance scans should replace biopsies for the diagnosis of diffuse brain stem gliomas: a report from the Children's Cancer Group. *Neurosurgery* 1993;**33**:1026–30.

7 Theeler BJ, Groves MD. High-grade gliomas. *Curr Treat Options Neurol* 2011;**13**:386–99.

8 Stupp R, Mason WP, van den Bent MJ *et al.* Radiotherapy plus concomitant and adjuvant temozolomide for glioblastoma. *N Engl J Med* 2005;**352**:987–66.

9 Cohen KJ, Heideman RL, Zhou T *et al.* Temozolomide in the treatment of children with newly diagnosed diffuse intrinsic pontine gliomas: a report from the Children's Oncology Group. *Neurooncology* 2011;**13**:410–16.

10 Chassot A, Canale S, Varlet P *et al.* Radiotherapy with concurrent and adjuvant temozolomide in children with newly diagnosed diffuse intrinsic pontine glioma. *J Neurooncol* 2012;**106**:399–407.

11 Jakacki RI, Yates A, Blaney SM *et al.* Phase 1 trial of temolozomide and lomustine in newly diagnosed high-grade gliomas of childhood. *Neurooncology* 2008;**10**:569–76.

12 Iwamoto FM, Fine HA. Bevacizumab for malignant gliomas. *Arch Neurol* 2010;**67**:285–8.

13 Gururangan S, Chi SN, Young Poussaint T *et al.* Lack of efficacy of bevacizumab plus irinotecan in children with recurrent malignant glioma and diffuse brainstem glioma: a Pediatric Brain Tumor Consortium study. *J Clin Oncol* 2010;**28**:3069–75.

14 Pollack IF, Hamilton RL, James CD *et al.* Rarity of PTEN deletions and EGFR amplification in malignant gliomas of childhood: results from the CCG 945 cohort. *J Neurosurg* 2006;**105**(5 suppl):418–24.

15 Hartmann C, Meyer J, Balss J *et al.* Type and frequency of IDH1 and IDH2 mutations related to astrocytic and oligodendroglial differentiation and age: a study of 1,010 diffuse gliomas. *Acta Neuropathol* 2009;**118**:469–74.

16 Haas-Kogan DA, Banerjee A, Poussaint T *et al.* Phase II trial of tipifarnib and radiation in children with newly diagnosed intrinsic pontine gliomas. *Neurooncology*2011; **13**:298–306.

17 Pollack IF, Stewart CF, Kocak M *et al.* Phase II study of gefitinib and irradiation in children with newly diagnosed brainstem gliomas: a report from the Pediatric Brain Tumor Consortium. *Neurooncology* 2011;**13**:290–7.

18 Pollack IF, Jakacki RI, Blaney SM *et al.* Phase I trial of imatinib in children with newly diagnosed brainstem and recurrent malignant gliomas: a Pediatric Brain Tumor Consortium report. *Neurooncology* 2007;**9**:145–60.

Summary of previous studies

Three early small randomized studies evaluated the role of chemotherapy in patients with relapsed disease. The first, published in 1984, included high-grade glioma, ependymoma, medulloblastoma, and miscellaneous other tumors [1]. Patients were randomized to MOPP (54 patients) or OPP (52 patients). MOPP was the standard regimen: mustine days 1 and 8, vincristine days 1 and 8, procarbazine day 1–10, and prednisolone days 1–10 every 28 days. OPP was the same regimen excluding the mustine. Due to early deaths or insufficient data, a large number were non-evaluable. Overall, 3/8 patients with astrocytoma had complete response (CR) or partial response (PR) after MOPP (CR 1; PR 2) versus 0/10 after OPP. Although the study was insufficiently powered for any statistical conclusions, the MOPP regimen, which was more toxic, produced more responses than the OPP regimen in children with recurrent astrocytoma.

In a later study run by the Pediatric Oncology Group published in 1992, carboplatin and iproplatin were compared in a randomized study containing a wide range of pediatric brain tumors [2]. Overall complete or partial response rate with carboplatin was 9% and 6% with iproplatin. There appeared to be a higher response rate to iproplatin in those children who were cisplatin naïve: 20% versus 3% for those with prior exposure compared to 10% and 9% respectively for patients treated with carboplatin. By histological subtype, the response rates for carboplatin and iproplatin respectively were low-grade astrocytoma 0/7, 1/15, high-grade astrocytoma 1/14, 0/12, medulloblastoma 1/15, 1/14, ependymoma 1/12, 0/7, brainstem glioma 0/14, 0/14. It was concluded that both drugs had very limited activity and differed only in relation to toxicity profile, with carboplatin being significantly more myelosuppressive than iproplatin.

The third study, carried out by the Children's Cancer Group (CCG) and published in 1999, evaluated the potential benefit of adding mannitol to enhance drug access across the blood–brain barrier when combined with single-agent etoposide [3]. Ninety-nine patients were registered; histological subtypes included 15 low-grade astrocytoma, 20 high-grade glioma, 22 brainstem glioma, and 42 primitive neuroectodermal tumor (PNET). Ultimately only 87 had evaluable imaging and local review showed a total of 12 partial and no complete responses. Response rates with etoposide plus mannitol were 17% compared to 10% with etoposide alone, with no significant differences in survival. It was concluded that the overall response rate to single-agent etoposide was low and mannitol did not improve its efficacy.

There were three studies specifically looking at high-grade glioma or brainstem glioma. The first study, published in 1989, was performed between 1976 and 1981 by the CCG evaluating the role of adding prednisolone, CCNU, vincristine (PCV) chemotherapy to standard-dose radiation therapy in high-grade astrocytoma. Brainstem and spinal cord tumors were excluded [4]. Patients were stratified into those with anaplastic astrocytoma or glioblastoma multiforme. Eligible patients were randomized within 4 weeks of surgery and all patients received standard radiation therapy 52.5 Gy. Younger children, between 2 and 3 years old, received a reduced dose of 45 Gy. Patients randomized to chemotherapy received six courses of PCV. Total duration of treatment was planned for 58 weeks. While 72 patients were enrolled in the study, only 58 were randomized – 28 to radiotherapy plus chemotherapy and 30 to radiotherapy alone. Event-free survival was 46% in the combined arm versus 18% for radiotherapy alone (p<0.05) while OS was 43% and 17% respectively (p=0.1). The difference appeared most marked for those with glioblastoma; 5-year EFS was 42% for those receiving chemotherapy versus 6% for those treated with radiotherapy alone (p=0.01). It was concluded that adjuvant chemotherapy with this regimen might prolong EFS particularly in glioblastoma multiforme but the numbers were too small to provide a reliable answer to the question posed.

A study carried out between 1985 and 1990 by the CCG evaluated in more detail the potential role of chemotherapy as an adjunct to radiation therapy. In this trial pre- and postoperative eight in one chemotherapy was compared to PCV [5]. Standard treatment consisted of local radiation therapy 54 Gy/30 F with 8 concurrent weekly injections of vincristine followed at week 10 by eight cycles of PCV given every 6 weeks. The experimental arm consisted of two courses of eight in one chemotherapy given 2 weeks apart followed by the same radiation therapy commencing 2 weeks after the second cycle and subsequently eight courses of eight in one chemotherapy given every 6 weeks. The projected duration of maintenance was 48 weeks in both treatment arms. One hundred and eighty-five patients were randomized, 13 were subsequently excluded. Overall the 5-year EFS was 33%; 26% in the PCV arm compared with 33% in the eight in one experimental arm. The median time to progression was 14 months in both arms. It was concluded that there was no significant difference in the outcome with the exception of more marrow suppression in the eight in one regimen.

Finally, a study carried out between 1992 and 1996 by the Pediatric Oncology Group and published in 1999 evaluated the role of hyperfractionated radiation therapy in brainstem glioma [6]. One hundred and thirty-two patients were entered, of whom 67 received conventional radiation therapy and 65 hyperfractionated radiation. Two patients, one in each arm, were ineligible. Treatment was started not more than 28 days from diagnosis and the study compared 180 cGy/fraction daily to a total of 54 Gy with 117 cGy/fraction given twice a day to a total of 70.2 Gy. The radiation field included tumor volume plus a 2 cm margin. Concurrent cisplatin was given as a continuous infusion over 120 h at weeks 1, 3, and 5 combined with steroids. A pathological diagnosis was obtained in 22 patients; 10 had anaplastic astrocytoma or glioblastoma multiforme. The median time to progression was 6 months (range 2–15 months) with conventional radiation therapy compared to 5 months range (1–12 months) with hyperfractionation. Overall survival rates at 1, 2, and 3 years were 30%, 7%, and 3.5% for conventional radiation compared to 27%, 7%, and 4.5%. It was concluded that in this patient population, hyperfractionated radiation therapy provided no short- or long-term advantage.

References

1 Cangir A, Ragab AH, Steuber P, Land VJ, Berry DH, Krischer JP. Combination chemotherapy with vincristine (NSC-67574), procarbazine (NSC-77213), prednisone with or without nitrogen mustard (NSC-762) (MOPP v OPP) in children with recurrent brain tumours. *Med Pediatr Oncol* 1984;**12**:1–3.

2 Friedman HS, Krischer JP, Burger P *et al.* Treatment of children with progressive or recurrent brain tumours with carboplatin or iproplatin: a Paediatric Oncology Group randomised phase II study. *J Clin Oncol* 1992;**10**:249–56.

3 Kobrinsky NL, Packer RJ, Boyett JM *et al.* Etoposide with or without mannitol for the treatment of recurrent or primarily unresponsive brain tumours: a Children's Cancer Group Study. CCG-9881. *J Neuro-Oncol* 1999;**45**:47–54.

4 Sposto R, Ertel IJ, Jenkins RDT *et al.* The effectiveness of chemotherapy for treatment of high-grade astrocytoma in children: results of a randomised trial. *J Neuro-Oncol* 1989;**7**:165–77.

5 Finlay JL, Boyett JM, Yates AJ *et al.* Randomised phase III trial in childhood high grade astrocytoma comparing vincristine, lomustine and prednisone with the eight-drugs-in-1-day regimen. *J Clin Oncol* 1995;**13**:112–23.

6 Mandell LR, Kadota R, Freeman C *et al.* There is no role for hyperfractionated radiotherapy in the management of children with newly diagnosed diffuse intrinsic brainstem tumours: results of a Pediatric Oncology Group phase III trial comparing conventional v. hyperfractionated radiotherapy. *Int J Radiat Oncol Biol Phys* 1999;**43**:959–64.

New studies

The authors have been unable to identify any new randomized trials in children with glioma published since the previous edition of this book.

CHAPTER 10

Non-Hodgkin lymphoma

Ross Pinkerton
Royal Children's Hospital, Brisbane, QLD, Australia

Commentary by Ross Pinkerton

The evolution of curative strategies for the more common childhood non-Hodgkin lymphomas (NHL) has been influenced by advances in adult cancer, children's cancer and, more recently, international initiatives. In the case of Burkitt lymphoma (BL), it is notable that the lessons from work in Africa in the 1960s by Burkitt, Ziegler and McGrath regarding the value of limited-agent, dose-intense chemotherapy were not widely applied for over a decade, during which time the focus in the USA and Europe was on modification to regimens in use at that time for acute lymphoblastic leukemia (ALL), diffuse large B-cell lymphoma (DLBCL) and Hodgkin disease (HD). When the Children's Cancer Study Group (CCSG) study [1] confirmed what by the time the trial was under way many already believed, namely, that short-duration alkylator-based regimens were superior for mature B-cell lymphoma, this strategy became widely accepted.

A recent Cochrane review attempted to assess the evidence regarding chemotherapy, surgery, radiotherapy, and immunotherapy in BL [2]. This included 13 randomized trials from as far back as 1971. As might have been expected, it was not possible to pool data for any outcomes due to differences between the interventions used. In the context of the dramatic overall improvements in the outcome of high-risk groups over the past 20 years, associated with intensified therapy, the author's conclusion that the "use of less intensive protocols appears to produce similar responses compared to standard regimens" would seem to ignore compelling, if nonrandomized, evidence.

The older studies that are summarized in the previous section largely focused on modifications of chemotherapy designed to improve outcome and often included several different histological subtypes. Up to the 1980s large cell lymphoma (LCL) comprised a number of subtypes but with improved immunohistochemistry, cytogenetics and molecular pathology, LCL is now divided into specific groups including diffuse large cell lymphoma (DLCL), mediastinal large B cell lymphoma (MLBCL), peripheral T-cell lymphoma (PTCL), and anaplastic large cell lymphoma (ALCL).

Earlier studies have shown that relatively minor alterations on the standard CHOP (cyclophosphamide, doxorubicin, vincristine, prednisone) regimen, for example, addition of high-dose methotrexate (MTX) or doxorubicin, had little impact on outcome in Burkitt lymphoma and it was only with the significant dose escalation and increased dose density developed by the St Jude, French Society for Paediatric Oncology (SFOP) and Berlin-Frankfurt-Münster (BFM) groups that outcome in advanced disease improved. Although this strategy was only proven in a single randomized trial at St Jude [3], the striking improvement compared to historical controls when applied by the UK CCSG, SFOP, BFM, Italian and subsequently many other groups lead to the SFOP "backbone" being regarded internationally as the gold standard for advanced disease [4]. There

Evidence-Based Pediatric Oncology, Third Edition. Edited by Ross Pinkerton, Ananth Shankar and Katherine K. Matthay.
© 2013 John Wiley & Sons, Ltd. Published 2013 by John Wiley & Sons, Ltd.

remains debate, however, about the necessity for such intensive treatment in patients with localized disease and there are undoubtedly many children who could be cured with standard CHOP.

Although there have been concerns about the acute toxicity and almost inevitable hospital admission between cycles using intensive regimens, it is the late sequelae which has been most debated. Infertility in males and potential cardiac toxicity are major concerns but it is now becoming clearer that in the SFOP regimen with a total cumulative dose of $<4\,g/m^2$ of cyclophosphamide, fertility is likely to be preserved and the relatively low dose of anthracycline is also unlikely to result in significant toxicity. Nonetheless, it is still relevant to seek new early prognostic indicators to allow dose reduction and omission of offending agents, as has been attempted in single-arm studies using COMP (cyclophosphamide, vincristine, methotrexate, prednisone; omitting anthracycline) [5] or AOP (doxorubicin, vincristine, prednisone; omitting cyclophosphamide) [6] and also to consider the potential role of rituximab [7].

To date, in BL, clinical staging and lactate dehydrogenase (LDH) remain the most useful arbiters of outcome but new cytogenetics and molecular pathological characteristics and positron emission tomography (PET) response may in the future play a role. It is also clear that the Murphy staging system, which has been invaluable over the past 30 years, is now no longer really applicable to some subtypes of NHL or to certain primary sites. There is a particular need to review the system in relation to ALCL and also the potential subdivision of previous poor prognostic group in Burkitt lymphoma. The concept of grouping based on prognosis using clinical staging simply as a description of disease location rather than reflecting prognosis *per se* has been introduced in other children's cancers such as neuroblastoma and rhabdomyosarcoma [8] and has enabled newer prognostic factors to be incorporated once their value has been clearly proven. It is, however, important to be cautious in drawing firm conclusions about "new factors" as these are too often based on single center or single group studies and should always be evaluated prospectively in large series of patients before being used routinely. It is also important to be aware that treatment strategy has always been a key prognostic factor and must be taken into account. With improved therapy some previous prognostic factors may lose significance, as was the case for stage III group A and B based on disease extent which appeared

to be of relevance in the early SFOP studies only to disappear with the more intensive approach [9, 10].

Of the four new randomized trials reviewed in this edition, two involved BL and two ALCL. No new studies for T-cell non-Hodgkin lyymphoma (TNHL) were published although a number of T-cell ALL (T-ALL) trials also included TNHL (see Chapters 18–21). It is notable that the studies were carried out by large international collaborations – one European/American (FABLMB group) and the other predominantly European (EICNHL group). This highlights the need for such large-scale collaboration if trials are to be adequately powered. The compromise of including more than one histological subtype is no longer valid unless the question clearly applies to all groups and the study is large enough for each subgroup to be analyzed independently.

In the FABLMB trial, three studies were conducted concurrently but applied to different prognostic subgroups. Group A was patients with localized disease with an excellent prognosis. There were insufficient numbers within this group to perform a randomized trial and this part of the study involved a simple 6-week regimen (COPAD; cyclophosphamide, vincristine, prednisone, doxorubicin) which was compared with published data from French, UK, and American experience. This confirmed that such minimal adjuvant chemotherapy was adequate for this group of patients [11]. The other two parts considered the question of how intensive treatment has to be to obtain the excellent results being achieved in the USA (Orange study) [12], UK (CCSG NHL 9000 series) [13], and France (SFOP LMB 95) [14]. As with any cancer where the cure rate is excellent, there is always reluctance to "de-escalate" and very sensitive stopping rules with close monitoring by an independent data monitoring committee are obviously essential.

The FABLMB trial was somewhat easier for the US participants to accept as the question was largely one of dose escalation. Many of the regimens in use at that time, such as COMP, were less intensive than the standard SFOP group B regimens. The trial was, however, a spectacular success with regard to international recruitment (over 1000 patients) and data handling and has resulted in a new standard regimen with the reduced dose of both alkylating agent and anthracycline and duration of treatment.

For the high-risk group C patients, the question not only related to chemotherapy intensity but also was designed to confirm that in comparison with historical series, the omission of central nervous system (CNS) irradiation did not compromise outcome. It is notable that not very long ago, CNS-positive B-cell ALL (B-ALL), especially with marrow disease, had a bleak outcome with few survivors, and standard therapy included both craniospinal irradiation and high-dose treatment with autologous or allogeneic rescue. The excellent outcome overall achieved in the FABLMB trial demonstrated that very intensive systemic and CNS-directed chemotherapy can obviate the need for CNS irradiation. It is worth reflecting that a strategy of intensified intrathecal (IT) therapy was applied in the 1970s in African BL which could explain the surprising outcome in some early published series of African children with initially involved CNS disease [15].

With regard to the reduction in therapy in group C patients, there was some hesitation by those already using the intensive arm. However, again, many groups were using regimens closer to the less intensive arm and there was no evidence at the time regarding the required doses of cytarabine and etoposide in this condition. It was also anticipated that the higher dose of methotrexate and the additional course between standard blocks would reduce the risk of lower doses reducing effectiveness. In the event, the data monitoring committee closed the trial in view of a statistically significant advantage to high-dose cytosine, arabinoside, etoposide (CYVE). An event-free survival (EFS) of 60% in those with combined CNS and bone marrow disease was, nonetheless, a dramatic improvement compared with historical data but confirmed this as the subgroup in which there remains considerable room for improvement and the need to consider novel approaches.

Major questions remaining in B-cell non-Hodgkin lymphoma (BNHL) include whether further "de-escalation" is possible in intermediate-risk disease, particularly whether antibody therapy such as anti-CD20 (rituximab) can replace some of the chemotherapy, and whether its addition to standard therapy could make further impact in the remaining 40% of treatment failures in high-risk disease. Following the COG pilot study of COPADM R [16], it is planned to include this regimen in a new randomized trial in Europe to determine if the addition of rituximab can improve outcome in high-risk patients.

The second most common subgroup in childhood is T-lymphoblastic lymphoma but there has been no recent randomized trial published in full. TNHL is often included in large trials for T-ALL but unfortunately numbers are invariably too small for conclusions to be drawn. This is particularly important as although the disease may be almost identical immunophenotypically, the behavior and outcome differ. Evaluation of minimal residual disease (MRD) after initial chemotherapy has proved of great prognostic value in ALL but the technique is only applicable to those with marrow involvement and in NHL no series has been large enough to replicate the ALL data. More recently, studies of initial minimal detectable disease (MDD) indicate that the latter may be of relevance but requires prospective evaluation [17]. With current treatment regimens there is little difference in outcome between Murphy stage III or IV disease. The recent suggestion that an early T precursor ALL with expression of stem cell or early myeloid markers (ETPALL) is a distinct entity with poor outcome requires investigation in TNHL [18]. This is a sizeable group of patients in whom a novel approach could have significant impact.

The unpublished COG A5971 trial has demonstrated that for T-ALL/NHL, the standard BFM95 regimen was not improved by intensification using cyclophosphamide and doxorubicin. POG9404 determined the value of adding high-dose methotrexate at the dose of $5\,g/m^2$ to the Dana Farber protocol. It was notable that this improved outcome in T-ALL (5-year EFS 80% versus 74%) but had no impact in TNHL (82% versus 88%). In the latter group numbers were relatively small (n = 137). No explanation was found for the apparently poorer outcome in those receiving high-dose methotrexate but in T-ALL the benefit was mainly seen in high-risk patients where CNS relapse was reduced [19].

The COG AALL0434 trial randomizes patients to receive Capizzi methotrexate without rescue versus high-dose methotrexate. Intermediate-risk patients are also randomized to receive nelarabine. This drug is one of the most interesting to emerge in recent years although neurotoxicity may limit its role [20]. TNHL are stratified into separate subgroups, the basis of initial MDD. Patients are randomized to Capizzi versus Capizzi plus nelarabine; those with >1% MDD are allocated to Capizzi. Those who fail to achieve a radiological partial response (PR) at the end of induction are allocated to receive Capizzi and nelarabine. No cranial irradiation is used, in contrast to 9404 and other earlier studies. The BFM has showed clearly that with high-dose methotrexate and intrathecal therapy, it is not necessary to use radiation in TNHL although this has not been confirmed in randomized trials.

The question of whether a regimen as long and as intensive as BFM95 is really necessary for localized T-cell disease will probably never be answered. The original CCG trial [1] showed no difference between LSA2L2 and COMP in this subgroup although neither arm had EFS comparable to that achieved with BFM90. To determine how much shorter or less intensive treatment could be would require very large numbers. It is generally accepted that current leukemia regimens have better EFS in localized disease and although overall survival may not differ in comparison with simpler protocols, there is a lower overall burden of treatment by avoiding the need for intensive treatment following relapse. The sample size for any future comparative study in localized disease would be impractical and the late effect concerns probably do not now justify such an investment. However, from the child and family's perspective, anything that would further reduce duration of treatment and the number of outpatient visits and inpatient episodes would no doubt be welcomed.

Diffuse large B cell lymphoma (DLBCL) is generally aligned with BNHL in most current protocols. The treatment of DLBCL in adults has differed somewhat from the approach in children and there are undoubtedly lessons to be learned from this experience. It is becoming clear that the very intensive approach for BL may not be required in this disease. In adults, dramatic improvement in DLBCL has been documented with dose-dense regimens such as CHOP14 and addition of etoposide or rituximab. Although a much simpler regimen, the total dose of anthracycline and alkylating agent does make the regimen potentially less attractive in children [21].

The POG trial completed in 2000 is of limited value in current practice as it included a range of "large cell lymphoma"; ALCL, DLBCL, and PTCL. It failed to show in advanced disease any advantage to intensification of the minimally intensive APO regimen. It was notable that the overall survival was 80% with EFS of 67%, indicating that with this broad group there may be room for dose reduction. There is a need for large-scale co-operation in DLBCL, potentially covering a wider age range, including adolescents and young adults, to answer this question.

With contemporary immunohistochemistry and molecular genetics, ALCL contributes 10% of NHL in children. Little has been learned in the past from studies when the tumor was included in an assortment of other tumor types. With the development of a single COG group and European collaboration in the form of the EICNHL group, the first large randomized studies are now emerging. Recent focus has also been on the development of a more clinically relevant system of prognostic grouping. The unusual site distribution of ALCL, i.e. lung and skin involvement, which is atypical for lymphomas in children, makes the Murphy classification of limited value. A large retrospective study of cases in Europe [22] led to a risk grouping that has been applied prospectively in the EIC trials. Very good-risk disease, i.e. resected stage I and isolated skin disease, received no adjuvant chemotherapy. Poor risk comprised those with skin, mediastinum or visceral disease, and intermediate risk all others.

One potential problem with the development of international collaboration is the attachment to traditional ways of using chemotherapy. In Europe, high-dose methotrexate in NHL has been used in various doses, schedules and combinations with IT therapy. The BFM trial had explored the value of prolonged infusion methotrexate in BNHL [23] and a similar question was asked by the EICNHL in ALCL. In the case of ALCL, it was not in relation to efficacy but rather the necessity to use a dose >1 g/m² and the need for additional intrathecal methotrexate. The approach of using a low dose over 24 h with IT therapy was used by the BFM group, while higher dose over a shorter period without additional intrathecal therapy was the standard practice of the French SFOP group. This trial has shown that the latter is equally effective, is less toxic and probably more cost-effective (even allowing for the higher dose of methotrexate) due to the omission of IT therapy. It is also more acceptable to the patient, avoiding lumbar punctures and causing less mucositis.

The role of vinblastine in ALCL has been an intriguing one since the demonstration by the SFOP group that survival post relapse appeared to be at least as good using a simple weekly, single-dose regimen as a variety of much more aggressive multiagent protocols [24]. Both EICNHL and COG have carried out similar trials, adding vinblastine to their respective standard regimens. The COG ANHL0131 study used the standard APO regimen as induction over 5 weeks and randomization of 15 cycles of APO with or without weekly vinblastine. The trial closed in 2009 when the DMC concluded that the experimental arm was unlikely to show benefit. There was also concern about the additional toxicity when administered with the APO regimen and the initial 6 mg/m² dose had to be reduced to 4 mg/m².

The EIC trial regimen was based on BFM90. Patients were randomized to receive or not receive vinblastine during both initial chemotherapy and maintenance phases. As in the COG trial, dose reductions were common. No difference was seen in CR rate but there was a striking increase in remission duration where vinblastine was given. The mechanism of action of vinblastine in this disease may be antiangiogenic rather than cytotoxic. This may explain the cytostatic effect with MRD being kept in check until cessation of maintenance therapy. The inconvenience of weekly injections and its potential toxicity make more prolonged maintenance therapy an unacceptable option. Data are now emerging that MRD monitoring using quantitative polymerase chain reaction (PCR) may be of value [25]. Also, evidence that levels of anaplastic lymphoma kinase (ALK) autoantibody may correlate with outcome raises the likelihood that immunotherapy may have an important role to play. Furthermore, the development of effective anti-CD30 antibodies is another exciting option in a fascinating disease [26].

It is likely that over the next few years, trials in children will focus on the role of monoclonal antibodies and it is becoming increasingly difficult for practitioners to resist simply following the adult practice in high-grade NHL. There are particular subgroups, such as sclerosing mediastinal B-cell lymphoma, where antibody therapy may have a valuable role to play. Treatment approaches in DLCL may also become more refined. The modified risk grouping for BNHL may allow study of novel approaches in poor-risk disease. This could potentially include a resurgence of repeated low-morbidity, high-dose therapy with more effective stem cell mobilization. The use of MDD and MRD monitoring will require evaluation on large trials, further reinforcing the need to build on the achievements of international collaborations to date.

References

1 Anderson JR, Wilson JF, Jenkin DT et al. Childhood non-Hodgkin's lymphoma. The results of a randomised therapeutic trial comparing a 4-drug regimen (COMP) with a 10-drug regimen (LSA2-L2). N Engl J Med 1983;**308**:559–65.

2 Okebe JU, Skoetz N, Meremikwu MM et al. Therapeutic interventions for Burkitt lymphoma in children. Database Cochrane Rev 2011;7:CD 005198.

3 Jenkin RD, Anderson JR, Chilcote RR et al. The treatment of localised non-Hodgkin's lymphoma in children: a report from the Children's Cancer Study Group. J Clin Oncol 1984;**2**:88–99.

4 Hochberg J, Cairo MS. Insight into the biology and treatment of pediatric lymphomas: clues from international studies. Pediatr Blood Cancer 2009;**52**:153–4.

5 Amos Burke GA, Imeson J, Hobson R, Gerrard M. Localized non-Hodgkin's lymphoma with B-cell histology: cure without cyclophosphamide? A report of the United Kingdom Children's Cancer Study Group on studies NHL 8501 and NHL 9001. Br J Haematol 2003;**121**:586–91.

6 Attias D, Weitzman S. The efficacy of rituximab in high-grade pediatric B-cell lymphoma/leukemia: a review of available evidence. Curr Opin Pediatr 2008;**20**:17–22.

7 Meinhardt A, Burkhardt B, Zimmermann M et al., for the Berlin-Frankfurt-Munster Group. Phase II window study on rituximab in newly diagnosed pediatric mature B-cell non-Hodgkin's lymphoma and Burkitt leukemia. J Clin Oncol 2010;**28**:3115–21.

8 Monclair T, Brodeur GM, Ambros PF et al., for the INRG Task Force. The International Neuroblastoma Risk Group (INRG) staging system: an INRG Task Force report. J Clin Oncol 2009;**27**:298–303.

9 Phillip T, Pinkerton R, Biron P et al. Effective multiagent chemotherapy in children with advanced cell lymphoma: who remains the high risk patient? Br J Haematol 1987;**65**:159–64.

10 Patte C, Auperin A, Michon J et al. The Société Française d'Oncologie Pédiatrique LMB89 protocol: highly effective multi-agent chemotherapy tailored to the tumour burden and initial response in 561 unselected children with B-cell lymphomas. Blood 2001;**97**:3370–9.

11 Gerrard M, Cairo MS, Weston C et al. Excellent survival following two courses of COPAD chemotherapy in children and adolescents with resected localized B-cell non-Hodgkin's lymphoma: results of the FAB/LMB 96 international study. Br J Haematol 2008;**141**:840–7.

12 Cairo MS, Krailo MD, Morse M et al. Long term follow-up of short intensive multiagent chemotherapy without high-dose methotrexate ('Orange') in children with advanced non-lymphoblastic non-Hodgkin's lymphoma: a Children's Cancer Group report. Leukemia 2002;**16**:594–600.

13 Atra A, Imeson JD, Hobson R et al. Improved outcome in children with advanced stage B-cell non-Hodgkin's lymphoma (B-NHL): results of the United Kingdom Children's Cancer Study Group (UKCCSG) 9002 protocol. Br J Cancer 2000;**82**:1396–402.

14 Reiter A, Schrappe M, Parwaresch R *et al.* Non-Hodgkin's lymphomas of childhood and adolescence: results of a treatment stratified for biologic subtypes and stage – a report of the Berlin-Frankfurt-Munster Group. *J Clin Oncol* 1995;**13**:359–72.

15 Ziegler JL, Magrath IT, Deisseroth AB *et al.* Combined modality treatment of Burkitt's lymphoma, *Cancer Treatment Rep* 1978;**62**:2031–4.

16 Griffin TC, Weitzman S, Weinstein H *et al.* A study of rituximab and ifosfamide, carboplatin, and etoposide chemotherapy in children with recurrent/refractory B-cell (CD20+) non-Hodgkin lymphoma and mature B-cell acute lymphoblastic leukemia: a report from the Children's Oncology Group. *Pediatr Blood Cancer* 2009;**52**:177–81.

17 Shiramizu B, Goldman S, Kusao I *et al.* Minimal disease assessment in the treatment of children and adolescents with intermediate-risk (Stage III/IV) B-cell non-Hodgkin lymphoma: a Children's Oncology Group report. *Br J Haematol* 2011;**153**:758–63.

18 Coustan-Smith E, Mullighan CG, Onciu M *et al.* Early T-cell precursor leukaemia: a subtype of very high-risk acute lymphoblastic leukaemia. *Lancet Oncol* 2009;**10**:147–56.

19 Asselin BL, Devidas M, Wang C *et al.* Effectiveness of high-dose methotrexate in T-cell lymphoblastic leukemia and advanced-stage lymphoblastic lymphoma: a randomized study by the Children's Oncology Group (POG 9404). *Blood* 2011;**118**:874–83.

20 Gokbuget N, Basara N, Baurmann H *et al.* High single-drug activity of nelarabine in relapsed T-lymphoblastic leukaemia/lymphoma offers curative option with subsequent stem cell transplantation. *Blood* 2011;**118**:3504–11.

21 Brusamolino E, Rusconi C,Montalbetti L *et al.* Dose dense R-CHOP supported by PEG filgrastim in patients with diffuse large B cell lymphoma: a phase 2 study of feasibility and toxicity. *Haematologica* 2006;**91**:496–502.

22 Le Deley MC, Reiter A, Williams D *et al.*, for the European Intergroup for Childhood Non-Hodgkin Lymphoma. Prognostic factors in childhood anaplastic large cell lymphoma: results of a large European intergroup study *Blood* 2008;**111**:1560–6.

23 Woessman W, Seidemann K, Mann G *et al.* The impact of the methotrexate administration schedule and dose in the treatment of children and adolescents with B-cell neoplasms: a report of the BFM Group Study NHL-BFM95. *Blood* 2005;**105**:948–58.

24 Brugieres L, Pacquement H, Le Deley MC *et al.* Single-drug vinblastine as salvage treatment for refractory or relapsed anaplastic large-cell lymphoma: a report from the French Society of Pediatric Oncology. *J Clin Oncol* 2009;**27**:5056–61.

25 Kalinova M, Krskova L, Brizova H, Kabickova E, Kepak T, Kodet R. Quantitative PCR detection of NPM/ALK fusion gene and CD30 gene expression in patients with anaplastic large cell lymphoma – residual disease montitoring and a correlation with the disease status. *Leuk Res* 2008;**32**:25–32.

26 Younes A. CD-30- targeted antibody therapy. *Curr Opin Oncol* 2011;**23**:587–93.

Summary of previous studies

The evolution of randomized studies in childhood NHL is characterized by an initial period when all histological subtypes were grouped together and questions addressed included the nature and duration of chemotherapy and the potential role of radiation. Following the clear demonstration of the importance of histology-directed therapy, later trials, particularly in relation to nonlocalized disease, distinguished between histological subtypes.

The trial which influenced all subsequent strategies was published in 1983 by Anderson *et al.* [1]. The Children's Cancer Group study CCG551 compared the COMP regimen with a modified LSA2L2. The latter had been developed as a treatment for childhood lymphoblastic leukemia. Both regimens lasted 18 months and included localized irradiation to bulk disease. CNS radiation was used only for those presenting with CNS disease or those suffering a CNS relapse within 6 months of starting treatment. One hundred and fifty-one children with nonlocalized disease and 60 with localized disease were randomized; 34% had lymphoblastic histology, 51% undifferentiated Burkitt/ non-Burkitt and 14% histiocytic. For the localized group there was no difference in outcome. However, significant differences were noted for those with non-localized disease (Murphy stage III–IV). Patients with lymphoblastic lymphoma had a significantly higher failure-free survival at 24 months when treated with the LSA2L2 regimen (76%) than treated with COMP (26%). The opposite was true for nonlymphoblastic disease where failure-free survival was 57% for those treated with COMP compared with 28% for those treated with LSA2L2.

This was a landmark study demonstrating the importance of treating NHL in children according to histological subtype. Follow-up in this first report was relatively short, particularly as later relapse may be more common in those with lymphoblastic disease. A subsequent follow-up report several years later [2] confirmed the significant difference in patients with nonlocalized disease. With median follow-up of 8 years, EFS for lymphoblastic lymphoma was 64% for LSA2L2 versus 35% for COMP. However, COMP produced better results for those with undifferentiated lymphoma (5-year EFS 50% versus 29% for LSA2L2). A further subanalysis of patients on CCG551 considering only those with localized disease emphasized that the outcome did not appear to be influenced by the regimen used [3].

The role of radiation was the subject of an early trial published in 1980 from St Jude [4]. Forty-six patients with stage III and IV disease, irrespective of histology, were treated with the CHOP regimen and then randomized to receive involved field radiation therapy. The dose was 20–25 Gy whole abdomen or hemithorax with 10–15 Gy boost to the primary site. Those who achieved a complete response were also subsequently randomized to receive 24 Gy cranial radiation and intrathecal therapy [4]. This study demonstrated no advantage to the addition of local radiation therapy but the isolated CNS relapse rate was higher (25%) in those receiving no CNS directed therapy versus for those who did (6%). The latter was not statistically significant due to the small numbers enrolled in this trial. The range of histological types also limits interpretation of this study.

A later study addressing the role of radiation therapy specifically in those with localized disease was undertaken by POG [5]. One hundred and twenty-nine patients received the CHOP regimen followed by 6 months maintenance therapy, including intrathecal chemotherapy. Patients were randomized to receive radiation therapy during the induction phase; 27 Gy to the involved field, 15 Gy to whole abdomen for abdominal tumors with boost and primary bone tumors receiving 37.5 Gy. There was no significant difference in this group with stage I and II disease; 4-year EFS was 88% for those receiving chemotherapy alone and 87% for those receiving chemotherapy plus radiotherapy.

Trials in children with localized disease irrespective of histological subtype demonstrated that treatment duration could be shortened. For example, in CCG 551/501, 115 patients with nonlymphoblastic histology were randomized to receive 6 versus 18 months of the COMP regimen. The shorter regimen had no adverse affect on outcome [6]. Similarly, an analysis of two sequential POG trials between 1983 and 1991 using the CHOP regimen followed by maintenance therapy (6MP/MTX plus triple intrathecal chemotherapy) demonstrated no difference in outcome in 182 children randomized to a short 9-week protocol (n=113) or 8 months treatment (n=69) [7]. It is notable that this report suggested that the relapse rate in the children with lymphoblastic lymphoma was higher with the shorter regimen than the 8-month protocol although numbers were too small to draw firm conclusions.

Studies that have focused on lymphoblastic lymphoma have compared chemotherapy regimens and evaluated the benefit of treatment intensification. The POG 7905 trial demonstrated that in 85 patients with lymphoblastic lymphoma, ACOP (doxorubicin, cyclophosphamide, vincristine, prednisone) produced results equivalent to LSA2L2 although in this study outcome with both regimens was relatively poor; 3-year disease-free survival (DFS) 53% (ACOP) and 58% (LSA2L2) respectively and for stage IV disease 14% and 12% respectively [8]. Outcome appeared to be superior for LSA2L2 in stage III disease although patient numbers were small. The CCG 502 trial evaluated intensification of the COMP regimen with addition of doxorubicin and asparaginase (ADCOMP). For 281 children randomized, the outcome with ADCOMP was still inferior to LSA2L2; 5-year EFS 64% versus 74% respectively [9]. Two later trials, which included T-ALL, demonstrated that the addition of higher dose asparaginase [10] or high-dose cytarabine [11] failed to improve outcome when included in a leukemia type protocol.

An European Organization for Research into Treatment of Cancer (EORTC) study compared *E.coli* asparaginase versus Erwinia asparaginase in T-cell lymphoma and leukemia and while T-cell leukemia patients appeared to have a higher EFS with the *E. coli* compound, this was not demonstrable in NHL patients because of very small numbers [12]. The *E. coli* formulation was, however, associated with a higher incidence of coagulopathy and toxicity.

A study from the UK published in 1984 evaluated the role of local radiation therapy when added to a complex multiagent regimen in children with T-cell leukemia/lymphoma [13]. This study showed a highly significant advantage in those randomized to receive 15 Gy mediastinal radiotherapy. Failure-free survival for children with T-cell leukemia was 51% versus 21% (p=0.01) while it was 66% versus 18% (p=0.01) for those with

TNHL. The nature of the chemotherapy regimen would, however, now be regarded as suboptimal which could account for the apparent benefit.

Studies in B-cell lymphoma have mainly focused on the treatment of children with Murphy stage III and IV disease. Until the late 1990s the approach in the USA was mainly building on the backbone of the COMP or APO regimens. In the CCG 503 trial, an anthracycline was added to the COMP regimen and 284 patients were randomized to receive COMP or DCOMP [14]. Toxicity was significantly worse in those receiving daunorubicin and 11/12 treatment-related deaths occurred with DCOMP. There was no difference in relapse rates and the 10-year EFS was 55% for COMP versus 57% for DCOMP.

Two POG trials have evaluated intensification of the APO regimen in diffuse large cell lymphoma. In POG 8165, 58/120 patients were randomized to receive 800 mg/m^2 of cyclophosphamide [15]. The 5-year EFS for APOC was 62% versus 72% for APO. In the POG 9315 trial, 90/180 children were randomized to the addition of high-dose cytarabine (2 g/m^2) and intermediate-dose methotrexate 1 g/m^2. Intensification had no impact on event-free survival: 4-year EFS 67% in both arms [16].

The relative heterogeneity of histopathological subtypes (inclusion of ALCL, for example) in the POG trials makes interpretation somewhat complex. In contrast, the approach in the major European groups such as the French SFOP and German BFM has been to focus on patients with mature B-cell lymphoma. The French SFOP study reported in 1991 [17] demonstrated that the intensive LMB (Lymphome Maligne B) protocol could be reduced from 7 months to 4 months with no adverse effect on outcome in patients with stage III and IV disease. Two hundred and sixteen children received the LMB induction and consolidation regimen and, following CYM1, 166/192 who achieved CR were randomized to standard or shortened therapy. Eighteen-month EFS was 89% and 87% respectively for the 4-month and 7-month regimens.

In 1997 the randomized trial comparing COMP with the St Jude total B regimen carried out by POG was published [18]. This key study demonstrated that high doses of cyclophosphamide, particularly given in a fractionated manner over a number of days, in addition to prolonged infusion of high-dose methotrexate (regimen B), significantly improved outcome when compared with a more standard-dose COMP regimen (regimen A) to which high-dose methotrexate was added. This study was restricted to diffuse undifferentiated small noncleaved Burkitt/non-Burkitt and stage III disease. Sixty-five children were randomized to receive the standard COMP regimen and 58 the more dose-intensive total B regimen. The complete response rate with the standard regimen A was 81% compared with 95% for regimen B. Event-free survival was 64% and 79% (p=0.027) respectively. This was the first randomized demonstration of the value of dose-intensive therapy.

The BFM group has addressed the issue of methotrexate dose and schedule [19], comparing two methotrexate schedules at doses of 1 or 5 g depending on risk group. In each risk group, patients were randomized to receive MTX over either 4 or 24 h. Both randomized groups received intrathecal therapy at the beginning of the infusion. One hundred and eighty children were randomized to receive a 4-h infusion and 184 to the 24-h infusion. Reducing the infusion time of methotrexate from 24 to 4 h reduced toxicity and appeared to be equally effective in patients with localized disease risk groups I and II who received $1 \, g/m^2$. The outcome was also similar to those who were given $5 \, g/m^2$ in the BFM 90 study. However, for risk groups III and IV with more advanced disease, there was a significantly higher failure rate with the shorter infusion time. In these patients who received $5 \, g/m^2$, when given as a 4-h infusion the 1-year progression-free survival was 77% compared with 93% for the 24-h infusion.

References

1 Anderson JR, Wilson JF, Jenkin DT et al. Childhood non-Hodgkin's lymphoma. The results of a randomised therapeutic trial comparing a 4-drug regimen (COMP) with a 10-drug regimen (LSA2-L2). N Engl J Med 1983;308:559–65.

2 Anderson JR, Jenkin RD, Wilson JF et al. Long-term follow-up of patients treated with COMP or LSA2L2 therapy for childhood non-Hodgkin's lymphoma: a report of CCG-551 from the Children's Cancer Group. J Clin Oncol 1993;11(6):1024–32.

3 Jenkin RD, Anderson JR, Chilcote RR et al. The treatment of localised non-Hodgkin's lymphoma in children: a report from the Children's Cancer Study Group. J Clin Oncol 1984;2:88–99.

4 Murphy SB, Hustu H. A randomised trial of combined modality therapy of childhood non-Hodgkin's lymphoma. Cancer 1980;45:630–7.

5 Link MP, Donaldson SS, Costan WB, Shuster JJ, Murphy SB. Results of treatment of childhood localised non-Hodgkin's lymphoma with combination chemotherapy with or without radiotherapy. N Engl J Med 1990;322:1169–74.

6 Meadows AT, Sposto R, Jenkin RD et al. Similar efficacy of 6 and 18 months of therapy with four drugs (COMP) for localised non-Hodgkin's lymphoma of children: a report from the Children's Cancer Study Group. J Clin Oncol 1989;7:92–9.

7 Link MP, Shuster JJ, Donaldson SS, Berard CW, Murphy SB. Treatment of children and young adults with early stage non-Hodgkin's lymphoma. N Engl J Med 1997;337:1259–66.

8 Hvizdala EV, Berard C, Callihan T et al. Lymphoblastic lymphoma in children – a randomised trial comparing LSA2-L2 with the A-COP therapeutic regimen: a Paediatric Oncology Group Study. J Clin Oncol 1998;6:26–33.

9 Tubergen DG, Krailo MD, Meadows AT et al. Comparison of treatment regimens for pediatric lymphoblastic non-Hodgkin's lymphoma: a Children's Cancer Study Group study. J Clin Oncol 1995;13:1368–76.

10 Amylon MD, Shuster J, Pullen J et al. Intensive high-dose asparaginase consolidation improves survival for pediatric patients with T cell acute lymphoblastic leukemia and advanced stage lymphoblastic leukemia: a Paediatric Oncology Group study. Leukemia 1999;13:335–42.

11 Millot F, Philipee N, Benoit Y et al. Value of high dose cytarabine during interval therapy of BFM based protocol in increased risk children with acute leukemia and lymphoblastic lymphoma. J Clin Oncol 2001;19:1936–42.

12 Duval M, Sucia S, Rialand X et al. Comparison of escherichia coli asparaginase with erwinia asparaginase in the treatment of childhood lymphoid malignancies. Blood 2002;99:2734–9.

13 Mott MG, Chessells JM, Willoughby ML et al. Adjuvant low dose radiation in childhood T cell leukaemia/lymphoma. Br J Cancer 1984;50:457–62.

14 Sposto R, Meadows A, Chilcote R et al. Comparison of long-term outcome of children and adolescents with disseminated non-lymphoblastic non-Hodgkin's lymphoma treated with COMP or daunomycin-COMP: a report from the Children's Cancer Group. Med Pediatr Oncol 2001;37:432–41.

15 Laver J, Mahmoud H, Pick T et al. Results of a randomised phase III trial in children and adolescents with advanced stage diffuse large cell non-Hodgkin's lymphoma: a Pediatric Oncology Group study. Leuk Lymphoma 2002;43:105–9.

16 Laver JH, Kraveka JM, Hutchison RE et al. Advanced stage large cell lymphoma in children and adolescents: results of a randomised trial incorporating intermediate-dose methotrexate and high dose cytarabine in the maintenance phase of the APO regimen: a Paediatric Oncology Group Phase III trial. J Clin Oncol 2005;23:541–7.

17 Patte C, Philip T, Rodary C et al. High survival rate in advanced-stage B-cell lymphomas and leukaemias without CNS involvement with a short intensive polychemotherapy: results from the French Paediatric Oncology Society of a randomized trial of 216 children. J Clin Oncol 1991;9:123–32.

18 Brecher ML, Schwenn MR, Coppes MJ et al. Fractionated cyclophosphamide and back to back high dose methotrexate and cytosine arabinoside improves outcome in patients with stage III high grade non cleaved cell lymphomas: a randomised trial of the Pediatric Oncology Group. Med Ped Oncol 1997;29:526–33.

19 Wossmann W, Seidemann K, Mann G et al. Impact of the methotrexate administration schedule and dose in the treatment of children and adolescents with B-cell neoplasms: a report of the BFM group study NHL-BFM95. Blood 2005;105:948–53.

New studies

Study 1

Patte C, Auperin A, Gerrard M *et al.*, for the FAB/LMB96 International Study Committee. Results of the randomized international FAB/LMB96 trial for intermediate risk B-cell non-Hodgkin lymphoma in children and adolescents: is it possible to reduce treatment for the early responding patients? *Blood* 2007;**109**:2773–80.

Objectives

To assess the possibility of reducing treatment in children/adolescents with intermediate-risk BNHL without jeopardising survival.

Study design

An international multicenter randomized trial conducted by three groups: the French Society for Paediatric Oncology (SFOP), the United Kingdom Children's Cancer Study Group (UKCCSG), and the Children's Cancer Group of the USA (CCG). It was a planned 5-year study that opened in May 1996 and closed in June 2001. Data were transferred from a total of 161 pediatric cancer centers every 6 months to an international database held at the Institut Gustave-Roussy, France.

The SFOP was responsible for interim and final analysis of this component of the LMB trial. An independent international data and safety monitoring committee that included three pediatric oncologists and one statistician reviewed interim analysis and 6-month data. Eligibility included nonimmunosuppressed patients, under the age of 18 years for the SFOP and UKCCSG or under 21 years for the CCG, with newly diagnosed mature B-cell lymphoma, either Burkitt, Burkitt-like or diffuse large B-cell lymphoma. Slides were reviewed both nationally and by an international panel of cytopathologists. Group B, intermediate-risk, patients included those with nonresected stage I and II disease, all stage III and all stage IV CNS negative according to the Murphy classification. The upper limit of bone marrow involvement to define the B-cell leukemia, rather than stage IV bone marrow disease, was 25% rather

than the 75% used in previous LMB studies. All patients were treated with a prephase of low0dose cyclophosphamide, vincristine, and prednisolone (COP) and patients with at least a 20% response at day 7 received the first induction course, COPAdM (cyclophosphamide, vincristine, prednisolone, doxorubicin, and high-dose methotrexate [3 g/m²] with intrathecal methotrexate). Patients were evaluated after the first COPAdM course and in the case of no disease progression, were randomized to receive full course in COPAdM2 or the trial regimen in which the dose of cyclophosphamide was reduced by 50%. COPAdM2 was given as soon as count recovery occurred. The standard regimen comprised 3 g/m² cyclophosphamide divided in six fractions and administered every 12 hours and the study arm 1.5 g.m².

All patients received two consolidation courses of CYM (cytosine and high-dose methotrexate) and standard regimen received one maintenance course of M1 (cyclophosphamide, vincristine, prednisolone, doxorubicin, and high-dose methotrexate). In the investigational arm, M1 was deleted completely. At the initial randomization after COPAdM1, patients were allocated between four arms: two arms with reduced-dose cyclophosphamide and two without M1. Randomization was performed in blocks of four with equal allocation and stratified for national group (CCG, SFOP, UKCCSG), histology (DLBCL or not), stage, and LDH levels.

Statistics

The primary endpoint of the trial was event-free survival defined as the minimum time between randomization and progressive disease or relapse or second malignancy or death from any cause or the last follow-up contact point with patients who did not experience any event. Secondary endpoints were survival and failure-free survival.

Survival was defined as the time between randomization and death from any cause or the last follow-up contact for patients who were alive. Failure-free survival (FFS) was defined as the minimum time between randomization and biopsy-positive residual disease following the first CYM course, i.e. no complete response at third evaluation or any other event as defined in the EFS. The term FFS was applied to account for patients with biopsy-proven residual disease who may have achieved and remained in remission after intensified therapy either on or off study. Therefore, FFS analysis was restricted to comparison between reduced dose of cyclophosphamide in the second COPAdM course and full-dose cyclophosphamide but not between no M1 versus M1. The comparisons between treatment were based primarily on the profile Cox likelihood confidence bounds for the log hazard ratio β. The criterion for detecting reduction in treatment efficacy was that the lower 80% profile likelihood confidence for β exceeded 0. Three interim analyses were performed.

The trial was planned with a 5-year accrual to link with at least 460 evaluable patients for the randomized comparison. In the event of a 7% reduction in EFS from 90% to 83% observed in the 460 patients, the probability that the lower one-sided 80% confidence bound exceeded 0 was 90% at the final analysis using the methods of Rubenstein adapted for survival functions that exhibit a cured fraction. Survival functions for time and to event endpoints were estimated with the Kaplan–Meier method. The 95% confidence intervals (CI) of the actual rates were calculated with the Rothman method. Cox models that included the treatment factors and stratification factors were used to analyse each endpoint. The interactions between major characteristics (stage, LDH, histology, primary mediastinal, DLBCL and treatment reductions) were all tested on the Cox models. Analyses were carried out according to the intention-to-treat principle on eligible patients. There were 20 patients declared ineligible following randomization. Analysis was also performed on all randomized patients. P-values are all two-sided. Details of the logistics of the randomization process were not described.

Results

Seven hundred and sixty-two patients were registered, of whom 105 were not randomized, 49 were not eligible due to no response to COP, protocol modifications or death, and 56 for various reasons, mainly parental or physician refusal. Pathology was reviewed by the international panel in 606 (92%) of 657 randomized patients and of these, 16 were declared ineligible after pathology review. Ultimately the analysis was based

on 637 patients. There were very few protocol deviations. Three patients in the reference arm did not receive M1 because of toxicity and one patient in each of the three reduced arms received the reference regimen, one by error and two after parental consent was withdrawn.

The median follow-up was 54 months. Amongst randomized patients, the 4-year overall survival (OS), EFS and FFS were 95%, 92% and 90% respectively. By stage, the 4-year EFS was 98% in stages I and II, 90% in stage III, and 86% in stage IV CNS-negative patients. The 4-year EFS was 96% and 86% respectively for patients with LDH below or above twofold the upper limit of institutional normal value. According to histological subtypes, the 4-year EFS rates were 93%, 93%, and 71% respectively for patients with Burkitt, diffuse large B-cell not primary mediastinal, and primary mediastinal DLBCL respectively. In the first comparison, the 4-year EFS was 93% and 91% in the groups with full versus half-dose cyclophosphamide in the second COPAdM respectively. The hazard ratio of event in the group randomized to half-dose cyclophosphamide compared to full dose was 1.27 (p=0.4). In the second comparison, the 4-year EFS rates were 92% versus 92% in the two groups with and without M1 respectively while the 4-year OS rates were 94% and 95% respectively. The hazard ratios of event and death were respectively 1 and 0.9 in those randomized to no M1 compared to those receiving M1. There was no significant interaction between the two therapy reductions on EFS (p=0.55) or OS (p=0.50) and furthermore, there was no significant interaction between the therapy reductions and prognostic factors, especially LDH levels, stage, and histology.

Toxicity

The first and second COPAdM courses with full dose of cyclophosphamide had similar toxicity profiles but there were significant differences in the second COPAdM courses between full- and half-dose cyclophosphamide, with lower toxicity in the latter. However, the rates of grade IV infections were not significantly different between these two courses.

Conclusions

It was concluded that children and adolescents with intermediate-risk BNHL who have an early response and achieve complete remission after the first consolidation course can be cured with a four-course treatment with a total dose of only 3.3 g/m² of cyclophosphamide and 120 mg/m² of doxorubicin.

Study 2

Cairo MS, Gerrard M, Sposto R *et al.*, on behalf of the FAB LMB96 International Study Committee. Results of a randomised international study of high-risk central nervous system B non-Hodgkin lymphoma and B-acute lymphoblastic leukaemia in children and adolescents. *Blood* 2007;**109**:2736–43.

Objectives

To determine the optimal treatment intensity for high-risk childhood BNHL comparing two regimens varying in total dose and dose intensity.

Study design

Eligibility criteria for inclusion were patients with B-ALL, DLBCL, BL or Burkitt-like lymphoma (BLL) according to the revised European and American lymphoma classification. Age range was 6 months or older and younger than 18 years (UKCCSG and SFOP) or 21 years (CCG), Staging was performed according to the Murphy classification. High-risk patients (group C) were those with bone marrow disease >25% L3 blasts or CNS disease defined by any of the following: L3 cerebrospinal fluid (CSF) blasts, cranial nerve palsy, clinical spinal cord compression, isolated intracerebral mass, or cranial and/or spinal parameningeal extension. Exclusions to study enrollment included any of the following: immunodeficiency, HIV positivity, prior organ transplant, prior malignancy or prior chemotherapy. An international cytopathology panel reviewed cases and was composed of at least two of the pathologists from each of the three pediatric co-operative groups. The study opened in May 1996 and closed to accrual in June 2001.

All patients received initial cytoreduction with low-dose cyclophosphamide, vincristine, and prednisolone (COP). The response to COP was designated as complete response (CR), incomplete response (IR; 21–99% tumor reduction), and nonresponse (<20% tumor reduction). Those patients with a nonresponse to COP were nonrandomly assigned to the standard high-dose intensity arm C1. On day 8 of COP or after the second COP, all patients received COPAdM1 and COPAdM2. These comprised cyclophosphamide, vincristine, prednisolone, doxorubicin and high-dose methotrexate (8 g/m²). Patients who presented with initial involvement of the central nervous system received additional double intrathecal chemotherapy on day 1 of each consolidation cycle and in between consolidation courses (absolute neutrophil count [ANC] >0.5×10⁹/L and platelets >50×10⁹/L) received an additional course of high-dose methotrexate plus triple intrathecal chemotherapy. In 1997 because of the high incidence of severe mucositis, infusion time of doxorubicin was changed from 48 h to 6 h in both COPAdM1 and COPAdM2.

Randomization was carried out within each national group following COPAdM2 using stratified blocked randomization with equal allocation, block size of four, strata defined by all combinations of national group (UKCCSG, CCG and SFOP), histology (DCBCL or not), and CNS disease at diagnosis (present or absent). The randomization was, in cases without initial CNS disease, two standard courses of cytarabine and etoposide (CYVE) or two courses of reduced doses of cytarabine (3 g/m₂/dose versus 2 g/m₂/dose × 4 days and etoposide 200 mg/m²/ dose versus 100 mg/m²/dose × 4 days) (mini CYVE) in combination with standard-dose continuous cytarabine infusion. Randomization for patients with initial CNS disease was the same. Treatment duration also differed between the two arms: those randomized to standard C1 arm received four maintenance courses: M1 – COPAdM3; M2 – cytarabine plus etoposide; M3 – cyclophosphamide, vincristine, prednisolone and doxorubicin; and M4 – cytarabine and etoposide. Those allocated to experimental arm C2 only received one maintenance course (M1).

Statistics

The primary endpoint for analysis was EFS which was defined as the minimum time to death from any cause: relapse, progressive disease, second neoplasm or biopsy-positive residual disease following CYVE 2 or mini CYVE 2. EFS was measured from the beginning of chemotherapy for the analysis of all eligible patients and from the date of randomization for comparison with two randomized groups. The secondary endpoint was OS which was the time to death from any cause measured from the start of therapy or the date of randomization, as appropriate. In the randomized comparison, the criteria for detecting a reduction in treatment efficacy was that the lower 80% profile likelihood confidence bound of the ratio of hazard functions of the reduced versus standard treatment groups as estimated by a stratified Cox proportional hazard model exceeded 1. This is equivalent to the use of a one-sided stratified log-rank test with 20% type 1 error. Interim monitoring was based on the method of Lan–DeMets. This criterion provided 90% power against a 12% reduction in the 4-year EFS probability from a hypothesized baseline of 88%. All analyses followed the intention-to-treat philosophy. An international independent data and safety monitoring committee comprising three pediatric oncologists and a statistician reviewed interim results annually.

Results

While 235 eligible patients were enrolled in the study, 34 patients were excluded: ineligible pathology (17), prior treatment (7), late enrollment (9) or inadequate consent (1). Two CNS-positive patients who were enrolled and treated mistakenly as group B are included in the overall analysis but not in the randomized comparison.

Two hundred and seventeen patients were evaluated for response to COP. Following the initial course of COP, 33 patients achieved a CR (15%), 171 had IR (81%) and nine had a nonresponse. The probability of 4-year EFS and OS for all patients entered into the study was 79% and 82% respectively. In patients who responded following COPAdM2 and who were randomized to the standard treatment arm, the 4-year EFS was 90% versus 80% in those randomized to reduced-intensity treatment (one-sided stratified log-rank test p=0.06, stratified Cox estimated hazard ratio 1.8; lower 80% profile likelihood confidence bound 1.3).

Overall survival at 4 years in these two randomized groups was 93% versus 83% respectively (p=0.03). In April 2001 the data and safety monitoring committee halted randomization to the reduced treatment arm on the basis of reduced efficacy. This reduction in efficacy was evident in both CNS-negative patients (94% versus 86%) and CNS-positive patients (84% versus 72%). In subgroup analysis, the probabilities of 4-year EFS for all patients grouped by bone marrow involvement only,

CNS involvement only and combined bone marrow and CNS involvement were 88%, 82%, and 61% respectively. The probability of 4-year EFS was 97% among complete responders to day 7 COP, 30% among nonresponders and 78% in incomplete responders. There was no significant difference in EFS due to diagnosis (DLBCL versus B-ALL) or LDH ≤2 versus >2 normal upper limit) or age (5-year categories) in the entire cohort.

Toxicity

Stomatitis and infection were the most frequent toxicities occurring with grade 3 or 4 severity at least once in 81% and 95% of patients. These were most commonly seen during the first two courses of COPAdM. There was a significant reduction in grade 3 and 4 stomatitis, infections and other nonhematological toxicity in patients who received the reduced-intensity treatment. There was also a significant reduction in the average days of hospitalization in patients treated with reduced-intensity CYVE (mean 5 days, p<0.001).

Conclusions

It was concluded that in patients in complete remission after three cycles of chemotherapy who were randomized to reduced-intensity therapy, the survival outcomes were significantly inferior, particularly in those with either combined bone marrow and CNS disease or a poor response to COP (p<0.001). Standard-intensity therapy was therefore recommended for all patients with high-risk BNHL (B-ALL with or without CNS involvement).

Study 3

Brugieres L, Le Deley M, Rosolen A *et al*. Impact of the methotrexate administration dose on the need for intrathecal treatment in children and adolescents with anaplastic large-cell lymphoma: results of a randomised trial of the EICNHL Group. *J Clin Oncol* 2009;27:897–903.

Objectives

To compare the effectiveness and safety of two methotrexate doses and administration schedules in children with anaplastic large cell lymphoma (ALCL).

Study design

This was an international randomized trial run under the auspices of the EICNHL Group. Ten national groups conducted it in 12 countries. Eligible candidates were biopsy-proven ALCL <22 years of age. Slides had to be available for national pathology review. Patients with isolated skin disease, completely resected stage I disease or CNS involvement were not eligible. Additional exclusions were previous treatment, congenital immunodeficiency, AIDS, previous organ transplantation or prior malignancy. The diagnosis of ALCL was based on morphology and immunophenotype and if possible on molecular criteria. Mandatory antibodies were CD30, CD15, EMA, ALK1, CD79A, CD20, CD3, CD43, and CD45RO. Patients were staged according to the St Jude and Ann Arbor staging systems. They were classified as high risk if they had at least one risk factor defined as the presence of skin and/or mediastinal, and/or visceral involvement (defined as lung, liver or spleen involvement) and as standard risk if they had no such risk factors.

Chemotherapy was based on the NHLBFM90 protocol; all patients received a 5-day prephase with dexamethasone, low-dose cyclophosphamide and one triple intrathecal injection. This was followed by six alternating courses, comprising course A (dexamethasone, methotrexate, ifosfamide, cytarabine, and etoposide) and course B (dexamethasone, methotrexate, cyclophosphamide, and doxorubicin). Arm MTX1 included methotrexate $1 \, g/m^2$ in 24-h infusion (leucovorin rescue was at 42, 48, and 54 h) with triple intrathecal injection on day 1, Arm MTX3 included methotrexate $3 \, g/m^2$ as a 3-h infusion (6-hourly leucovorin rescue starting at 24 h until the MTX level was <0.15 $\mu m/L$) with no intrathecal injection. Additionally, high-risk patients could enter a second randomized trial before the first course B which randomly assigned patients to receive or not receive a vinblastine injection ($6 \, mg/m^2/dose$) during the five later courses and then weekly for a total duration of treatment of 1 year. This second randomization is not the subject of the present report.

Tumor response was evaluated after each course; a comprehensive evaluation had to be performed once all signs of disease had disappeared or no later than the sixth course. Complete remission was defined as disappearance of disease for at least 4 weeks. A residual lesion at the end of treatment was not considered a treatment failure if it was <30% of the initial tumor mass. Relapses had to be confirmed by biopsy.

Statistics

Random assignment was balanced and stratified according to country and risk group (standard risk versus high risk). Five different data centers managed the random assignment. A centralized randomization software was used in all five data centers except in Italy, where their minimization program or stratified random assignments were with permuted blocks of size 4. In the Italian data center, predefined, stratified balanced random assignment lists were used to allocate treatments.

The primary endpoint was EFS, defined as the time from random assignment to first failure (progression, relapse, second malignancy or death) or the last follow-up visit for patients in complete remission. Secondary endpoints were OS, CR, CNS relapse, and acute toxicity. OS rates were estimated from date of randomization to the date of death of whatever cause or date of last follow-up clinic visit. Toxicity was assessed using the National Cancer Institute Common Toxicity Criteria version 2.0. Grade 4 hematological and grades 3–4 nonhematological toxicity were considered as serious toxicity.

The issue raised in the trial was formulated as a noninferiority question in terms of EFS. Considering the factorial design of the trial, the sample size was determined for the vinblastine trial to demonstrate a reduction of a risk of events by adding vinblastine in high-risk patients. A total of 204 high-risk patients were required for the vinblastine trial. Assuming that the high-risk patients eligible for the vinblastine random assignment accounted for 64% of those eligible for the methotrexate randomization, it was expected to accrue 320 patients onto the methotrexate trial during accrual onto the vinblastine trial. With the given sample size, it was recognized that a noninferiority conclusion could never be proven, so it was planned only to provide CI for differences in EFS in the two arms. Three planned interim analyses were performed using the Flemings plan and discussed with the independent data monitoring committee.

The final analysis was performed with a one-sided p=0.0412. The main analysis of EFS was to be performed on a modified intention-to-treat population excluding only patients in whom the diagnosis of ALCL had been rejected after review. Two secondary analyses were performed, one with no exclusions and the second on a per protocol population that excluded patients who were not eligible for random assignment, patients for whom the diagnosis of ALCL had been rejected, and patients with major modification of the allocated treatment. Hazard ratios (HR) were estimated using Cox models adjusted by the risk group (standard risk versus high risk) and country and stratified by the treatment allocated by the second random assignment (i.e. not randomly assigned, no vinblastine, or vinblastine). Prespecified secondary analyses using Cox models were performed to study variations in the treatment effect according to risk group, treatment allocated by the second random assignment, and country. Toxicity rates between MTX1 and MTX3 arms were compared using mixed models controlling the number of the course (1 to 6) and the adjunction or not of vinblastine and considering the patient effect as a random effect. Data were entered and checked with PIGAS software and analyzed with SAS software version 8.2.

Results

Between November 1999 and December 2005, 487 patients were screened for study entry; 112 were excluded. Following pathology review, ultimately 352 patients were included in the main analysis – 175 assigned to MTX1 and 177 to MTX 3. Median age was 11, range 4 months to 19 years. Risk group stratification was standard 38% (n=133) and high risk 62% (n=218). Overall 47% had mediastinal involvement, 21% lung, 14% liver, 18% spleen, 19% skin, 16% soft tissue mass, 19% bone lesion, and 12% bone marrow involvement. A major protocol violation was observed in four patients, two patients in both arms. The treatment was significantly modified as a result of toxicity in four additional patients. These eight patients were included in the main analysis but were excluded from the protocol analysis. A modification of the MTX dose or IT injections in less than three courses was observed in nine and 10 patients in the MTX1 and MTX3 arms respectively. The median follow-up was 3.8 years.

Disease disappeared completely from all the initially involved sites in 88% (n=309) of patients. Only two patients had a CNS relapse as a first event. The overall 2-year EFS rate was 74%. Thirty-two deaths were reported: 21 as a result of disease progression and 11

from treatment toxicity. There was no significant difference between the two randomized groups for any of the main and secondary efficacy endpoints. Complete remission rates were 89% and 87% respectively in the MTX1 and MTX3 arms and the 2-year EFS curves were superimposable at 74%. The 2-year OS rates were 90% and 95% in the MTX1 and MTX3 arms respectively.

Toxicity

Severe toxicity was reported after 75% of courses and consisted mostly of grade 4 hematological toxicity (72% of courses) and grade 3–4 mucositis (13%). These were significantly more frequent after MTX1 courses. Incidence of grade 3 or 4 infections was low and comparable for both arms. However, if all grades of infection are considered, the incidence was significantly higher after MTX1 (50%) compared with the MTX3 courses (52%) ($p < 0.0001$).

Conclusions

These results indicated that the methotrexate schedule originally used in the NHL BFM 90 protocol including intrathecal therapy can be safely replaced by a less toxic schedule giving a shorter infusion at higher dose of methotrexate without intrathecal therapy. This alternative regimen is also less toxic with regard to myelosuppression mucositis and infection. A subsequent study has described in greater detail the toxicities in this trial.

Study 4

Le Deley M, Roselen A, Williams DM *et al.* Vinblastine in children and adolescents with high-risk anaplastic large-cell lymphoma: results of the randomised ALCL99 vinblastine trial. *J Clin Oncol* 2010;**28**:3987–93.

Objectives

To determine the impact of adding vinblastine to a 4-month chemotherapy regimen based on the NHL BFM 90 protocol in children with high-risk anaplastic large cell lymphoma.

Study design

This was a prospective randomized multicenter trial conducted between 1999 and 2006 in 12 countries by 10 co-operative groups that were mainly European with a single Japanese group. The ALCL99 vinblastine study was part of a factorial design trial including another trial comparing the efficacy and safety of two methotrexate doses and administration schedules during six induction courses of chemotherapy (MTX trial).

Eligible patients included age <22 years with biopsy-proven ALCL classified as high risk (mediastinal, lung, liver or spleen involvement or biopsy-proven skin disease). Patients with isolated skin disease or involvement of CNS were not eligible. Also excluded were those with disease progression after the first course of chemotherapy, prior treatment, evidence of congenital immunodeficiency, AIDS, previous organ transplantation or previous malignancy. The diagnosis of ALCL was based on morphological and immunophenotypic criteria and where possible molecular definition (evidence of anaplastic lymphoma kinase fusion genes). A review by the national pathologist was requested before random assignment for all patients who were anaplastic lymphoma kinase 1 (ALK 1) negative on immunostaining, Additionally all patients were to be reviewed by an international panel blinded to treatment allocation. Pretreatment evaluation included physical examination, computed tomography (CT) scan of chest and abdomen, isotope bone scan, bone marrow aspirations and biopsies and CSF cytospin. The patients were staged according to the St Jude and Ann Arbor staging systems.

Chemotherapy was based on the NHL BFM 90 protocol. All patients received a 5-day prephase followed by six alternating induction courses: courses A and B given every 21 days (see Study 3 for details). Tumor response was evaluated after each course of treatment; a complete remission was defined as disappearance of disease for at least 4 weeks and unconfirmed CR was defined as a reduction in tumor size exceeding 70%. Relapse required confirmation with biopsy.

Statistics

Random assignment was performed after the first induction course to allow for pathology review for patients not fulfilling classic diagnostic criteria. Random assignment was balanced and stratified according to country and to the treatment allocated by the first random assignment for methotrexate trial (factorial design). Five different data centers managed the random assignment. Centralized randomization software was used in all five with slightly different methodology in different centers, with a minimization

program or stratified random assignment with permuted blocks of size 4 and predefined stratified balanced random assignment lists. The primary endpoint was EFS, defined as the time from random assignment to first failure (progression, relapse, second malignancy or death) or last follow-up. Secondary endpoints were OS, CR, and acute toxicity. OS was estimated from the data random assignment to death of whatever cause or last follow-up. Toxicity was defined according to the National Cancer Institute Common Toxicity Criteria. Survival rates were estimated using the Kaplan–Meier method with Rothman 95% CIs. Median follow-up time was estimated using Schemper's method. Hazard ratios for EFS and deaths (OS) were estimated using Cox models adjusted on country and on treatment allocated at first assignment (MTX1/MTX3). The trial was designed to demonstrate an improvement from 62% to 80% in 2-year EFS probability (HR=0.47). A total of 59 events and 204 patients were required to reach a power of 80% with a type 1 error of 5% (two-sided log-rank test). Three planned interim analyses were performed after observing 25%, 50%, and 75% of events using Fleming's plan and discussed with the independent data monitoring committee. The main analysis was performed on the intention-to-treat population.

Results

Between 1999 and 2006, 529 patients were screened for study entry. Overall, 217 of 254 potential eligible patients were included, 107 in the no vinblastine arm and 110 in the vinblastine arm. All patients except one were observed for at least 2 years from random assignment. Central pathology review was performed in 207 of the 217 patients and the diagnosis of ALCL was rejected in seven patients: one Hodgkin disease, three ALK-negative peripheral T-cell lymphoma, one ALK-negative B-cell lymphoma, one ALK-positive immunoblastic B-cell lymphoma, one CD 30+ cutaneous lymphoproliferation. The WHO classification histological subtypes were common type 107, mixed 58, small cell 14, lymphohistiocytic seven, Hodgkin like six, and giant cell three.

A major protocol violation was observed in four patients: three patients in the vinblastine arm did not receive any of the planned vinblastine and one in the no-vinblastine arm received the whole maintenance therapy. Ten of 110 patients in the vinblastine arm did not receive any maintenance as a result of progression or death (n=5), protocol violation (n=3), or other reasons (n=2). The median duration of treatment was 53 weeks; 17 patients received more than 70 weeks therapy. Prolonged treatment durations arose through misinterpretation of the term duration of treatment versus duration of maintenance. Overall, only 33 of 100 patients received at least 90% (5.4 mg/m²/week) of the planned total dose. Dose reduction was mainly as a result of hematological toxicity.

Overall, 205 evaluable patients achieved CR or unconfirmed CR before the end of induction treatment. An event was reported in 66 of 217 patients: 10 progression during treatment, 55 relapses, and one toxic death. The 2-year EFS and OS were 71% and 94% respectively for the whole trial population. With regard to treatment arm, complete remission rate was 85% (n=91) in the no-vinblastine arm versus 84% (n=93) in the vinblastine arm, progressive disease 5.6% (n=6) versus 3.6% (n=4). Progression during therapy was seen in six versus four patients, while relapse (from completion of induction to >1 year after randomization) occurred in 26 versus 29 patients in the no-vinblastine and vinblastine arms respectively. Overall, the number of events differed little between the two arms but the median interval from random assignment to progression/relapse differed greatly between the two arms: 13 months for vinblastine versus 6 months for

no vinblastine (p<0.001). During the first year there was a significantly lower risk of events in the vinblastine arm compared with the no vinblastine (HR=0.31, p=0.002) whereas the risk was significantly increased in this arm after the first year (HR=5, p=0.003). This resulted in no significant difference at 2 years: 72% versus 70% respectively. No significant interaction was detected between the effect of vinblastine and the dose of methotrexate, the other component of the randomized trial.

Toxicity

During induction there were no differences in the incidence of toxicity except for grade 4 anemia 8% vinblastine versus 5% no vinblastine (p=0.05) and grade 3 or 4 stomatitis 13% versus 9% (p=0.05). One patient in the vinblastine arm experienced grade 3 peripheral neuropathy during induction. While only three patients stopped vinblastine maintenance as a result of toxicity, the dose was reduced in 31% of courses (793/2563 courses), mainly as a consequence of hematological toxicity.

Conclusions

The addition of vinblastine during induction and as maintenance for total treatment duration of 1 year significantly delayed the occurrence of relapse but did not reduce the risk of failure.

CHAPTER 11

Hodgkin lymphoma

Ross Pinkerton
Royal Children's Hospital, Brisbane, QLD, Australia

Commentary by Cindy L. Schwartz

Pediatric Hodgkin lymphoma (HL) is highly responsive to both chemotherapy and radiation therapy, resulting in excellent survival that now exceeds 90%. Although biologically similar if not identical to HL affecting young or middle-aged adults, late effects such as musculoskeletal (MSK) hypoplasia in radiation fields, cardiopulmonary dysfunction, infertility, secondary malignancy, and thyroid disease appear to be more prominent in younger patients. This has resulted in pediatric/adolescent treatment paradigms that have diverged from those used in adult populations.

Radiation was the first therapy recognized to have efficacy in HL. Initially, high-dose radiation (35–40 Gy) to extended fields was standard. Unfortunately, hypoplasia was a major consequence of high-dose radiation in the child. MOPP (mustine, vincristine, procarbazine, prednisone) and ABVD (doxorubicin, bleomycin, vinblastine, dacarbazine) were then developed as effective agents for adults and children with advanced HL. Recognizing the adverse effects of full-dose radiation in children, pediatricians pioneered the addition of chemotherapy to the algorithm of care for all stages of disease as a method of reducing radiation dose and field.

Randomized trials have compared (1) dose and field of radiation, (2) chemotherapy regimens, and (3) chemotherapy versus chemoradiotherapy. The significant cure rate has often limited compliance with such

trials, as physicians and patients select therapies based on adult data or conjecture. In addition, the excellent results achieved necessitate accrual of large cohorts to ensure sufficient power to detect improvements in outcome. This has limited the development of randomized trials, with many large trial consortia relying on single-arm studies in HL. While these studies have shown improved outcomes with successive protocols, they reflect rather than develop strategies for care. It is the randomized trials that allow us to compare overall strategies, ensuring that the paradigms of care are optimal for children.

Radiation therapy

The emergence of MSK hypoplasia in young children treated for HL with full-dose radiation led to the early pediatric clinical trials whose goal was to prevent MSK hypoplasia by use of low-dose, limited-field radiation. The trials by Bayle-Weisgerber et al. [1] and Gehan et al. [2] evolved in an era prior to the universal use of chemotherapy in children with HL. Both groups evaluated chemotherapy in specific cohorts (see below) but also attempted to understand the optimal field size for pediatric radiation therapy (RT). Bayle-Weisgerber et al. [1] compared para-aortic RT plus splenectomy to splenolumbar RT in a total of 21 patients without discernible difference in outcome in this underpowered study. Gehan et al. [2] reported the results of two

Evidence-Based Pediatric Oncology, Third Edition. Edited by Ross Pinkerton, Ananth Shankar and Katherine K. Matthay.
© 2013 John Wiley & Sons, Ltd. Published 2013 by John Wiley & Sons, Ltd.

parallel studies for stage I or II disease, each a comparison of MOPP plus involved-field RT to radiation alone (involved field [IF] in one study, extended field [EF] in the other). The comparison of the two RT approaches was therefore not a formally randomized study but the difference in 5-year relapse-free survival (RFS) was 67% versus 41% for EF versus IF, suggesting a benefit of EF when used as the sole therapy. These data lost relevance in pediatric HL as chemotherapy became a mainstay of treatment, with MOPP chemotherapy. In both studies, the chemotherapy arm vastly surpassed the efficacy of radiation (RFS 93% and 97% in the two trials) although the radiation-only arms had an overall survival (OS) of 95–96% versus 89–90% for the MOPP arms, most likely a consequence of the reduced burden of treatment. Similar outcomes in adult trials led to an adult care strategy that provided RT to all with low-stage disease despite lesser event-free survival (EFS), knowing that chemotherapy salvage would boost the OS to an acceptable level. The pediatric paradigm diverged from the adult paradigm as evidence mounted that low-dose radiation in combination was highly efficacious and reduced the risk for hypoplasia.

Cramer and Andrieu [3] also studied IF versus mantle in patients with IA–IIA disease in conjunction with chemotherapy (MOPP), but the study was too small (13 patients) to be interpreted (as was their small randomized comparison of MOPP/RT versus CVPP[chlorambucil, vinblastine, procarbazine, prednisolone]/RT). The more important contribution of their work was the confirmation of the efficacy of combining chemotherapy with low-dose radiation. Perhaps the most important study of this era [4] gave only low-dose RT for those with good response to therapy in their excellent comparison of MOPP versus MOPP/ABVD. This critical study confirmed that children did not need high-dose (35–40 Gy) radiation in the context of combination therapy. Although remission could be induced with higher dose RT for slow responders, they noted that the adverse long-term prognosis was not averted.

Combination therapy

The Gehan et al. [2] study noted above showed the improvement in EFS achieved when MOPP chemotherapy was added to either IF or EF RT. Bayle-Weisgerber et al. [1] performed a small randomized trial of radiation with and without vinblastine; limited accrual

resulted in an inadequately powered result. However, their sequential studies showed improvement in outcome with the addition of MOPP to radiation.

Chemotherapy was soon recognized to also be associated with significant long-term toxicity for children: gonadal toxicity and secondary malignancy with alkylating agents, cardiac toxicity with doxorubicin, and pulmonary toxicity with bleomycin. From 1976 to 1982, Sullivan et al. [5] compared MOPP with bleomycin (MOPP-B) to cyclophosphamide, vincristine, procarbazine, prednisolone (COPP) with doxorubicin (A-COPP) in an attempt to improve outcome with doxorubicin versus bleomycin. Acute hematological toxicity was reduced, presumably by replacing the lomustine with cyclophosphamide. More complete responses (92% versus 84%) were induced with A-COPP, and the 5-year disease-free survival (DFS) was higher with A-COPP as well (87.8% versus 77.3%) but the 10-year DFS rates were similar, revealing the adverse impact of anthracycline-induced cardiomyopathy as an emerging late toxicity. Overall results were improving with the addition of chemotherapy, but additional agents also resulted in additional toxicities.

Oberlin et al. [4] showed that MOPP and MOPP/ABVD were equally efficacious in favorable HL when used with low-dose radiation. This began an approach that has remained prevalent in pediatric HL care in which multiple agents are used in reduced doses to avoid thresholds for known toxicity. Sackmann-Muriel et al. [6] also evaluated approaches to the reduction of therapy. In low-risk disease, they showed that three and six cycles of CVPP with IF RT were equally effective, thus reducing the cumulative dose of alkylator to limit risk of sterility and secondary malignancy. For advanced stage disease, an attempt to replace exposure to cyclophosphamide and procarbazine with doxorubicin and etoposide was unsuccessful, showing a reduction in EFS from 87% to 67%. Similar outcomes have been noted in single-arm trials when etoposide has been used to completely replace alkylating agents [7]. This same effect has not been noted if etoposide replaces some, but not all, of the alkylating agents in patients with advanced HL [8, 9].

Chemotherapy only

Combination chemotherapy was highly effective but long-term risks associated with even low-dose radiation remain. Secondary malignancy, particularly breast cancer in young women, is a significant risk with high-dose therapy. A recent report from O'Brien *et al.* [10] showed that risk persisted even with low-dose radiation. Atherosclerotic heart disease after radiation is another concern, with an unknown degree of mitigated risk after lower dose radiation. Pediatric chemotherapy regimens now contain 6–8 chemotherapy agents to avoid thresholds for chemotherapy-associated toxicity and to achieve sufficient efficacy to support the elimination of radiation in responsive cohorts.

The Children's Cancer Group (CCG) study reported by Hutchinson *et al.* [11] randomized patients with advanced-stage HL to either 12 cycles of alternating MOPP/ABVD or six ABVD with low-dose EF RT. This study did not show a statistically significant difference in outcome although the EFS was 77% versus 87% for the chemotherapy versus combined modality arms, with a relative risk of mortality of 0.69 for those receiving radiation. All instances of recurrence in the chemotherapy arm were at sites that would have been irradiated. Either the six MOPP were less effective than was the IF RT, or the effect of six ABVD was enhanced by delivery over 6 versus 12 months.

The Hutchinson study randomized patients to the different approaches at diagnosis. More recent studies have required a defined therapeutic response, usually complete response at the end of chemotherapy, to allocate patients to the randomized option of chemotherapy only. In low-stage disease, the Pediatric Oncology Group (POG) randomized patients with a complete or partial remission (CR or PR) after four cycles of alternating MOPP/ABVD to either two more cycles of chemotherapy or 25.5 Gy of IF RT [12]. Eight-year EFS was 83% versus 91% (not statistically significant) for chemotherapy versus combined modality therapy with no difference in OS. However, the study was small and only powered to detect a 15% difference in EFS. Results have been variably interpreted as either showing similar efficacy of two cycles of chemotherapy versus RT, sufficiency of four cycles of chemotherapy for low-stage disease, or as an underpowered study with a trend to benefit of radiation therapy. For advanced-stage disease, the Pediatric Oncology Group [13] randomized patients in CR to +/– RT after eight cycles of alternating MOPP/ABVD. There was no difference in EFS (79% versus 80%) or OS, suggesting that eight cycles of chemotherapy are sufficient if a CR has

been achieved; this was the only such study to show equivalent outcomes of chemotherapy and combined modality therapy. Patients achieving CR after three cycles had EFS of 94% versus 78% for those not in clinical CR at that time. This finding (and similar findings in low-risk HL by Kung *et al.* [12]) led to the future efforts of the POG and Children's Oncology Group (COG) to use early response to titrate therapy for each patient.

Lascar *et al.* [14] and Nachman *et al.* [15] also randomized patients achieving CR to +/– RT. Both studies found a benefit to radiation therapy. Lascar randomized patients in CR after six cycles of ABVD, while Nachman randomized them after 4–6 cycles of COPP/ABV for stages I–III, and after a nine-drug regimen for those with stage IV disease. In comparison to Weiner *et al.* [13], these studies used fewer chemotherapy cycles and were more restrictive. The Nachman study randomized more than 500 patients and, therefore, was powered to detect small differences in outcome. These studies again suggested that response at the end of therapy did not accurately identify the patients who could be spared radiation, although many patients clearly do well with chemotherapy only.

Based on the Kung and Weiner studies [12, 13], the POG initiated an algorithm of care designed to enhance efficacy with dose-dense chemotherapy (ABVE-PC) and to use an early response to limit cumulative therapy [8]. The COG has recently completed AHOD0031 [16], a randomized trial in which patients who achieved a rapid early response (60% two-dimensional tumor reduction) were randomized to IF RT versus no RT after four cycles of ABVE-PC. In this cohort, no benefit was noted for RT and augmentation of chemotherapy with a different chemotherapy regimen enhanced EFS for slow early responders who were fluorodeoxyglucose-positron emission tomography (FDG-PET) positive [16]. This allocation was by computed tomography (CT) scan, but FDG-PET scans were also performed in the majority of patients. COG data suggest that allocation of therapy by CT scan is more robust than by PET scan, although both imaging modalities are independently predictive of EFS, thus suggesting benefit to using both modalities [17]. Single-arm studies in Europe are also using FDG-PET with CT to stratify therapy based on early response [18]. The randomized COG AHOD0031 trial was unique in that it proved that early response can identify a cohort who can truly be spared radiation.

Current randomized approaches to HL in both Europe and the US will investigate the use of early response to tailor therapy to the individual, using dose-dense chemotherapy regimens (OPPA, ABVE-PC) to enhance the efficacy of therapy. Instead of choosing between toxicity and efficacy, the early response-based algorithm will allow us to simultaneously improve efficacy while limiting long-term toxicity.

References

1 Bayle-Weisgerber C, Lemercier N, Teillet F, Asselain B, Gout M, Schweisguth O. Results of therapy in a mixed group of 178 clinical and pathologically staged patients over 13 years. *Cancer* 1984;**54**:215–22.

2 Gehan EA, Sullivan MP, Fuller LM *et al.* The Intergroup Hodgkin's disease in children. A study of stages 1 and 11. *Cancer* 1990;**65**:1429–37.

3 Cramer P, Andrieu JM. Hodgkin's disease in childhood and adolescence: results of chemotherapy- radiotherapy in clinical stages 1A-IIB. *J Clin Oncol* 1985;**3**:1495–502.

4 Oberlin O, Leverger G, Pacquement H *et al.* Low-dose radiation therapy and reduced chemotherapy in childhood Hodgkin's disease; the experience of the French Society of Paediatric Oncology. *J Clin Oncol* 1992;**10**:1602–8.

5 Sullivan MP, Fuller LM, Berard C, Ternberg J, Cantor AB, Leventhal BG. Comparative effectiveness of two combined modality regimens in the treatment of surgical stage III Hodgkin's disease in children. An 8-year follow-up study by the Pediatric Oncology Group. *Am J Pediatr Hematol Oncol* 1991;**13**:450–8.

6 Sackmann-Muriel F, Zubizarreta P, Gallo G *et al.* Hodgkin's disease in children: results of a prospective randomised trial in a single institution in Argentina. *Med Pediatr Oncol* 1997;**29**:544–52.

7 Hudson MM, Krasin M, Link MP *et al.* Risk-adapted, combined-modality therapy with VAMP/COP and response-based, involved-field radiation for unfavorable pediatric Hodgkin's disease. *J Clin Oncol* 2004;**22**(22):4541–50.

8 Schwartz CL, Constine LS, Villaluna D *et al.* A risk-adapted, response-based approach using ABVE-PC for children and adolescents with intermediate- and high-risk Hodgkin lymphoma: the results of P9425. *Blood* 2009;**114**(10):2051–9.

9 Dörffel W, Lüders H, Rühl U *et al.* Preliminary results of the multicenter trial GPOH-HD 95 for the treatment of Hodgkin's disease in children and adolescents: analysis and outlook. *Klin Paediatr* 2003;**215**(3):139–45.

10 O'Brien MM, Donaldson SS, Balise RR, Whittemore AS, Link MP. Second malignant neoplasms in survivors of pediatric Hodgkin's lymphoma treated with low-dose radiation and chemotherapy. *J Clin Oncol* 2010;**28**(7):1232–9.

11 Hutchinson RJ, Fryer CJH, Davis PC *et al.* MOPP or radiation in addition to ABVD in the treatment of pathologically staged advanced Hodgkin's disease in children: results of the Children's Cancer Group phase III trial. *J Clin Oncol* 1998;**16**:897–906.

12 Kung FH, Schwartz CL, Ferree CR *et al.*, for the Children's Oncology Group. POG 8625: a randomised trial comparing chemotherapy with chemotherapy for children and adolescents with Stages I, IIA, IIA¹ Hodgkin disease. *J Pediatr Hematol Oncol* 2006;**28**:362–8.

13 Weiner MA, Leventhal B, Brecher ML *et al.* Randomised study of intensive MOPP-ABVD with or without low-dose total-nodal radiation therapy in the treatment of stages 11B, 111A2, 111B and IV Hodgkin's disease in paediatric patients: a Paediatric Oncology Group study. *J Clin Oncol* 1997;**15**:2769–79.

14 Lascar S, Gupta T, Vimal S *et al.* Consolidation radiation after complete remission in Hodgkin's disease following six cycles of doxorubicin, bleomycin, vinblastine and dacarbazine chemotherapy: is there a need? *J Clin Oncol* 2004;**22**:62–8.

15 Nachman JB, Sposto R, Herzog P *et al.* Randomised comparison of low-dose involved field radiotherapy and no radiotherapy for children with Hodgkin's disease who achieve a complete response to chemotherapy. *J Clin Oncol* 2002;**20**:3765–71.

16 Friedman DL, Wolden S, Chen L, Trippet T, de Alarcon P, Schwartz CL. AHOD0031: a phase III study of dose-intensive therapy and radiotherapy for intermediate risk Hodgkin lymphoma: a report from the Children's Oncology Group. Presentation at ASH, Orlando, FL, December 2010.

17 Schwartz CL, Friedman DL, McCarten K *et al.* Predictors of early response and event free survival in Hodgkin lymphoma (HL): PET versus CT imaging. Proceedings of the ASCO Annual Meeting, 2011.

18 Körholz D, Claviez A, Hasenclever D *et al.* The concept of the GPOH-HD 2003 therapy study for pediatric Hodgkin's disease: evolution in the tradition of the DAL/GPOH studies. *Klin Paediatr* 2004;**216**(3):150–6.

Summary of previous studies

Two reviews published in the mid-1980s by two French groups outlined the development of treatment strategies in children and adolescents [1, 2]. Bayle-Weisgerber [1] reviewed experience from the Institute Gustave-Roussy in Paris from 1965 to 1978. A total of 212 children under the age of 15 with clinical stage I and II disease were included. Of the five studies published during this period, two were small randomized studies. One conducted between 1964 and 1971, that included 35 patients, compared EF radiation therapy with or without 2 years of weekly vinblastine. Only eight patients were randomized to the chemotherapy arm and although no difference was shown, the study was insufficiently powered to address the question. The second randomized trial took place between 1972 and 1976 and included 30 patients who were randomly assigned to para-aortic radiation plus splenectomy versus splenolumbar radiation therapy. Ten and 11 patients respectively were randomized to each arm and again no difference was shown in overall survival but the study size was very small and minimal details were provided about the studies themselves.

A year later, Cramer and Andrieu from the Hôpital St Louis in Paris reviewed their experience of treating 72 children and adolescents between 1972 and 1980. Two small randomized studies were included, the first for good-risk patients with stage I–IIA where mantle or mantle excluding mediastinal radiation was compared with involved field radiation. For patients with more advanced disease, mantle or mantle excluding mediastinum was compared with mantle or mantle excluding mediastinum plus lumbo-aortic field. In both studies radiation was preceded by 3–6 courses of MOPP chemotherapy. Very small numbers of patients were enrolled and although no difference was demonstrated, the studies were insufficiently powered. Both these reports, however, were important in that the non-randomized component in both reviews began to demonstrate the effectiveness of combination chemotherapy with low-dose IF radiation therapy which formed the basis of most pediatric protocols in subsequent years.

In 1992 Oberlin et al. from the Institute Gustave-Roussy published an important randomized trial, which compared four cycles of ABVD to two cycles of MOPP alternated with two cycles of ABVD in favorable Hodgkin disease (IA and IIA). All patients received reduced-dose (20 Gy) IF radiotherapy following a good response to treatment [3]; 82% achieved a complete response with chemotherapy. The overall disease-free survival at 6 years was 89% for stage I and II patients. One hundred and thirty-two patients (n=136) with IA or IIA disease were randomized, 67 to MOPP plus ABVD and 65 to ABVD alone. Detailed reasons for nonrandomization were not provided but there was no significant imbalance between the two arms. The risk of relapse at 4 years was 13% for MOPP/ABVD and 10% for ABVD alone. One patient treated with MOPP/ABVD plus IF RT subsequently developed acute myeloid leukemia. It was concluded that the treatments were comparable in low-stage disease and the efficacy of low-dose radiation with 20 Gy was evident.

A further study comparing chemotherapy strategies published by Sullivan et al. in 1991 was carried out by the Pediatric Oncology Group between 1976 and 1982 [4]. Patients with stage III disease were randomized to receive a "sandwich" regimen with either MOPP-B (bleomycin + MOPP) or A-COPP (doxorubicin + COPP) and IF RT. In both arms radiation therapy was given after two courses of chemotherapy. One hundred and thirty-two patients were entered in the study but 48 were excluded for a variety of reasons; 39 received A-COPP and 45 received MOPP-B. At 10 years, the duration of remission was 70% for MOPP-B and 67% for A-COPP (p=0.22). It was concluded that in this group, treatment was equally effective when an anthracycline replaced an alkylating agent.

A study run by a combination of POG, the Children's Cancer Study Group (CCSG), and the Cancer and Leukemia Group B (CALGB) was reported by Gehan et al. [5]. Patients with stage I and II disease were enrolled in parallel studies comparing IF RT plus six courses of MOPP versus IF RT alone (POG) and in the other, EF RT alone versus six courses of MOPP plus IF RT (CCSG and CALGB). Specific good-risk groups that were excluded comprised stage I unilateral neck disease except those with lymphocyte-depleted histology, all unilateral inguinal stage I and stage I mediastinal disease with nodular sclerosing histology. Although 220 patients were randomized, 26 were excluded after randomization. The 5-year RFS for IF RT plus MOPP was 97% versus 41% for IF alone (p<0.01). This difference was less but still evident with EF RT: 93% (MOPP+IF RT) versus 67% (EF RT) (p<0.01). There was, however, no difference in overall survival between patients randomized to IF versus IF RT+MOPP or EF RT versus IF RT+MOPP. While it was concluded that combination chemotherapy with IF RT provided superior RFS, it had little impact on overall survival. It was emphasized that the overall burden of treatment must be taken into account when considering the lack of difference in overall survival.

A further POG study published in 1997 by Weiner et al. [6] was designed to determine whether the addition of low-dose nodal radiation in patients with advanced-stage HL receiving alternating MOPP/ABVD chemotherapy improved event-free or overall survival when compared with chemotherapy alone. Chemotherapy comprised four 1-month cycles of MOPP alternating with four 1-month cycles of ABVD for a total of 8 months chemotherapy with or without radiation. Response was evaluated after three and six cycles of chemotherapy, at completion of chemotherapy, and after radiation therapy. Any abnormalities at the end of treatment were required to be biopsied and if positive, patients came off study. The radiation field was determined by the pretreatment evaluation. All lymphoid tissue, including spleen, received 21 Gy apart from liver, lung, parenchyma, pericardium, and kidney, which received up to 10.5 Gy. Eighty-nine patients were randomized to chemotherapy alone and 90 to combined modality treatment. There were 38 stage IIB, 22 stage IIIA, 52 stage IIIB, 20 stage IVA and 27 stage IVB. Overall 5-year EFS was 79% ± 6% and survival 92% ± 4%. The 5-year EFS for those who received combination chemotherapy plus radiation therapy was 80% ± 8% compared to 79% ± 9% for chemotherapy alone (p=0.60) with 5-year overall survival of 87% and 96% (p=0.97). It was concluded that the addition of radiation therapy after eight cycles of chemotherapy was of no significant benefit.

An Argentinian study published in 1997 described the pediatric cohort in an adult and pediatric study [7]. Risk group was based on a prognostic index scoring system which took into account age, B symptoms, stage, and number of involved regions. The study question differed in relation to risk group; namely, the duration of chemotherapy in favorable disease (three versus six courses) and two different regimens in intermediate risk (CVPP versus AOPE). Twenty-six patients were in the favorable group, using conventional staging; this comprised 21 stage IA and IIA, three stage IB or IIB and two stage IIIA. There were 64 patients in the intermediate group, comprising 32 stage IA or IIA, 12 stage IB or IIB, 18 stage IIIA or IIIB and two stage IVA. The remaining patients (n=24) fell into the unfavorable group; these were all given intensive multiagent chemotherapy plus IF RT. The favorable group was randomized at presentation between the three or six courses of CVPP chemotherapy, which comprised cyclophosphamide, vinblastine, procarbazine, and prednisolone. The intermediate group was randomized between CVPP, three courses given prior to the IF RT to three courses of AOPE (doxorubicin, vincristine, etoposide, and prednisolone). Three courses of the same regimen were given after radiotherapy. Radiation dose depended on response to initial chemotherapy. If there was >70% reduction in imageable disease, a dose of 30 Gy was given otherwise it was 40 Gy. The study demonstrated that for the favorable group of patients, there was no difference in overall complete response rate (94% versus 100%) or 80-month EFS (85% versus 87%; p=0.08) for three and six courses respectively. In the intermediate group the response rate was 98% for CVPP versus 86% for AOPE but there was a significantly poorer 80-month EFS for the AOPE regimen, being 67% ± 10% compared with 87% ± 5% for CVPP (p=0.04). It was concluded that the shorter course was equally effective for patients with good-risk disease and that the etoposide-based regimen appeared to be inferior to the standard alkylating agent-based regimen.

Between 1986 and 1990 the Children's Cancer Group carried out a study which addressed one of the key issues in childhood Hodgkin disease, namely whether radiation therapy could be omitted in the setting of effective systemic chemotherapy [8]. This trial involved patients with stage III and IV disease who were all pathologically staged. Stage IIIA patients with no large mediastinal mass and disease limited to splenic celiac or portal nodes were excluded, as were those with <5 splenic nodules as these patients were regarded as having a favorable outcome. At presentation, patients were randomized to receive either 12 28-day cycles of chemotherapy alternating between MOPP and ABVD (regimen A) or six 28-day cycles of ABVD alone followed by low-dose regional field radiation therapy to regions of initial involvement (regimen B). Radiation dose was 21 Gy and field based on disease extent at presentation. Those with lung involvement received 10.5 Gy. Patients with significant residual nodal enlargement after chemotherapy were eligible to receive higher doses of radiation but it was recommended that this was only following pathological verification. While 125 patients entered the study, 14 were excluded and ultimately, 71 stage III and 40 stage IV were randomized, 57 to MOPP/ABVD alone and 54 to combined chemoradiation. The 4-year overall survival was 87% for the total population; 84% for regimen A and 90% in regimen B (p=0.45). Four-year EFS was 77% versus 87% (p=0.09) for regimens A and B respectively. Four patients receiving anthracyclines developed grade 3 or 4 cardiac toxicity and eight patients grade 3 or 4 pulmonary toxicity. It was concluded that although the overall survival was identical, the EFS appeared to be lower in those who did not receive EF RT although this did not reach statistical significance. It was suggested that both age and previous medical history should be taken into consideration when determining therapy on the basis of potential late complications. Additionally, the authors concluded that MOPP could be safely eliminated from front-line chemotherapy regimens in children with advanced-stage Hodgkin lymphoma.

A subsequent study run by the Children's Oncology Group between 1995 and 1998 again attempted to address the issue of the need for radiation therapy specifically in children who had achieved a complete response to chemotherapy [9]. Patients with both localized and advanced disease were included and stratified into three risk groups. Patients with stage IV disease (group 3) received a multiagent regimen including cytosine/etoposide, COPP/ABV, and ACOMP (doxorubicin, cyclophosphamide, vincristine, methylprednisolone, prednisone) with G-CSF support. Patients in risk groups 1 and 2 received four and six courses of alternating COPP/ABV

chemotherapy respectively. All those who received a radiological complete remission were randomized between no further therapy or low-dose (LD) IF RT. The latter dose was 21 Gy plus 10.5 Gy to the lungs for those with lung disease. Gallium scanning was used to define complete remission in patients with a >70% reduction in tumor mass, i.e. a gallium scan that changed from positive to negative was included as a complete remission. Eight hundred and thirty-four patients were enrolled in the study; 34 were excluded and 650 achieved a complete response and were eligible for randomization. Only 501 were, in fact, randomized and two-thirds of patients who declined randomization did not receive radiation therapy. Among patients who achieved a complete response to initial chemotherapy, 92% of those randomized to receive LD IF RT were alive and disease free 3 years after randomization, versus 87% for patients randomized to receive no further therapy (p=0.057). With an "as-treated" analysis, 3-year EFS after randomization for the radiation cohort was 93% versus 85% for patients receiving no further therapy (p=0.0024). Three-year OS for patients treated with and without LD IF RT was 98% for patients who received radiation and 99% for patients who did not receive radiation. The 3-year EFS did not differ between treatment groups (IF RT versus no IF RT). For most favorable group 1, EFS was 97% versus 91%, group 2 87% versus 83%, and group 3 90% versus 81%. This study again was somewhat inconclusive and investigators suggested that combined modality therapy remains the standard of care although there may be a significant fraction of patients who can be cured with chemotherapy alone.

Finally, a single-center trial from the Tata Memorial Hospital in Mumbai was performed from 1993 to 1996, which also aimed to determine whether the addition of IF RT improved outcome following ABVD chemotherapy [10]. The study included both children and adults and a total of six cycles of standard ABVD was given. Complete responders were randomly assigned to either observation or radiation therapy. The recommended dose was 30 Gy with 10 Gy boost to bulky disease. Two hundred and fifty-one patients were enrolled; 179 achieved complete remission with 56 stage I, 43 stage II, 68 stage III and 12 stage IV. The median age was 18 years. Eighty-four patients were randomized to the observation arm while 95 received radiation. Almost half of all patients were children under the age of 15. Eighty-four percent of patients received IF RT, a smaller percentage received EF with inverted-Y (11%) or mantle field (4%) for extensive nodal disease. The 8-year EFS with radiation therapy was 88% compared to 76% with chemotherapy alone (p=0.01). For children under 15 years of age, this was 97% versus 53% (p=0.02). Overall survival was also better in the group receiving radiotherapy: 100% versus 89% (p=0.04). It was concluded that the addition of radiation therapy improved outcome following ABVD chemotherapy in this particular patient population.

References

1 Bayle-Weisgerber C, Lemercier N, Teillet F, Asselain B, Gout M, Schweisguth O. Results of therapy in a mixed group of 178 clinical and pathologically staged patients over 13 years. *Cancer* 1984;**54**:215–22.

2 Cramer P, Andrieu JM. Hodgkin's disease in childhood and adolescence: results of chemotherapy- radiotherapy in clinical stages 1A-IIB. *J Clin Oncol* 1985;**3**:1495–502.

3 Oberlin O, Leverger G, Pacquement H *et al.* Low-dose radiation therapy and reduced chemotherapy in childhood Hodgkin's disease; the experience of the French Society of Paediatric Oncology. *J Clin Oncol* 1992;**10**:1602–8.

4 Sullivan MP, Fuller LM, Berard C, Ternberg J, Cantor AB, Leventhal BG. Comparative effectiveness of two combined modality regimens in the treatment of surgical stage III Hodgkin's disease in children. An 8-year follow-up study by the Pediatric Oncology Group. *Am J Pediatr Hematol Oncol* 1991;**13**:450–8.

5 Gehan EA, Sullivan MP, Fuller LM *et al.* The Intergroup Hodgkin's disease in children. A study of stages 1 and 11. *Cancer* 1990:**65**:1429–37.

6 Weiner MA, Leventhal B, Brecher ML *et al.* Randomised study of intensive MOPP-ABVD with or without low-dose total-nodal radiation therapy in the treatment of stages 11B, 111A2, 111B and IV Hodgkin's disease in paediatric patients: a Paediatric Oncology Group study. *J Clin Oncol* 1997;**15**:2769–79.

7 Sackmann-Muriel F, Zubizarreta P, Gallo G *et al.* Hodgkin's disease in children: results of a prospective randomised trial in a single institution in Argentina. *Med Pediatr Oncol* 1997;**29**:544–52.

8 Hutchinson RJ, Fryer CJH, Davis PC *et al.* MOPP or radiation in addition to ABVD in the treatment of pathologically staged advanced Hodgkin's disease in children: results of the Children's Cancer Group phase III trial. *J Clin Oncol* 1998;**16**:897–906.

9 Nachman JB, Sposto R, Herzog P *et al.* Randomised comparison of low-dose involved field radiotherapy and no radiotherapy for children with Hodgkin's disease who achieve a complete response to chemotherapy. *J Clin Oncol* 2002;**20**:3765–71.

10 Lascar S, Gupta T, Vimal S *et al.* Consolidation radiation after complete remission in Hodgkin's disease following six cycles of doxorubicin, bleomycin, vinblastine and dacarbazine chemotherapy: is there a need? *J Clin Oncol* 2004;**22**:62–8.

New studies

Study 1

Al-Tonbary Y, Sarhan MM, El-Ashray R, Salama E, Sedky M, Fouda A. Comparative study of two mechlorethamine, vincristine, procarbazine and prednisone derived chemotherapy protocols for the management of paediatric Hodgkin lymphoma (HL): a single-center 5-year experience. *Leukaemia Lymphoma* 2010;51:656–63.

Objectives

To compare two protocols (OAP and COMP) as chemotherapy in children with all stages of Hodgkin lymphoma.

Study design

This was a single-center study from Mansoura, Egpyt. Alternate patients were allocated to receive OAP or COMP. Even-numbered patients were given COMP and uneven-numbered OAP. OAP consisted of vincristine 1.5 mg/m^2 IV days 1, 8, 15; doxorubicin 60 mg/m^2 IV days 1, 15; and prednisolone 40 mg/m^2 PO daily days 1–14. The COMP protocol consisted of cyclophosphamide 600 mg/m^2 IV day 1; vincristine 1.4 mg/m^2 IV days 1 and 8; methotrexate 40 mg/m^2 IV days 1 and 8; and prednisolone 40 mg/m^2 PO days 1–14. Procarbazine was omitted from both regimens due to its expense locally and its association with long-term effects. No radiotherapy was used because of lack of access to this modality.

Follow-up for the assessment of response was performed after the second or third cycle of therapy and the criteria used according to the National Cancer Institute (NCI)/World Health Organization (WHO) classification. Toxicity was also evaluated according to NCI criteria and if toxicity was more than grade 2 or 3, this was an indication for discontinuation of chemotherapy and changing to the alternative regimen.

Statistics

The *t* test was used to compare between two independent means and the chi-square test to compare between independent proportions. Survival functions were estimated by the Kaplan–Meier method and compared by log-rank test. Overall survival was calculated from time of diagnosis to death or last follow-up. Disease-free survival was calculated in patients with complete remission from time of diagnosis until event recurrence. No sample size calculations or power prediction were given.

Results

A total of 119 patients were treated between 2002 and 2006; 74 were male and the median age was 8 years (1–16 years). Median follow-up was 19.5 months (3–74.6 months). Stage distribution was 51% stage I, 23% stage II, 20% stage III, and 6% stage IV. Sixty patients were assigned the OAP protocol and 59 COMP. Complete response was achieved in 81% (n=48) of patients treated with COMP versus 53% (n=32) of those receiving OAP. Partial response was 23% (n=14) in OAP and 5% (n=3) in COMP. Induction of second remission after first failure was more successful in those who had received OAP and subsequently received COMP (50%) compared to the other way round, where it was only 3%.

Overall survival for all patients was 68.1% (95% confidence interval [CI] 3.739–4.753; standard error [SE] 0.259) and was higher in those receiving COMP: 76% (95% CI 3.952–5.322; SE 0.35) versus 60% (95% CI 3.097–4.563, SE 0.374) (p=0.057). Disease-free survival was 62% (95% CI 3.363–4.604) overall; 69.8% (95% CI 3.597–5.192; SE 0.407) for COMP versus 53% (95% CI 2.565–4.418; SE 0.473) for OAP (p=0.014). The relapse rate was almost equal in both arms but occurred earlier in OAP.

Toxicity

Acute toxicity was minor with both protocols and did not require hospitalization. Chronic toxicity was recurrent in three patients treated with the COMP protocol in the form of toxic hepatitis or liver cell failure. Complications were more prominent with the OAP protocol where four patients (6.8%) developed doxorubicin-induced cardiac dysfunction and 20%

toxic hepatitis. A total of eight cycles of chemotherapy was administered in both arms, and the total dose of doxorubicin was therefore $480\,mg/m^2$.

Conclusions

Patients treated with the COMP protocol achieved a better response and less toxicity but ultimately overall survival did not differ between the two regimens.

Study 2

Kung FH, Schwartz CL, Ferree CR *et al.* for the Children's Oncology Group. POG 8625: a randomised trial comparing chemotherapy with chemotherapy for children and adolescents with Stages I, IIA, IIA[1] Hodgkin disease. *J Pediatr Hematol Oncol* 2006;28:362–8.

Objectives

To determine if six courses of chemotherapy alone could achieve the same or better outcome than four courses of the same chemotherapy followed by radiation in pediatric and adolescent patients with Hodgkin disease.

Study design

This was a prospective, randomized multicenter study run by the Children's Oncology Group (POG 8625). Patients under 21 years of age with biopsy-proven, pathologically staged I, IIA or IIIA Hodgkin lymphoma were assigned to four courses of alternating MOPP/ABVD prior to formal restaging. At that time patients in complete or partial remission were randomized to receive either two further courses (1 MOPP, 1 ABVD) or IF RT 25.5 Gy. Partial response was defined as ≥50% decrease in the sum of the products of the perpendicular diameters of all lesions. Patients who failed to achieve a complete or partial response were treated with alternative therapy. It was planned to electively exclude from randomization those patients who were Tanner stage IV–V with stage I–IIA disease and small mediastinal mass <1/3 the M/T ratio without pulmonary chest wall or pericardial involvement. These patients were treated with standard-dose radiation therapy alone and no chemotherapy. Patients with stage I unilateral high neck or stage I unilateral femoral

inguinal nodal involvement of lymphocyte-predominant histology were also excluded and were treated with IF RT or chemotherapy alone. All patients were pathologically staged by laparotomy, splenectomy, liver, and bone marrow biopsies, and node sampling at several subdiaphragmatic sites.

Statistics

The primary objective of the study was the intention-to-treat comparison of event-free survival of children with early HD assigned to chemotherapy or chemoradiation. Children registered at diagnosis were assigned to treatment 1 or 2 by a call to the statistical office after response to the first four courses was determined. The randomization was balanced according to whether the child had stage I, II or IIIA disease, whether or not the MT ratio was >or< than 1/3 and whether the response to the first four courses was CR or PR. Using the Fisher exact test, a baseline comparability analysis was performed to check for imbalances between randomized treatment groups. Proportions of responders by treatment group were compared using the Fisher exact. EFS for treatment comparison was measured from the date of randomization until relapse, second malignancy, death or last contact. With a planned randomization sample of 150–160 patients, the study was designed to detect a 15% difference in 3-year EFS (75% versus 90%) with 80% power using a two-sided log-rank test and 0.05 significance level. OS and EFS estimates were computed by the Kaplan–Meier method with standard errors determined according to Peto and Peto.

Results

Between 1986 and 1992, 247 patients from 52 institutions were enrolled in the study; 169 were randomly assigned and 49 were nonrandomly assigned to treatment. An additional 29 patients were initially registered with the intent of being randomized but failed to call back for randomization for a range of reasons, including progressive disease, toxic death, and patient/physician refusal. Of 169 randomly assigned patients, 10 were ineligible, eight had B symptoms, one had non-Hodgkin lymphoma and one was incorrectly staged. Therefore 159 eligible patients were analyzed. Median age was 13 (3–20 years), sex ratio 1: 1.4, F: M. Overall there were 26 stage I, 83 stage II, and 53 stage IIIA. Forty-one patients had a large mediastinal mass

(M/T ratio >1/3). Sixty-two percent had nodular sclerosing histology, 26% mixed cellularity, 3% lymphocyte predominant and 1% lymphocyte depleted and in 8% the histological subtype was not specified. Seventy-eight patients were assigned to chemotherapy only (treatment 1) and 81 to chemoradiotherapy (treatment 2). In mid-1991 because of a shortage of supply, dacarbazine was deleted from the ABVD regimen and 28 patients were treated with ABV.

At the point of randomization after four courses of MOPP/ABVD, the CR rate was 64% and PR rate 26%; therefore 64% of randomized patients were classified as early responders and eligible for randomization. The addition of two courses of MOPP/ABVD (treatment 1) or LD RT (treatment 2) increased the overall CR rate to 89%. For those randomly assigned and alive without an event, the median follow-up was 8.25 years (4 months –12.7 years). The 8-year OS rate was 95.4% ± 12.2% and EFS 86.9% ± 3.7%. EFS rates for treatment 1 (n=78) and treatment 2 (n=81) were 82.6% ± and 91% ± 4.5% respectively while the OS rates were 93.6% ± 3.9% and 96.8% ± 2.7% (p=0.785) respectively. There was no difference in either EFS or OS between the two arms. The conclusions were unchanged when the patients who did not receive dacarbazine were excluded. The EFS for early complete responders was significantly higher than in nonresponders: 92.7% versus 76.7% (p=0.006). However, EFS and OS curves were no different for patients with CR at the end of therapy compared with patients with PR at the end of therapy: 86.8% versus 87.5% (p=0.443) and 96.2% versus 100% (p=0.629).

Toxicity

Grade 4 neutropenia developed in 47% in treatment 1 and 54% in treatment 2 some time during therapy. No clinically relevant cardiac or lung toxicity was reported. Two second malignancies occurred after treatment of recurrent disease, acute myeloid leukemia and non-Hodgkin lymphoma, both after bone marrow transplants.

Conclusions

There was no statistical difference in EFS or OS between those receiving chemotherapy alone or chemoradiation. For pediatric patients with asymptomatic low-stage and intermediate-stage Hodgkin disease, outcome was indistinguishable between chemotherapy or chemoradiotherapy. The correlation between early response to treatment and outcome led to the COG paradigm of response-based risk-adapted therapy for HD.

PART 2

Leukemia

CHAPTER 12
Acute myeloid leukemia commentary

Robert J. Arceci

Johns Hopkins University, Baltimore, MD, USA

Whilst tremendous overall improvements have been witnessed in the survival of children with cancer over the past several decades, the outcome for children and adolescents with acute myeloid leukemia (AML) remains a significant challenge [1]. The greatest increase in cure rates occurred in the era leading up to 1990 when survival rose from less than 20% to the 40–45% range. Over the next 20 years, the overall survival (OS) increased to the 45–60% range. However, more refined methods for defining molecular prognostic factors have improved our ability to stratify treatments for different risk groups with substantially different outcomes. For example, children with AML characterized by t(8;21) or inv(16) chromosomal alterations have a 5-year OS of 80–90%. In contrast, AML with a high FLT3-ITD mutation to normal allele ratio is associated with an extremely poor prognosis when treated with conventional chemotherapy.

Furthermore, an ever increasing number of molecular signatures are continuing to demonstrate the profound heterogeneity that characterizes AML. The most important future challenges are thus to define completely the molecular events that result in the development and physiology of AML, to integrate these diverse datasets into a description of the functional pathways resulting from the molecular changes and, finally, to exploit therapeutically such knowledge. Improvements in the short- and long-term outcomes for patients with AML will not likely arise from a shuffling of the conventional chemotherapy deck of cards but by changing the rules of the game.

Induction

The first significant advance in inducing remission in patients with AML included the combination of 7 days of cytosine arabinoside (ARAC) at 100 mg/m² by continuous infusion along with three initial days of daunomycin at 45 mg/m²/day. In children and young adults, this regimen led to remission rates of 60–70% [2,3]. Subsequent trials have attempted to improve on this regimen through a variety of ways.

Both the type and dose of anthracyclines have been modified. The BFM 93 trial randomized patients to receive cytarabine and etoposide plus either daunorubicin (ADE) or idarubicin (AIE). The hypothesis was that idarubicin along with its longer acting metabolites and central nervous system (CNS) penetration would be more effective. Neither the complete response (CR) rate nor the event-free survival (EFS) were, however, different between the two regimens [4]. The Children's Cancer Group (CCG) 2941 study attempted to build on the intensive timing DCTER regimen of the CCG 2891 study by introducing idarubicin (IDADCTER). However, two intensely timed courses of IDADCTER resulted in unacceptable hematotoxicity and hepatotoxicity [5]. Thus, the CCG 2961 study used IDADCTER followed by DCTER as a first course of therapy. This regimen resulted in a remission rate of 88% that was similar to historical controls [6]. The use of mitoxantrone instead of daunorubicin or idarubicin has also been studied but with no significant improvement in remission rates [7,8]. The MRC 12 trial compared etoposide and ARAC plus either mitoxantrone (MAE) or

Evidence-Based Pediatric Oncology, Third Edition. Edited by Ross Pinkerton, Ananth Shankar and Katherine K. Matthay.
© 2013 John Wiley & Sons, Ltd. Published 2013 by John Wiley & Sons, Ltd.

daunorubicin (ADE) during remission induction and demonstrated a reduction in relapse risk and in treatment-related mortality with MAE. There was no significant difference in OS compared with ADE [9].

Several studies in adults have randomized higher doses of daunorubicin such as 90 mg/m^2 compared to 45 mg/m^2 for 3 days along with standard 7 days of 100 mg/m^2 ARAC with resulting significant improvements in both remission and overall survival [10, 11, 12]. However, the issue of late cardiotoxicity was not evaluated. This dose of anthracycline has not been tested in children. Thus, with no compelling data as to whether one particular anthracycline results in improved remission rates, daunorubicin or equitoxic doses of other anthracyclines have continued to be used for children. Liposomal encapsulated anthracyclines have demonstrated less cardiotoxicity in studies in adults and have the advantage of circumventing the multidrug resistance transporter P-glycoprotein, and thus may provide a novel, and potentially less toxic, anthracycline. In addition, the use of cardioprotectants has not been studied in randomized trials of children with AML.

Another approach to improving CR rates has been to increase the dose of ARAC in order to potentially increase intracellular levels or to alter the dosing schedule of ARAC. Several studies have demonstrated improvements in CR rates using prolonged courses of ARAC, such as 10 days compared to 3 days [13]. Other trials have tested anywhere from modest to quite large increases in the dose of ARAC, i.e. from 100 mg/m^2 to 200 mg/m^2 to 3000 mg/m^2 twice a day [7, 8]. The POG 9421 study compared ARAC at 100 mg/m^2 continuous infusion for 7 days versus ARAC at 1000 mg/m^2 twice a day for 7 days and observed no difference in the CR rates (87.9% versus 91% respectively) [14]. The subsequent SJCRH AML97 trial compared a variety of chemotherapeutic drugs, depending on cytogenetic risk group or FAB classification, with ARAC at 3000 mg/m^2 every 12 h on days 1, 3, and 5 versus ARAC at 100 mg/m^2 every 12 h on days 1–10 of induction [15]. No significant difference was observed in remission rates (80% after one course and 94% after induction 2) or in the level of minimal residual disease (MRD) at the end of induction [15].

Other attempts to improve remission rates have included the addition of chemotherapeutics, such as etoposide or thioguanine. The MRC 10 trial compared daunorubicin and ARAC plus either etoposide (ADE) or thioguanine (DAT) with no significant difference in remission rates, but with different toxicity profiles, such as hepatotoxicity with the thioguanine [16]. No disease-free survival was observed either. The introduction in the COG 03P1 trial of the calicheamicin conjugated, anti-CD33 monoclonal antibody (gemtuzumab ozogamicin or GO) at 3 mg/m^2 for a single dose to ADE chemotherapy was shown to be feasible and resulted in an 87% CR rate; however, this was not considered significantly different from historical controls [17]. The results of the randomized COG 0531 comparing ADE with GO or without GO have been completed but outcomes are not yet reported. The MRC AML15 trials randomized remission induction to four different regimens (ADE 10+3+5 versus daunorubicin and ARA-C (DA) 3+10+GO versus fludarabine, ARA-C, GCSF and idarubicin (FLAG-Ida) plus or minus GO) with remission rates of 82% and 83% for the GO or no GO containing regimens [18].

Another critical aspect of improving CR rates has been the use of aggressive supportive care measures, particularly in terms of pre-emptive use of antibiotics and antifungal agents and blood product transfusions. The use of hematopoietic colony-stimulating factors, such as granulocyte colony-stimulating factor (G-CSF), has been tested in a number of randomized trials in adults with AML [19, 20]. While the period of neutropenia has been modestly reduced, usually by several days, CR rates and overall survival have not improved. The introduction of G-CSF into the CCG 2891 trials resulted in a reduced number of infection-related deaths, but this was not randomized and the comparison was to the group treated before the introduction of G-CSF [21]. Thus, the interpretation is potentially biased, perhaps by improvement over time in early deaths during the course of a study. The BFM AML98 trials randomized patients during the first two cycles of therapy to receive or not receive G-CSF [22, 23]. The results showed no significant differences in outcomes between the two groups, although a subset analysis showed that patients with AML that expressed the G-CSF receptor isoform IV had a significantly higher relapse rate [24]. Thus, G-CSF is not routinely recommended during the treatment of patients with AML as a standard approach.

Acute promyelocytic leukemia (APL) remains an exception in the world of AML, in that the introduction of all-trans-retinoic acid (ATRA) has significantly improved both the remission rates (greater than 90%) and overall survival (75–90%) [25, 26, 27]. The use of arsenic trioxide and GO in regimens to treat APL has also shown excellent response rates and antileukemic activity, providing the possibility that treatment of APL with nonconventional chemotherapy could some day become a reality [28, 29, 30]. However, a remaining problem in patients with high-risk, newly diagnosed APL is early death from hemorrhage, often intracranial [31]. No treatment has led to the eradication of this complication, although novel observations on the regulation of coagulation relevant receptors on APL cells may provide targets to initiate early preventive supportive treatment [32].

Complete response rates have indeed improved over the past 35 years, with decreased percentages of patients with refractory disease and treatment-related mortality. Lessons learned include the need for aggressive supportive care, intensification of treatment, the importance of minimal residual disease and the need for novel, more effective approaches to better individualize remission regimens. To this end, tyrosine kinase inhibitors, proteasome directed drugs, and chromatin remodeling strategies are all being tested in remission induction. The days of giving every patient the same induction therapy will hopefully become an approach of the past.

Postremission therapy

Consolidation

Postremission therapy usually includes a variety of regimens, differing numbers of courses, and the use of allogeneic transplantation. While the same postremission therapy was often given to all patients, subsequent studies have stratified treatment based on an assessment of different prognostic factors. This has resulted in the avoidance of hematopoietic stem cell transplantation (HSCT) for patients with AML having a good outcome with chemotherapy and using HSCT for patients with high-risk disease; trials testing novel, targeted drugs for patients with AML characterized by relevant gene mutations are also ongoing. However, several key unanswered questions remain.

For instance, the optimal number of postremission courses of therapy has not been ascertained, although several studies have led to some definitive conclusions. The CCG 2961 study gave a total of three intensive courses of chemotherapy, resulting in an overall survival of 52%, which was comparable to other studies with greater number of treatment courses from that period, suggesting that more courses may not be necessary [33]. The MRC 12 trial randomized five versus four courses of therapy and showed no difference in relapse-free or overall survival [9].

Attempts have also been made to identify treatment approaches that could improve overall outcomes. For instance, the POG 9421 study randomized patients after remission induction therapy to receive or not receive high-dose cyclosporine A (CsA) as an inhibitor of the MDR1 P-glycoprotein drug efflux pump. This type of targeted therapy did not, however, result in a prolongation of remission or an improvement in overall survival [14]. The CCG 2961 trial randomized the second course of consolidation therapy to either IdaDCTER/DCTER or fludarabine/cytarabine/idarubicin. No significant outcome differences were observed in EFS or OS [6]. The AML-BFM-1998 study prescribed a course of consolidation with high-dose ARAC and mitoxantrone (HAM) and showed a 92% OS and 84% EFS for patients with AML having a t(8;21) translocation. The subsequent AML-BFM-2004 study did not include this second HAM course and the OS (80%) was significantly lower as well as the EFS (59%). Of interest, these results did not hold true for patients with AML having an inv(16) good-risk rearrangement [34].

The introduction of more targeted approaches such as with GO have been randomized with conflicting results. For example, the MRC AML 15 trial tested whether GO given during remission induction and in postremission therapy improved outcomes [18]. The results demonstrated that there was no overall difference between the groups receiving or not receiving GO, with the exception of patients with favorable-risk AML who showed a statistically significant improvement in survival. There was borderline significant improvement in those with intermediate-risk AML and no advantage for patients with high-risk AML. One criticism of the results of this study was that the group of patients with favorable-risk AML who did not receive GO had a lower than expected overall survival. The ECOG 1900 trial randomized adult patients following remission induction to receive two courses of high-dose ARAC followed by either GO or autologous rescue. No significant difference was observed between the two groups, regardless of risk group classification [35]. A randomized study of postremission GO or no GO in adults over 60 years of age also showed no difference in any outcome measures [36]. The randomized SWOG study of GO versus no GO in adults with AML used an induction regimen of daunomycin, ARAC, and GO for one group and daunomycin plus ARAC for the second group. This study was closed early because no significant differences were observed in terms of CR and DFS as well as an increase in treatment-related mortality for the group receiving GO (ClinicalTrials.gov). The COG trial 0531 randomized GO during induction and in the postremission setting, but the results have not been reported.

Attempts have also been made to stimulate immune-mediated antileukemic effects. For example, the CCG 2961 trial randomized patients in the postremission setting to receive a relatively short course of interleukin (IL)-2 versus no IL-2 with no differences noted even though the group receiving IL-2 had biochemical responses [6, 37].

Ongoing efforts to improve postremission treatment for children with AML include strategies using tyrosine kinase inhibitors, demethylating agents, immunostimulation, and stem cell-directed therapies. The ability to target and follow minimal residual disease as well as understand the molecular changes that occur or are selected for during relapse provide additional grounds for optimism.

Hematopoietic stem cell transplantation

With improvement in the effectiveness of chemotherapeutic regimens, particularly for patients with favorable-risk AML, post-remission HSCT is no longer recommended. The use of allogeneic HSCT for patients with intermediate-risk AML is more controversial. An intention-to-treat analysis of approximately 470 young adults treated on the Bordeaux Grenoble Marseille Toulouse (BGMT) trial reported a significant survival advantage for patients with intermediate-risk AML who underwent matched family donor HSCT [38]. A retrospective analysis of pediatric trials, including POG 8821, CCG 2891, COG 2961 and MRC AML 10, suggested a benefit from matched family donor HSCT, but no benefit for patients with favorable-risk AML [39]. In both of the above analyses, there were too few patients with high-risk AML to make definitive

conclusions. The MRC AML 12 trial reported no advantage for patients with favorable- and intermediate-risk AML, but did observe a statistically significant benefit for 12% of patients with poor-risk AML [9]. In contrast, the MRC AML 15 trial has reported that 70% of patients with intermediate-risk AML can benefit from matched family donor HSCT; the 30% of these patients who showed no benefit had higher white blood cell counts, poor performance status, and secondary AML [18].

In the recently opened COG 1031 trial, the combination of cytogenetic, molecular and MRD is being used to define a low-risk group that includes AML with mutations of CBF, CEBPA and NPM as well as those with no MRD at the end of induction while a high-risk group (27% of all patients) includes patients with adverse karyotypic abnormalities, high FLT3-ITD to wild-type allelic ratio or MRD positivity at end of induction. Only patients in the high-risk group are stratified to receive an allogeneic HSCT from the best HLA match available donor.

It is quite clear that the benefit of HSCT depends on the classification of risk and likely on the underlying biology of particular AML subtypes. In addition, non-ablative HSCT regimens linked to immunostimulatory antileukemia strategies may provide future benefits to patients with high-risk disease.

Maintenance

Maintenance therapy is usually not a part of most pediatric AML studies because randomized trials have demonstrated no benefit for it in AML with currently used, intensive regimens. Several earlier studies, such as CCG 213 and LAME 91, showed not only no advantage to maintenance therapy, but rather reduced overall survival for those receiving maintenance treatment [8, 40, 41]. The BFM AML 87 trial, however, reported a benefit of maintenance therapy for low-risk patients not undergoing HSCT [4]. The BFM studies continue to prescribe maintenance therapy.

An exception to the lack of benefit of maintenance therapy in AML is that of APL for which maintenance therapy with ATRA plus or minus chemotherapy has been shown to significantly improve outcomes [25]. Of potential interest is a recent report of a randomized study in adults reporting that maintenance therapy does not improve EFS for patients with APL who achieve a complete molecular remission at the end of consolidation [42]. This question has not yet been evaluated in children.

Autologous stem cell transplantation

Several randomized studies have demonstrated no advantage of autologous HSCT compared to chemotherapy in pediatric patients with AML [16, 43, 44, 45]. However, such studies have reported equivalent results to chemotherapy, thus raising the issue that in some circumstances autologous HSCT could replace additional rounds of chemotherapy after remission induction and consolidation. Whether *ex vivo* selective leukaemia eradication from the autologous graft or post-transplant immunostimulatory antileukaemia could be of benefit remains to be seen.

The one application in which autologous HSCT should be considered is in relapsed APL. Several retrospective studies have reported similar 5-year EFS in patients with relapsed APL who underwent autologous versus allogeneic HSCT [46, 47]. Such improved survival is likely to be dependent on the patient and the stem cell autologous product being negative for the APL/RAF fusion transcript by sensitive polymerase chain reaction (PCR) methods [48].

Central nervous system prophylaxis

Optimal outcomes for patients with AML require eradication of all disease, including the central nervous system (CNS). And although CNS involvement at diagnosis is more common in AML than in acute lymphoblastic leukemia (ALL), it does not appear to have a significant impact on outcome, possibly due to the high doses of chemotherapy used such as ARAC. CNS involvement is also more common in patients with monocytic or myelomonocytic AML as well as those who have very high peripheral white blood cell counts [49, 50]. Although not tested in most studies using a randomized approach, most treatment regimens include several intrathecal doses of ARAC and/or methotrexate (MTX); CNS relapses occur in approximately 2–8% [7, 8, 13, 51, 52, 53]. The BFM AML 87 study did, however, randomize children without CNS disease at diagnosis to receive cranial radiation or no cranial radiation [4, 54]. A significant decrease in the 5-year cumulative incidence of systemic relapse was observed in the group that received cranial radiation. However, the randomization was stopped before the conclusion of the trial, and when an analysis of only the patients who underwent randomization was done, the difference in relapse risk was no longer significant. When the results of 1800 cGy on BFM AML 98 were compared to 1200 cGy on BFM 2004, no difference in CNS relapses was observed [55]. Thus, cranial radiation is no longer routinely used for CNS prophylaxis in the treatment of children with AML.

References

1 Pui CH *et al*. Biology, risk stratification, and therapy of pediatric acute leukemias: an update. *J Clin Oncol* 2011;**29**(5):551–65.

2 Buckley JD *et al*. Remission induction in children with acute non-lymphocytic leukemia using cytosine arabinoside and doxorubicin or daunorubicin: a report from the Children's Cancer Study Group. *Med Pediatr Oncol* 1989;**17**(5):382–90.

3 Yates J *et al*. Cytosine arabinoside with daunorubicin or Adriamycin for therapy of acute myelocytic leukemia: a CALGB study. *Blood* 1982;**60**(2):454–62.

4 Creutzig U *et al*. Treatment strategies and long-term results in paediatric patients treated in four consecutive AML-BFM trials. *Leukemia* 2005;**19**(12):2030–42.

5 Lange BJ *et al*. Pilot study of idarubicin-based intensive-timing induction therapy for children with previously untreated acute myeloid leukemia: Children's Cancer Group Study 2941. *J Clin Oncol* 2004;**22**(1):150–6.

6 Lange BJ *et al*. Outcomes in CCG-2961, a Children's Oncology Group phase 3 trial for untreated pediatric acute myeloid leukemia: a report from the Children's Oncology Group. *Blood* 2008;**111**(3):1044–53.

7 Lie SO *et al*. Long-term results in children with AML: NOPHO-AML Study Group – report of three consecutive trials. *Leukemia* 2005;**19**(12):2090–100.

8 Perel Y *et al*. Treatment of childhood acute myeloblastic leukemia: dose intensification improves outcome and maintenance therapy is of no benefit – multicenter studies of the French LAME (Leucemie Aigue Myeloblastique Enfant) Cooperative Group. *Leukemia* 2005;**19**(12):2082–9.

9 Burnett AK *et al*. Attempts to optimize induction and consolidation treatment in acute myeloid leukemia: results of the MRC AML12 trial. *J Clin Oncol* 2010;**28**(4):586–95.

10 Fernandez HF *et al*. Anthracycline dose intensification in acute myeloid leukemia. *N Engl J Med* 2009;**361**(13):1249–59.

11 Lowenberg B *et al*. High-dose daunorubicin in older patients with acute myeloid leukemia. *N Engl J Med* 2009;**361**(13):1235–48.

12 Ohtake S *et al*. Randomized study of induction therapy comparing standard-dose idarubicin with high-dose daunorubicin in adult patients with previously untreated acute myeloid leukemia: the JALSG AML 201 study. *Blood* 2011;**117**(8):2358–65.

13 Gibson BE *et al*. Treatment strategy and long-term results in paediatric patients treated in consecutive UK AML trials. *Leukemia* 2005;**19**(12):2130–8.

14 Becton D *et al.* Randomized use of cyclosporin A (CsA) to modulate P-glycoprotein in children with AML in remission: Pediatric Oncology Group study 9421. *Blood* 2006;**107**(4):1315–24.

15 Rubnitz JE *et al.* Minimal residual disease-directed therapy for childhood acute myeloid leukaemia: results of the AML 02 multicentre trial. *Lancet Oncol* 2010;**11**(6):543–52.

16 Hann IM *et al.* Randomized comparison of DAT versus ADE as induction chemotherapy in children and younger adults with acute myeloid leukemia. Results of the Medical Research Council's 10th AML trial (MRC AML10). Adult and Childhood Leukaemia Working Parties of the Medical Research Council. *Blood* 1997;**89**(7):2311–18.

17 Cooper TM *et al.* AAML03P1, a pilot study of the safety of gemtuzumab ozogamicin in combination with chemotherapy for newly diagnosed childhood acute myeloid leukemia: a report from the Children's Oncology Group. *Cancer* 2012;**118**(3):761–9.

18 Burnett AK *et al.* Identification of patients with acute myeloblastic leukemia who benefit from the addition of gemtuzumab ozogamicin: results of the MRC AML15 trial. *J Clin Oncol* 2011;**29**(4):369–77.

19 Heil G *et al.* A randomized, double-blind, placebo-controlled, phase III study of filgrastim in remission induction and consolidation therapy for adults with de novo acute myeloid leukemia. The International Acute Myeloid Leukemia Study Group. *Blood* 1997;**90**(12):4710–18.

20 Witz F *et al.* A placebo-controlled study of recombinant human granulocyte-macrophage colony-stimulating factor administered during and after induction treatment for de novo acute myelogenous leukemia in elderly patients. Groupe Ouest Est Leucemies Aigues Myeloblastiques (GOELAM). *Blood* 1998;**91**(8):2722–30.

21 Alonzo TA *et al.* Impact of granulocyte colony-stimulating factor use during induction for acute myelogenous leukemia in children: a report from the Children's Cancer Group. *J Pediatr Hematol Oncol* 2002;**24**(8):627–35.

22 Creutzig U *et al.* Less toxicity by optimizing chemotherapy, but not by addition of granulocyte colony-stimulating factor in children and adolescents with acute myeloid leukemia: results of AML-BFM 98. *J Clin Oncol* 2006;**24**(27):4499–506.

23 Lehrnbecher T *et al.* Prophylactic human granulocyte colony-stimulating factor after induction therapy in pediatric acute myeloid leukemia. *Blood* 2007;**109**(3):936–43.

24 Ehlers S *et al.* Granulocyte colony-stimulating factor (G-CSF) treatment of childhood acute myeloid leukemias that overexpress the differentiation-defective G-CSF receptor isoform IV is associated with a higher incidence of relapse. *J Clin Oncol* 2010;**28**(15):2591–7.

25 Fenaux P *et al.* A randomized comparison of all transretinoic acid (ATRA) followed by chemotherapy and ATRA plus chemotherapy and the role of maintenance therapy in newly diagnosed acute promyelocytic leukemia. The European APL Group. *Blood* 1999;**94**(4):1192–200.

26 Fenaux P *et al.* Long-term follow-up confirms the benefit of all-trans retinoic acid in acute promyelocytic leukemia. European APL group. *Leukemia* 2000;**14**(8):1371–7.

27 Tallman MS *et al.* All-trans-retinoic acid in acute promyelocytic leukemia. *N Engl J Med* 1997;**337**(15):1021–8.

28 Finizio O *et al.* Combination of all-trans-retinoic acid and gemtuzumab ozogamicin in an elderly patient with acute promyelocytic leukemia and severe cardiac failure. *Acta Haematol* 2007;**117**(3):188–90.

29 Aribi A *et al.* Combination therapy with arsenic trioxide, all-trans retinoic acid, and gemtuzumab ozogamicin in recurrent acute promyelocytic leukemia. *Cancer* 2007;**109**(7):1355–9.

30 Estey E *et al.* Use of all-trans retinoic acid plus arsenic trioxide as an alternative to chemotherapy in untreated acute promyelocytic leukemia. *Blood* 2006;**107**(9):3469–73.

31 Tallman MS *et al.* Clinical round table monograph. Early death in patients with acute promyelocytic leukemia. *Clin Adv Hematol Oncol* 2011;**9**(2):1–16.

32 O'Connell PA *et al.* Regulation of S100A10 by the PML-RAR-alpha oncoprotein. *Blood* 2011;**117**(15):4095–105.

33 Lange BJ *et al.* Outcomes in CCG-2961, a Children's Oncology Group phase 3 trial for untreated pediatric acute myeloid leukemia (AML): a report from the Children's Oncology Group. *Blood* 2008;**111**:1044–53.

34 Creutzig U *et al.* Second induction with high-dose cytarabine and mitoxantrone: different impact on pediatric AML patients with t(8;21) and with inv(16). *Blood* 2011;**118**(20):5409–15.

35 Fernandez HF *et al.* Autologous transplantation gives encouraging results for young adults with favorable-risk acute myeloid leukemia, but is not improved with gemtuzumab ozogamicin. *Blood* 2011;**117**(20):5306–13.

36 Lowenberg B *et al.* Gemtuzumab ozogamicin as postremission treatment in AML at 60 years of age or more: results of a multicenter phase 3 study. *Blood* 2010;**115**(13):2586–91.

37 Lange BJ *et al.* Soluble interleukin-2 receptor alpha activation in a Children's Oncology Group randomized trial of interleukin-2 therapy for pediatric acute myeloid leukemia. *Pediatr Blood Cancer* 2011;**57**(3):398–405.

38 Jourdan E *et al.* Early allogeneic transplantation favorably influences the outcome of adult patients suffering from acute myeloid leukemia. Societe Francaise de Greffe de Moelle (SFGM). *Bone Marrow Transplant* 1997;**19**(9):875–81.

39 Horan JT *et al.* Impact of disease risk on efficacy of matched related bone marrow transplantation for pediatric acute myeloid leukemia: the Children's Oncology Group. *J Clin Oncol* 2008;**26**(35):5797–801.

40 Wells RJ *et al.* Impact of high-dose cytarabine and asparaginase intensification on childhood acute myeloid leukemia: a report from the Children's Cancer Group. *J Clin Oncol* 1993;**11**(3):538–45.

41 Perel Y *et al.* Impact of addition of maintenance therapy to intensive induction and consolidation chemotherapy for childhood acute myeloblastic leukemia: results of a prospective randomized trial, LAME 89/91. Leucamie Aique Myeloide Enfant. *J Clin Oncol* 2002;**20**(12):2774–82.

42 Avvisati G *et al.* AIDA 0493 protocol for newly diagnosed acute promyelocytic leukemia: very long-term results and role of maintenance. *Blood* 2011;**117**(18):4716–25.

43 Woods WG *et al.* A comparison of allogeneic bone marrow transplantation, autologous bone marrow transplantation,

and aggressive chemotherapy in children with acute myeloid leukemia in remission: a report from the Children's Cancer Group. *Blood* 2001;**97**(1):56–62.

44 Ravindranath Y *et al.* Autologous bone marrow transplantation versus intensive consolidation chemotherapy for acute myeloid leukemia in childhood. Pediatric Oncology Group. *N Engl J Med* 1996;**334**(22):1428–34.

45 Woods WG *et al.* Intensively timed induction therapy followed by autologous or allogeneic bone marrow transplantation for children with acute myeloid leukemia or myelodysplastic syndrome: a Children's Cancer Group pilot study. *J Clin Oncol* 1993;**11**(8):1448–57.

46 Dvorak CC *et al.* Hematopoietic stem cell transplant for pediatric acute promyelocytic leukemia. *Biol Blood Marrow Transplant* 2008;**14**(7):824–30.

47 Bourquin JP *et al.* Favorable outcome of allogeneic hematopoietic stem cell transplantation for relapsed or refractory acute promyelocytic leukemia in childhood. *Bone Marrow Transplant* 2004;**34**(9):795–8.

48 De Botton S *et al.* Autologous and allogeneic stem-cell transplantation as salvage treatment of acute promyelocytic leukemia initially treated with all-trans-retinoic acid: a retrospective analysis of the European Acute Promyelocytic Leukemia Group. *J Clin Oncol* 2005;**23**(1):120–6.

49 Grier HE *et al.* Prognostic factors in childhood acute myelogenous leukemia. *J Clin Oncol* 1987;**5**(7):1026–32.

50 Pui CH *et al.* Central nervous system leukemia in children with acute nonlymphoblastic leukemia. *Blood* 1985;**66**(5):1062–7.

51 Creutzig U *et al.* Treatment strategies and long-term results in paediatric patients treated in four consecutive AML-BFM trials. *Leukemia* 2005;**19**(12):2030–42.

52 Smith FO *et al.* Long-term results of children with acute myeloid leukemia: a report of three consecutive Phase III trials by the Children's Cancer Group: CCG 251, CCG 213 and CCG 2891. *Leukemia* 2005;**19**(12):2054–62.

53 Ravindranath Y *et al.* Pediatric Oncology Group (POG) studies of acute myeloid leukemia (AML): a review of four consecutive childhood AML trials conducted between 1981 and 2000. *Leukemia* 2005;**19**(12):2101–16.

54 Creutzig U *et al.* Does cranial irradiation reduce the risk for bone marrow relapse in acute myelogenous leukemia? Unexpected results of the Childhood Acute Myelogenous Leukemia Study BFM-87. *J Clin Oncol* 1993;**11**(2):279–86.

55 Creutzig U *et al.* CNS irradiation in pediatric acute myeloid leukemia: equal results by 12 or 18 Gy in studies AML-BFM98 and 2004. *Pediatr Blood Cancer* 2011;**57**(6):986–92.

CHAPTER 13

Remission induction in acute myeloid leukemia

Ananth Shankar

University College London Hospitals NHS Foundation Trust, London, UK

Summary of previous studies

The improved survival outcome in children with acute myeloid leukemia (AML) can be linked to the progress made in the induction regimens used to improve remission rates. The Children's Cancer Study Group (CCSG) trial CCG 213 [1] that was conducted between January 1986 and February 1989 compared a standard remission induction regimen of cytosine arabinoside (ARAC) and daunorubicin (DNR) with a five-drug DCTER regimen comprising ARAC, DNR, etoposide (VP-16), dexamethasone (DEX), and thioguanine (TG). All patients below 22 years of age with a diagnosis of AML with the exception of children <2 years of age with acute monoblastic leukemia were enrolled on the trial. All patients were randomized at diagnosis to one of two induction regimens. Details of the randomization methodology were not provided in the report.

For regimen 1, the first cycle consisted of 7 days of continuous infusion of ARAC and bolus doses of DNR on the first 3 days of therapy. The second cycle was shortened to 5 days of ARAC and 2 days of DNR if bone marrow assessment after the first cycle showed <5% blasts; otherwise the second and/or the third cycle were identical to cycle 1. Regimen 2 consisted of the five-drug DCTER regimen. Depending on the response, two or three cycles were given. Patients initially randomized to regimen 1 crossed over to receive regimen 2 after two cycles if in remission or after three cycles irrespective of marrow status, and vice versa.

Central nervous system (CNS) prophylaxis consisted of intrathecal (IT) ARAC on the first day of each induction cycle and throughout the consolidation block (except during high-dose IV ARAC) for those not transplanted. Patients who had CNS disease at diagnosis received weekly IT ARAC during induction and monthly during consolidation. All patients who had HLA-matched donors were assigned to bone marrow transplantation if they were in remission (two or three cycles) or after two courses (five cycles) if they had <16% blasts in bone marrow.

Remission success was similar with both regimens. Five-year overall survival (OS) for patients in regimen 1 and 2 was 41% (95% confidence interval [CI] 35–47%) and 37% (95% CI 31–43%) respectively and 5-year event-free survival (EFS) rates was 32% (95% CI 26–38%) and 31% (95% CI 26–36%) respectively. However, patients in regimen 1 had a higher degree of bone marrow aplasia and deaths. Clearly, the addition of other chemotherapeutic agents to the standard regimen of ARAC and DNR did not improve OS or EFS in children and adolescents with AML.

In the subsequent CCG trial (CCG 2891) [2] that ran from October 1989 to May 1993, the five-drug DCTER regimen was adopted but patients were randomized to receive the courses at conventional intervals or more intensely to achieve faster bone marrow blast clearance. Patients younger than 21 years of age with AML were randomized at diagnosis to either the

Evidence-Based Pediatric Oncology, Third Edition. Edited by Ross Pinkerton, Ananth Shankar and Katherine K. Matthay.
© 2013 John Wiley & Sons, Ltd. Published 2013 by John Wiley & Sons, Ltd.

standard induction regimen or the intensive regimen. Both regimens used identical drugs and doses except that patients randomized to the intensive arm received the second cycle of DCTER 6 days after completion of cycle 1 irrespective of bone marrow or hematological status. Patients randomized to the standard arm underwent bone marrow reassessment on day 14 and proceeded to cycle 2 immediately if they had residual leukemia (>40% blasts). However, if leukemic clearance was satisfactory or if the bone marrow was hypoplastic, cycle 2 was withheld until blood counts recovered or there was clear evidence of disease progression. Patients who showed no response after two cycles were considered treatment failures and withdrawn from the trial. Standard timing was closed in May 1993 and granulocyte colony-stimulating factor (G-CSF) was introduced for all patients thereafter, during the induction phase. CNS prophylaxis consisted of four doses of IT ARAC administered at the start of each DCTER cycle. Patients who had CNS leukemia had an additional six doses of IT ARAC twice a week.

Of the 589 eligible patients, 294 were randomized to the standard induction arm and 295 to the intensive induction arm; 195/294 patients (70%) in the standard arm achieved a complete remission (CR) while 71 (26%) failed therapy and 11 (4%) died due to chemotherapy-related toxicity. For patients in the intensive induction arm, the CR rate, treatment failure rate and deaths due to chemotherapy toxicity were 75% (n=212/295), 14% (n=38) and 11% (n=31) respectively. Comparing the two induction arms, the failure rate was significantly higher in the standard induction arm (p=0.0003). The 3-year disease-free survival (DFS) from the end of induction for the intensive arm (n=212) patients was 55%±8% compared to 37%±8% (p=0.0002) for patients in the standard arm (n=195) and the actuarial survival at 3 years was 63%±9% versus 47%±9% (p=0.01) for the intensive and standard arm patients respectively. Myelosuppression was significantly higher for patients who received intensive induction than for those who received standard induction (43% versus 24%, p<0.00001), as was pulmonary, renal, hepatic, and gut toxicity. However, all deaths on both arms were related to either bleeding or infections. This landmark trial demonstrated that an intensively timed remission induction markedly improved DFS and OS in children and adolescents with AML.

The MRC AML 10 trial [3], which included both adults and children, involved slightly higher doses of DNR and more prolonged ARAC than used in the CCG trials and patients were randomized to receive either TG or VP-16 as the third drug. This intensive regimen was designed to achieve blast clearance after one course. CNS prophylaxis consisted of triple IT with ARAC, MTX, and hydrocortisone (HYSN), which was given as part of each course of treatment to a total of five. There was no significance difference in the CR rate between the DAT (81%; ARAC, DNR and TG) or the ADE (83%; ARAC, DNR and VP-16) arms and nor was there any difference in the number of courses needed to achieve CR. The percentages failing to achieve CR due to resistant disease were 11% with DAT versus 9% with ADE (p=0.07). DFS at 6 years from CR was 42% for DAT versus 43% for ADE (p=0.8); relapse rate at 6 years was 50% for DAT versus 49% for ADE (p=0.6) and OS from study entry for patients in the two arms was identical at 40% (±4%) at 6 years (p=0.9). Analysis of OS by AML FAB subtype did not show any difference between the two arms. Although hematological toxicity was higher with DAT, there was no difference in the induction death rates between DAT 8% and ADE 9% (p=0.9). This trial showed that both ADE and DAT regimens were equivalent with regard to efficacy and toxicity.

The Berlin-Frankfurt-Münster (BFM) 93 trial [4] compared two different anthracyclines (DNR and idarubicin) during remission induction therapy in childhood AML. Only children and adolescents (0–17 years) with previously untreated AML were entered on the study. Patients who had secondary AML, granulocytic sarcoma, myelodysplastic syndrome (MDS) or Down syndrome were excluded from the trial. All patients were randomized at diagnosis to an 8-day induction regimen with either ADE (ARAC on days 1 and 2, DNR on days 3–5, and VP-16 on days 6–8) or AIE (idarubicin on days 3–5, with ARAC and VP-16 as in the ADE regimen). High-risk patients were randomized to early HAM (high-dose IV ARAC and mitoxantrone followed by consolidation) or late HAM (consolidation followed by HAM).

All patients received consolidation therapy that consisted of 6 weeks of treatment with oral TG (days 1–43), oral prednisolone (days 1–28), IV vincristine (on days 1, 8, 15, 22), IV doxorubicin (days 1, 8, 15, 22),

IV ARAC (on days 3–6, 10–13, 17–20, 24–27, 31–34, and 38–41), IV cyclophosphamide (days 29 and 43) and IT ARAC on days 1, 15, 29, and 43. This was followed by intensification with high-dose ARAC and VP-16, 18 Gy cranial irradiation (in children >3 years) and maintenance therapy with oral TG and subcutaneous ARAC for a total of 18 months. Although patients who received idarubicin (IDA) during remission induction had a significantly better bone marrow blast cell reduction on day 15, 17% patients had >5% blasts compared to 31% on the DNR induction arm (p=0.01, X^2 test); the 5-year DFS and EFS rates were similar in both groups of patients. The infection rate was higher in the IDA arm (p trend =0.016), as was the duration of bone marrow aplasia that was 2 days longer. There was no evidence that IDA, despite its greater bone marrow blast clearance, improved the 5-year DFS or EFS in children with AML.

References

1 Wells RJ, Woods WG, Buckley JD et al. Treatment of newly diagnosed children and adolescents with acute myeloid leukemia: a Children's Cancer Group study. *J Clin Oncol* 1994;**12**:2367–77.

2 Woods WG, Kobrinsky N, Buckley JD et al. Timed-sequential induction therapy improves post remission outcome in acute myeloid leukemia: a report from the Children's Cancer Group. *Blood* 1996;**87**:4979–89.

3 Hann IM, Stevens RF, Goldstone AH et al. Randomized comparison of DAT versus ADE as induction chemotherapy in children and younger adults with acute myeloid leukemia. Results of the Medical Research Council's 10th AML trial (MRC AML10). Adult and Childhood Leukaemia Working Parties of the Medical Research Council. *Blood* 1997;**89**:2311–18.

4 Creutzig U, Ritter J, Zimmermann M et al. Improved treatment results in high-risk pediatric acute myeloid leukemia patients after intensification with high-dose cytarabine and mitoxantrone: results of Study Acute Myeloid Leukemia-Berlin-Frankfurt-Münster 93. *J Clin Oncol* 2001;**19**:2705–13.

New studies

Study 1

Lange BJ, Smith FO, Feusner J *et al*. Outcomes in CCG-2961, a Children's Oncology Group phase 3 trial for untreated pediatric acute myeloid leukemia: a report from the Children's Oncology Group. *Blood* 2008;111: 1044–53.

Objectives

The main aims of this study were:
- to compare the combination of fludarabine, cytarabine, and idarubicin (FAMP/AC/IDA) to a second course of the hybrid IdaDCTER/DCTER regimen in achieving a CR
- to determine whether the use of a single dose of interleukin (IL)-2 in patients with donors after consolidation with HIDAC (high-dose cytarabine and L-asparaginase) improved survival outcome.

Study design

Patients with *de novo* AML FAB subtypes M0–M2 and M4–M7 and who were <21 years at diagnosis were eligible for enrollment on the study. Patients with acute promyelocytic leukemia, juvenile myelomonocytic leukemia, Down syndrome, constitutional marrow failure syndromes, and treatment-related AML were excluded. Although patients who had myelodysplastic syndromes and granulocytic sarcoma were eligible for study enrollment, they were not included in this report. Patients who had <5% blasts on day 14±2 of induction received G-CSF till the neutrophil count (ANC) was >1×10^9/L. All who were in complete remission (<5% blasts with trilineage maturation) or partial remission (5–29% blasts with moderate hypocellularity with or without marrow recovery defined as ANC >1×10^9/L and platelets >100×10^9/L) after the IdaDCTER/DCTER remission induction therapy were eligible for randomization for course 2 that was either a repetition of course 1 or FAMP/AC/IDA. Patients who did not have a suitable donor were assigned to receive HIDAC and subsequently were randomized to rIL-2 or follow-up. CNS prophylaxis consisted of IT cytarabine or triple IT consisting of IT cytarabine, IT methotrexate, and IT hydrocortisone for patients who had persistent blasts in the cerebrospinal fluid (CSF) after the third lumbar puncture. After April 1998, drug doses of FAMP/AC/IDA and HIDAC were reduced in patients who had reduced renal function.

Statistics

The main outcome measures were remission status after courses 1 and 2, overall survival, event-free survival, disease-free survival, and treatment-related mortality. The study was designed to have 80% power to detect a 5% difference in remission rates between IdaDCTER and FAMP/AC/IDA intensification and to have an adequate power to detect a 10% difference in DFS in the patients randomized to IL-2 or follow-up. All analyses were based on an intention-to-treat principle. All data were analyzed that were collected up to October 30th 2006 and the median follow-up was 56 months. To compensate for early reporting of relapses and deaths, data were censored 6 months before the final analyses on October 30th 2006.

Results

Of the 901 patients enrolled on the study, only 738 patients underwent the first randomization (IdaDCTER; n=367: FAMP/AC/IDA; n=371), The 5-year DFS and OS rates in the randomized groups were 46%±5% and 59%±5% for the IdaDCTER group compared to 49%±5% (p=0.361) and 56%±6% (p=0.612) for the FAMP/AC/IDA group respectively. Although there were no differences in the EFS or OS rates between the two groups, patients in the FAMP/AC/IDA group had significantly fewer relapses but twice as many treatment-related deaths.

Of the 385 patients in continuous remission following HIDAC consolidation, 96 patients did not take part in the second randomization. Of the remaining 289 patients, 144 patients were randomized to receive IL-2 and 145 patients to follow-up alone without IL-2. Again, there was no significant difference in DFS or OS between the two groups. There was no treatment-related mortality (TRM) seen after IL-2.

Toxicity

Although the time to recovery of both neutrophils and platelets was significantly shorter in patients who received FAMP/AC/IDA, patients in this arm had significantly higher TRM that was attributed to bacterial infections. However, no excess of fungal- or viral-related deaths was seen in patients who received FAMP/AC/IDA.

Conclusions

It was concluded that although patients who received the FAMP/AC/IDA regimen had a lower incidence of relapses, this did not result in a better survival outcome because of higher TRM. Secondly, the use of IL-2 given in the dose and schedule of this study did not improve disease-free or overall survival.

Study 2

Rubnitz JE, Crews KR, Pounds S *et al*. Combination of cladribine and cytarabine is effective for childhood acute myeloid leukemia: results of the St Jude AML 97 trial. *Leukemia* 2009;23:1410–16.

Objectives

The main aim of this upfront window study was to determine whether combining cladribine (CLDB) with cytarabine (ARAC) would improve therapeutic efficacy by increasing intracellular ara-CTP levels and thereby improve survival outcome of children with acute myeloid leukemia.

Study design

The St Jude AML 97 trial was a prospective randomized upfront window study that ran from March 1997 to June 2002 and included children below 22 years with previously untreated AML except those with acute promyelocytic leukemia.

Patients were randomly assigned to receive either a daily short infusion of ARAC (arm A) or a continuous ARAC infusion (arm B). Patients in arm A received ARAC as a 2-h infusion (500 mg/m²/day) and CLDB as a 30 min infusion (9 mg/m²/day) for 5 days that began 24 h after the start of the first ARAC infusion. There was a 2-h interval between the end of each CLDB infusion and commencement of the next ARAC infusion. Arm B patients received ARAC (500 mg/m²/day)

as a 120-h continuous infusion and five daily 30-min CLDB infusions (9 mg/m²/day) which began 24 h after the start of the continuous ARAC infusion.

This was followed by two identical courses of induction chemotherapy (DAV1 and DAV2) consisting of daunorubicin (30 mg/m²/day as a continuous infusion on days 1–3), ARAC (250 mg/m²/day as a continuous infusion on days 1–5) and etoposide (200 mg/m² as continuous infusion on days 4 and 5). Response to the CLDB/ARAC treatment was assessed by a bone marrow examination on day 15 from start of treatment. Complete remission was defined as trilineage recovery with <5% blasts in the bone marrow (BM), platelet count >30 × 10⁹/L and neutrophil count >0.3 × 10⁹/L. Patients who had persistent disease on day 15 BM started DAV1 immediately. High-risk patients (megakaryoblastic AML, RAEB-T, secondary AML, patients with persistent AML after DAV1, etc.) were eligible for allogeneic stem cell transplantation (allo-HSCT) after DAV2. Low-risk patients (t (8;21) inv16) were not eligible for allo-HSCT. All other patients (standard risk) were eligible for HSCT if a matched sibling donor was available. Between March 1997 and January 1999, patients not receiving allo-HSCT underwent autologous stem cell transplantation (auto-HSCT) after a busulphan and cyclophosphamide-conditioning regime. In January 1999, auto-HSCT was replaced with two further consolidation courses consisting of high-dose ARAC (3 g/m² 12 hourly on days 1, 2, 8, 9) and L-asparaginase (6000 U/m²/dose after the fourth and eighth doses of ARAC) followed by mitoxantrone (10 mg/m²/day on days 1–5) and ARAC (1 g/m² 12 hourly on days 1–3). CNS prophylaxis consisted of monthly doses of age-adjusted triple IT chemotherapy: ARAC, MTX, and hydrocortisone (TIT) for 4 months. Patients with CNS leukemia had weekly TIT until the CSF was clear and then monthly doses of TIT for 4 months.

Statistics

The primary objective was to compare intracellular ara-CTP concentration in leukemic blasts after CLDB administration to that before CLDB administration across the two arms. Although it was initially planned to recruit 80 eligible patients with evaluable ara-CTP concentrations, this was later revised to 52 patients per arm to give 80% power and an overall type 1 error rate of 5%. The Kaplan–Meier method was used to calculate event-free and overall survival and the log-rank test was used to make comparisons of EFS and OS distributions.

Results

Of the 102 randomized patients, 50 patients were assigned to arm A and 46 to arm B (six declined to participate). Intracellular ara-CTP levels increased significantly from day 1 to day 2 (p=0.0002).

Ninety-six percent (44/46) of patients in arm B achieved a CR after only one course each of the upfront CLDB/ARAC and DAV induction compared to 76% (38/50) in arm A. Although the median blast percentage at day 15 did not differ between the two groups of patients, patients in arm A had a shorter interval to start induction course DAV1 than those in arm B (arm A 18 days versus 25 days in arm B; p=0.008).

Among all randomized patients, 76% of patients (n=13/17) with monoblastic AML (FAB M5) achieved a CR after window therapy compared to 49% (38/77) of non-FAB M5 patients (p=0.059). The results were even more striking amongst randomized *de novo* AML patients: 85% (n=11/13) versus 50% (n=32/64) (p=0.031).

Survival outcome

Although the two groups did not differ significantly with respect to minimal residual disease levels, EFS or OS, there was a trend towards better OS among patients in arm B than arm A (5-year OS 60.9%±7.2% versus 40.0%±6.8%; p=0.069).

Effects of amendments

Overall, there were no statistically significant differences in the EFS or OS between those treated before and after the protocol amendments. Within each arm, there were no significant differences in the pre- and post-amendment cohorts with respect to sex, age, cytogenetics, CNS involvement, initial white blood cell count or FAB subtype.

Toxicity

More patients in arm B experienced grade 3 or 4 toxicity with the upfront window therapy compared to patients in arm A (48% versus 24%; p=0.019). The two arms did not differ significantly in the number of patients experiencing toxicity during DAV1 and DAV2.

Conclusions

It was concluded that cladiribine infusion increased intracellular ara-CTP levels significantly and that cladribine combination with continuous infusion of ARAC is effective therapy for children with AML.

Study 3

Rubnitz JE, Inaba H, Dahl G *et al*. Minimal residual disease-directed therapy for childhood acute myeloid leukaemia: results of the AML 02 multicentre trial. *Lancet Oncol* 2010;**11**:543–52.

Objectives

The primary purpose of this trial was to determine whether the use of high-dose cytarabine during induction treatment in children with AML reduces the incidence of MRD positivity and thereby improves survival outcome.

Study design

The AML 02 was a prospective multicenter randomized study conducted between October 2002 and June 2008 and included patients with *de novo* AML (n=206), therapy-related or myelodysplastic-related AML (n=12) or mixed lineage leukemia (n=14). Age at diagnosis ranged from 2 days to 21.4 years. Patients with acute promyelocytic leukemia or Down syndrome were excluded. Zelen block randomization method with a block size of 6 was used to assign patients to high-dose (HD) or low-dose (LD) ARAC. Although treatment assignments were concealed until needed for the next enrolled patient, there was no masking as treatment assignments were revealed to physicians, participants, and data analysts.

Patients were randomly assigned to receive daunorubicin (50 mg/m^2 IV on days 2, 4 and 6) and etoposide (100 mg/m^2 IV on days 2–6) and either HD ARAC (3 g/m^2 IV 12 hourly on days 1, 3 and 5) or LD ARAC (100 mg/m^2 IV 12 hourly on days 1–10) during the first induction block. Bone marrow was reassessed for treatment response on day 22 and those with ≥1% blasts commenced the second induction block immediately whilst those patients who had <1% blasts commenced the second induction block on blood count recovery. During the second induction block, all patients received

LD ARAC, daunorubicin and etoposide (ADE) with or without gemtuzumab ozogamicin (GO). Patients with MRD ≥0.1% after induction block 2 received GO as induction 3. From February 2005, GO was given along with ADE in induction 2 to all patients with MRD ≥1% after the first induction block. The subsequent consolidation therapy was based on initial risk assessment and treatment response. Low-risk patients received three courses of ARAC-based chemotherapy while high-risk patients (> 25% blasts after induction 1 or persistent MRD positivity after three courses of treatment) were eligible for stem cell transplantation. All other patients were classified as standard risk and were eligible to receive HSCT only if they had a matched sibling donor. CNS prophylaxis consisted in total of five dose of IT ARAC; one dose at the start of each course of treatment. Those who had CNS disease at diagnosis received weekly IT ARAC until the CSF was clear (minimum four doses) and then four additional doses. From July 2003, IT ARAC was replaced with IT methotrexate, hydrocortisone and ARAC (triple IT therapy).

Statistics

The main aim of the trial was to compare the incidence of MRD positivity (MRD ≥0.1% on day 22 of induction) in patients randomized to HD ARAC versus LD ARAC based on the O'Brien–Fleming group sequential method of comparing two binomial distributions. The design specified enrollment of 186 patients evaluable for MRD and included four interim analyses and one final analysis. At a significance level of 5%, the study provided an overall power of 80% for a two-sided test to detect a difference of 20% between the two groups, assuming one group had an MRD-negative rate of 50%.

Results

Of the 232 eligible patients enrolled in the study, 230 were randomized to receive HD ARAC (n=113) or LD ARAC (n=117). Two patients were not randomized because of physician choice or parental refusal. Presenting features were similar in the two groups except that patients in the LD ARAC group had a greater proportion of patients with higher white blood cell count and a normal karyotype.

On day 22 of the first induction block, there was no significant difference in MRD positivity between the patients given HD ARAC and LD ARAC (34% versus

42%; p=0.17). The result was similar when the analysis was limited to patients who had *de novo* AML (33% versus 40%; p=0.22). Likewise, there was no difference in MRD positivity when analysis was repeated according to risk group categorization based on presenting features: low-risk group (12% in the HD ARAC group versus 14% in the LD ARAC group; p=1.0), standard-risk group (33% versus 40%; p=0.62) and high-risk group (53% versus 68%; p=0.31).

Patients randomized to either HD ARAC or LD ARAC during induction 1 had similar event-free survival rates (60.2% versus 65.7%; p=0.41), overall survival rates (68.8% versus 73.4%; p=0.41), cumulative incidence of relapse (17.5 versus 21.5; p=0.50) and cumulative incidence of death unrelated to relapse (11.9 versus 5.5; p=0.13) at 3 years. Similarly, when analyses were done within each risk category, there were no differences in EFS or OS between the two groups of patients.

Toxicity

Patients in the HD ARAC group had higher cumulative incidence of grade 2 or higher fungal infections (23.6%, standard error [SE] 4.2 versus 13.6%, SE 3.3; p=0.058) at 6 months. However, there were no differences in the incidence of grade 3 or higher toxicities during induction block 1 or in the cumulative incidence of bacterial infections between the two groups.

Conclusions

It was concluded that the use of high-dose cytarabine during the first induction block did not significantly lower the rate of MRD positivity and also did not improve event-free or overall survival rates.

Study 4

Gregory J, Kim H, Alonzo T *et al.* Treatment of children with acute promyelocytic leukemia: results of the first North American Intergroup trial INT0129. *Pediatr Blood Cancer* 2009;53:1005–10.

Objectives

To compare the complete remission rates, DFS and OS and toxicity of treatment with ATRA versus conventional chemotherapy during remission induction and/or maintenance phase treatment in children with previously untreated acute promyelocytic leukemia (APL).

Study design

This was a multicenter randomized trial that ran between April 1992 and February 1995. Eligibility criteria included age 0–18 years, a diagnosis of APL based on BM morphology, no previous chemotherapy except hydroxyurea, normal hepatic and renal function and an Eastern Co-operative Oncology Group performance status of 0 (normal activity) to 3 (bedridden >50% of the time). Cytogenetic evaluation of t(15;17) was mandatory although results did not affect participation in the study. However, patients without documentation of t(15;17) were not included in this report.

Patients were randomly assigned to receive either daunorubicin (45 mg/m^2 on days 1–3) plus cytarabine (ARAC 100 mg/m^2/day on days 1–7) or ATRA (45 mg/m^2/day until complete remission or to maximum of 90 days). For patients assigned to cytotoxic chemotherapy, a second induction cycle was with identical doses was given if day 14 BM had >50% abnormal promyelocytes or if disseminated intravascular coagulation was continuing. Patients who did not tolerate ATRA or who did not achieve CR by day 90 were switched to the cytotoxic chemotherapy arm. Patients who did not achieve a CR after two cycles of chemotherapy were deemed failures and were treated off protocol. No central nervous system prophylaxis was given in this study.

Consolidation

Patients in CR after cytotoxic chemotherapy or ARTA received two cycles of consolidation chemotherapy; the first cycle was identical to the induction chemotherapy and the second cycle included high-dose ARAC (2 g/m^2/dose 12 hourly on days 1–4) and daunorubicin (DNR; 45 mg/m^2 on days 1–2).

Maintenance therapy

Children in CR after both cycles of consolidation chemotherapy irrespective of the induction therapy were randomly assigned to a year of maintenance ATRA or to observation. Patients who were intolerant of ATRA at induction were directly assigned to observation.

If the white blood cell count (WBC) at diagnosis in patients randomized to ATRA was $\geq 10 \times 10^9$/L,

hydroxyurea was commenced at a dose 1 g/m2 q6h until the WBC count was $\leq 10 \times 10^9$/L, at which time ATRA was commenced. If during ATRA treatment the WBC rose to $>30 \times 10^9$/L, ATRA was interrupted and hydroxyurea commenced till the WBC count became $\leq 10 \times 10^9$/L before resuming ATRA.

Statistics

Two-sided Fisher's exact test was used for 2×2 table analysis and a two-sided Wilcoxon -rank-sum test was used for a two-sample comparison of continuous variables. OS and DFS were calculated using the Kaplan–Meier method and the life table curves were compared using log-rank tests.

Results

Fifty-three patients were included in the study, of whom 26 were randomly assigned to the chemotherapy arm and 27 to the ATRA arm. Patients in the ATRA arm had a higher CR rate than those who were treated with DNR and ARAC (22/27; 81% [ATRA] versus 17/26; 65% [DNR/ARAC]; p=0.22).

There were five induction failures in the ATRA arm (four had ATRA intolerance; one early death) compared to nine induction failures in the chemotherapy arm (six patients had resistant disease; three early deaths). All four patients who had ATRA intolerance crossed over to the chemotherapy arm and achieved CR.

Maintenance therapy

Ten patients were not randomized because of resistant disease or early deaths. An additional seven patients were not randomized and the reason was not clear in the report. Of the remaining 36 patients, 18 each were randomly assigned to ATRA maintenance or observation only.

Survival outcome

The 5-year DFS from time of CR for the ATRA and chemotherapy arms were 49%±10% versus 29%±11% (p=0.16) respectively. The 10-year DFS from the time of CR was identical to the 5-year DFS rates. The 5-year DFS from the start of maintenance for the ATRA and observation arms were 61%±11% and 15%±9% (p=0.0002) respectively.

The 5-year DFS from time of CR for the 36 patients who underwent randomization to ATRA versus observation were as follows: 0% for the DNR/ARAC and observation arm; 56%±17% in the DNR/ARAC+ATRA arm; 24%±14% in the ATRA and observation arm; and 67%±16% in the ATRA+ATRA arm (p<0.001). The 5-year DFS from time of CR for the 29 patients who were randomized to ATRA for induction or maintenance or both was 48%±9% compared to 0% for patients who never received ATRA (n=7; p<0.0001).

The 5-year OS for all patients was 69%±6%. When considering OS according to treatment arm, the 10-year OS for the ATRA and chemotherapy induction arms were 69%±9% and 57%±10% respectively (p=0.35). OS was also calculated for the 36 patients who were randomized to ATRA maintenance versus observation only. The 5-year OS rates for each of the four possible treatment combinations when considering induction and maintenance randomizations were 57%±19% in the DNR/ARAC+observation arm, 89%±10% in the DNR/ARAC+ATRA arm, 73%±13% in the ATRA+observation arm and 78%±14% in the ATRA+ATRA arm (p=0.29). The 5-year OS for patients who were randomized to ATRA at induction or maintenance or both (n=29) was 79%±8% versus 57%±19% who never received ATRA (n=7; p=0.07).

Conclusions

It was concluded that ATRA treatment significantly improved disease-free survival in children with acute promyelocytic leukemia.

CHAPTER 14

Acute myeloid leukemia consolidation

Ananth Shankar

University College London Hospitals NHS Foundation Trust, London, UK

New study

Study 1

Becton D, Dahl GV, Ravindranath Y *et al.*, for the Pediatric Oncology Group. Randomized use of cyclosporin A (CsA) to modulate P-glycoprotein in children with AML in remission: Pediatric Oncology Group Study 9421. *Blood* 2006;**107**:1315–24.

Objectives

To determine whether interference of the P-glycoprotein mediated drug efflux mechanism by the addition of cyclosporine A (CsA) to consolidation chemotherapy in children with acute myeloid leukaemia will prolong remission and improve overall outcome.

Study design

The Pediatric Oncology Group (POG) trial 9421 was a prospective randomized study conducted between February 1995 and August 1999. All patients with *de novo* acute myeloid leukemia (AML) of any subtype except FAB M3 subtype below 21 years of age were eligible for study enrollment. Other exclusions included secondary AML or prior diagnosis of a myelodysplastic syndrome. Although patients with Down syndrome were eligible for study entry as long as they were registered on the POG 9841 trial, they did not receive CsA during the consolidation block. Randomization for both the induction (standard dose cytarabine combined with daunomycin and thioguanine [DAT] versus high dose cytarabine, daunomycin and thioguanine

[HDAT]; DAT plus high-dose cytosine arabinoside [ARAC]) and consolidation blocks (with or without CsA) was done at trial registration. This report only describes the primary results of the POG 9421 AML study.

Induction 1 and 2

Patients were randomly assigned to standard DAT, treatment arms 1, 2, and 5 (daunorubicin 45 mg/m²/day IV days 1–3, cytarabine 100 mg/m²/day as a continuous IV infusion on days 1–7 and thioguanine 100 mg/m²/day orally on days 1–7) or HDAT, treatment arms 3 and 4 (identical doses of daunorubicin and thioguanine but cytarabine 1 g/m2/dose every 12 h on days 1–7). Patients underwent a bone marrow examination on day 15 and if blasts were <10%, commenced second induction on recovery of blood counts. Patients with residual leukemia, i.e. >10% blasts on day 15, commenced second induction immediately. Induction 2 was identical for both groups and consisted of high-dose cytarabine 1 g/m²/dose 12 hourly for 5 days.

Consolidation block

Patients without matched sibling donors received three consolidation blocks. Children randomized to treatment arms 1 (DAT), 3 (HDAT) or 5 (DAT) received etoposide 100 mg/m²/day IV on days 1–5 and mitoxantrone 10 mg/m²/day IV on days 1–4 and intrathecal cytarabine 40 mg/m² on day 1 whilst patients randomized to treatment

Evidence-Based Pediatric Oncology, Third Edition. Edited by Ross Pinkerton, Ananth Shankar and Katherine K. Matthay.
© 2013 John Wiley & Sons, Ltd. Published 2013 by John Wiley & Sons, Ltd.

arms 2 (DAT) and 4 (HDAT) received a reduced dose of etoposide (60mg/m^2/day IV on days 1–5) and mitoxantrone (6mg/m^2/day IV on days 1–4).

Cyclosporine randomization

Patients randomized to receive CsA (treatment arms 2 and 4) received it as a 2-h infusion (10 mg/kg) 2 h prior to first chemotherapy dose followed by continuous infusion of CsA 30 mg/kg/day for 98 h (total 100 h of CsA infusion). The aim was to achieve a steady-state serum CsA concentration of 3000–5000 ng/mL.

All patients received consolidation block 2 that was identical to induction block 2.

Statistics

With the designated sample of 560 patients and a power of 80% at a one-sided significance level of 0.05%, the study investigators were able to detect a difference of 13% (45% versus 58%) at 2 years after start of remission between patients who received consolidation with CsA and patients who received no CsA. DFS, EFS, and OS rates were calculated according to the Kaplan–Meier methods and findings were tested for significance by the log-rank test. The difference in remission rate was tested by the chi square test. All reported p-values were two-sided.

Results

Of the 565 eligible patients without Down syndrome, 83 children underwent protocol-directed bone marrow

transplantation. The 3-year DFS rates for patients in remission randomized to receive CsA (n = 209) was 40.6%±3.6% versus 33.9%±3.5% for patients randomized to the no CsA arm (n = 209; p = 0.24).

The estimated 3-year DFS rates for patients in arms 1, 2, 3, and 4 were 27.2%±4.6%, 41.1%±5.2%, 40.5%±5.1%, and 40.2%±5% respectively.

For the 418 patients who achieved CR and went on to consolidation with or without CsA, the 3-year DFS rates were 40.6% ± 3.6% and 33.9% ± 3.5% respectively (p=0.24).

Toxicity

Patients who were randomized to receive CsA had a higher incidence of hyperbilirubinemia, stomatitis, renal impairment ,and hypertension. Six patients randomized to receive CsA did not receive the drug with their final consolidation block because of persistent renal insufficiency (n = 2) or allergic reactions (n = 4).

Cyclosporine concentrations

Infants and young children frequently required 1–3 increments of 25% in the CsA infusions to maintain CsA concentrations >3000 ng/mL whereas teenagers required a temporary cessation of CsA infusion and resumption at a 25–50% lower rate.

Conclusions

It was concluded that the addition of cyclosporine A to consolidation chemotherapy did not prolong remission or improve overall survival in children with AML.

CHAPTER 15

Maintenance treatment in acute myeloid leukemia

Ananth Shankar

University College London Hospitals NHS Foundation Trust, London, UK

Summary of previous studies

The use of postremission low-dose maintenance treatment (MT) in childhood acute myeloid leukemia (AML) has yielded mixed results. The studies by Perel *et al.* [1] and Wells *et al.* [2] suggest that MT does not appear to improve overall survival (OS).

The Perel *et al.* study was a multicenter randomized trial conducted between December 1998 and June 1996. Previously untreated children and adolescents with AML with FAB subtypes M1–M6 were included in the trial. All patients with secondary AML, Down syndrome, and biphenotypic leukemia as well as those with FAB subtypes M0 and M7 were excluded from the trial. Remission induction (RI) consisted of 7 days of continuous IV infusion of cytosine arabinoside (ARAC) and 5 days of IV mitoxantrone. Children <1 year received two-thirds of these doses. Patients who had >20% blasts on day 20 bone marrow (BM) received a second continuous IV infusion of ARAC for 3 days and mitoxantrone (MTXN) for 2 days. All patients who achieved complete remission (CR) and had a human leukocyte antigen (HLA) identical family donor underwent allogeneic bone marrow transplantation (allo-BMT). Patients with no matched donors received two courses of consolidation therapy. The first consolidation block consisted of 4 days each of IV etoposide (VP-16) and IV ARAC as a continuous infusion and IV daunorubicin. The second consolidation course comprised two cycles

of IV ARAC infusions plus L-asparaginase administered 7 days apart. All patients >1 year of age also received amsacrine on days 4–6 between the two cycles of ARAC. MT commenced after the second consolidation course and consisted of daily oral 6-mercaptopurine and subcutaneous ARAC for 18 months.

In March 1991, children still in CR after the second consolidation course were randomized to either stop or continue MT for 18 months. Comparing the disease-free survival (DFS) and OS for the randomized patients, the 6-year DFS was 50%±15% for patients assigned to MT versus 60%±19% in the stop arm (p=0.25) while the 6-year OS was 58%±15% in the MT arm versus 81%±13% in the stop arm (p=0.04). When DFS and OS were compared for the whole group (including randomized and nonrandomized patients), patients who received MT had a poorer outcome (MT- DFS 50%±11% versus 63%±12% stop arm, p=0.48; and MT-OS 59%±11% versus 73%±11% stop arm; p=0.08). The probability of achieving a second CR was significantly higher for MT-negative patients than for MT-positive patients (19 of 28 versus 14 of 34; p=0.04). Exposure to maintenance may contribute to clinical drug resistance and treatment failure in patients who experience a relapse.

The CCG 213 trial [2] that ran from January 1986 to February 1989 included all patients <22 years of

---

Evidence-Based Pediatric Oncology, Third Edition. Edited by Ross Pinkerton, Ananth Shankar and Katherine K. Matthay.
© 2013 John Wiley & Sons, Ltd. Published 2013 by John Wiley & Sons, Ltd.

age with a diagnosis of AML except those <2 years of age with acute monoblastic AML. Patients not assigned to BMT received postinduction consolidation. Following consolidation, patients were randomized to receive MT or stop treatment. MT was identical to the second consolidation course and continued for 18 months.

Of the 225 patients who completed consolidation and were eligible for randomization, only 140 were randomized (MT 67, stop treatment 73). The 5-year OS and DFS for the MT group were 46% (95% confidence interval [CI] 33–59%) and 42% (95% CI 30–54%) respectively compared to 68% (95% CI 57–79%; p=0.01) and 52% (95% CI 40–64%; p=0.12) respectively for the stop treatment group. In all comparisons (i.e. randomized, nonrandomized and as treatment received), survival outcome was inferior for patients who received MT. Evidently, maintenance therapy in children and adolescents with AML was not beneficial.

The APL 93 trial [3] was a randomized European study (April 1993–October 1998) evaluating postremission therapy for patients with acute promyelocytic leukemia (APL). The main objectives of this trial were to determine the optimal timing of all-trans-retinoic acid (ATRA) treatment in childhood APL and its role during MT in APL. All patients with APL younger than 18 years were included in the trial. Patients were randomized at diagnosis to either an induction regimen of oral ATRA treatment followed by sequential chemotherapy (CT) (ATRA–CT) or ATRA+CT. In the former group, patients received oral ATRA till CR was achieved or a maximum of 90 days. Following CR, all patients received IV daunorubicin (DNR) along with continuous IV infusion of ARAC for 7 days (course 1). If the white blood cell (WBC) count rose rapidly during ATRA-only treatment, CT was commenced immediately. Patients randomized to ATRA+CT received the same dose of ATRA with identical CT that commenced on day 3 of ATRA treatment. Patients with a presenting WBC count $>5 \times 10^9$/L were not randomized but received ATRA+CT from day 1. Patients in CR after course 1 received two consolidation courses of CT; course 2 was identical to course 1 and course 3 consisted of DNR and ARAC 12 hourly×4 days. Patients in CR at the end of the consolidation phase were randomized to one of four postconsolidation arms: (1) no MT, (2) intermittent oral ATRA for 15 days every 3 months,

(3) daily oral 6-mercaptopurine plus weekly oral methotrexate or (4) CT+ATRA. Randomization for MT was done according to 2×2 factorial design stratified by initial induction therapy. Total duration of maintenance therapy was 2 years.

Of the 27 patients eligible for the MT randomization, only 21 were randomized (no MT 2, ATRA alone 6, CT alone 6, ATRA+CT 7). None of the seven patients in the ATRA+CT group relapsed but one in the no MT group and two in the ATRA alone group relapsed. Although no firm conclusions can be drawn from the randomized comparisons due to small patient numbers, the trial seemed to suggest that ATRA+CT during MT in children with APL improved survival outcome.

A later study, the GIMEMA-AIEOPAIDA trial [4], also evaluated the benefit of MT in childhood AML. The study population included all patients over the age of 1 year with newly diagnosed APL confirmed by either molecular genetics or cytogenetic evidence of PML-RARA fusion. Remission induction consisted of oral ATRA combined with IV infusion of IDA on days 2, 4, 6, and 8. ATRA was continued until hematological remission (HCR) was achieved or for a maximum of 90 days. All patients who were in HCR received three consolidation courses of IV infusion of ARAC on days 1–4 with IV IDA on days 1–4 (course 1); IV mitoxantrone on days 1–5 and IV VP-16 on days 1–5 (course 2); IV IDA on day 1, ARAC subcutaneously on days 1–6 and thioguanine (TG) on days 1–5 (course 3). Patients in molecular remission (polymerase chain reaction [PCR] negative for PML-RARA transcript) after the third consolidation course were randomized to one of four MT arms: (1) daily oral 6-mercaptopurine with weekly IM methotrexate; (2) ATRA for 15 days every 3 months; (3) arm 1 for 3 months followed by arm 2 for 15 days; and (4) no MT. From April 1997, randomization to arms 1 and 4 was closed and all subsequent randomizations were to either arm 2 or 3. The total duration of MT was 2 years. No patient received CNS prophylaxis. Patients who had persistent disease at the molecular level at the end of consolidation were eligible for allogeneic or autologous BMT.

Of the 91 children who were PCR negative at the end of consolidation (PML-RARA transcript negative), only 85 underwent randomization, of whom 31 were randomized to ATRA+CT and 32 to ATRA alone (as randomization was closed early, comparison was not possible between the four MT arms). The DFS for children randomized to the ATRA+CT arm was significantly better than the ATRA alone arm (77% versus 42%; p=0.01). Once again, MT with ATRA combined with CT improved survival outcome in children with APL although no conclusion can be drawn on the advantage of MT in APL due to early closure of the control arm.

References

1 Perel Y, Auvrignon A, Leblanc T *et al.*, for the Group LAME of the French Society of Pediatric Hematology and Immunology. Impact of addition of maintenance therapy to intensive induction and consolidation chemotherapy for childhood acute myeloblastic leukemia: results of a prospective randomized trial, LAME 89/91. Leucámie Aigüe Myéloïde Enfant. *J Clin Oncol* 2002;**2**:2774–82.

2 Wells RJ, Woods WG, Buckley JD *et al.* Treatment of newly diagnosed children and adolescents with acute myeloid leukemia: a Children's Cancer Group study. *J Clin Oncol* 1994;**12**:2367–77.

3 De Botton S, Coiteux V, Chevret S *et al.* Outcome of childhood acute promyelocytic leukemia with all-trans-retinoic acid and chemotherapy. *J Clin Oncol* 2004;**22**:1404–12.

4 Testi AM, Biondi A, Lo Coco F *et al.* GIMEMA-AIEOPAIDA protocol for the treatment of newly diagnosed acute promyelocytic leukemia (APL) in children. *Blood* 2005;**106**:447–53.

New studies

The authors have been unable to identify any new randomized trials regarding maintenance treatment in acute myeloid leukemia in children published since the previous edition of this book.

CHAPTER 16

Autologous bone marrow transplantation in acute myeloid leukemia

Ananth Shankar

University College London Hospitals NHS Foundation Trust, London, UK

Summary of previous studies

As the most effective consolidation therapy for children in first complete remission of acute myeloid leukemia (AML) remained contentious, the Associazione Italiana Ematologia and Oncologia Pediatrica (AIEOP) Co-operative Group Trial [1] was seminal in defining the role of autologous bone marrow transplantation (ABMT) in first remission in children with AML. Children <15 years of age with previously untreated AML, except those with Down syndrome, secondary AML or AML that developed on a background of myelodysplasia, were included in the study. Induction therapy consisted of 7 days of continuous infusion of cytosine arabinoside (ARAC) and 3 days of daunorubicin (DNR) infusion. If the day 21 bone marrow (BM) showed residual leukemia, a second course of ARAC and DNR was administered, otherwise the second course was delayed until recovery of peripheral blood counts. Consolidation of remission was with the DAT regimen (DNR IV on day 1, ARAC subcutaneously×5 days and oral thioguanine×5 days). Children without a matched sibling donor were randomized to ABMT or six courses of postremission chemotherapy. All randomized patients received a second course of DAT prior to ABMT or postremission chemotherapy. Seventy-two children were randomized to either ABMT (n=35) or postremission chemotherapy (n=37). The 5-year disease-free survival for the ABMT group was 21% (standard error [SE] 8%) compared to 27% (SE 8%) for the postremission chemotherapy group. ABMT was clearly shown as not being superior to postremission chemotherapy in improving disease-free survival outcome in children with AML.

The Pediatric Oncology Group (POG) trial [2] also focused on the same issue of whether ABMT offered any benefit for children with AML. In this study, all eligible patients <21 years of age with previously untreated AML or isolated granulocytic sarcoma were enrolled on the trial. Remission induction commenced with the DAT regimen (DNR 45 mg/m^2 on days 1–3, ARAC continuous infusion on days 1–7 and oral thioguanine on days 1–7). Intrathecal (IT) ARAC was given on days 1 and 8 of course 1 and additional doses on day 12 and 19 were given to those who had central nervous system (CNS) leukemia at diagnosis. Course 2 commenced on day 15 if the bone marrow showed residual leukemia but otherwise it began when blood counts had fully recovered. The second course consisted of high-dose ARAC for six doses. All patients in clinical and hematological remission were randomized to either six courses of intensive postremission chemotherapy or ABMT. Intensive postremission chemotherapy consisted of course 1: DNR on day 1 and ARAC in second induction course; course 2: DNR on days 1 and 2,

Evidence-Based Pediatric Oncology, Third Edition. Edited by Ross Pinkerton, Ananth Shankar and Katherine K. Matthay.
© 2013 John Wiley & Sons, Ltd. Published 2013 by John Wiley & Sons, Ltd.

ARAC as continuous infusion days 1–5; course 3: etoposide on days 1–3 and azacytidine on days 4–5; course 4: high-dose ARAC 12 hourly×6 doses; course 5: same as course 2, and course 6: same as course 3. The 3-year event-free survival (EFS) rates for patients in the intensive chemotherapy and ABMT groups were 36%±5.8% and 38%±6.4% respectively (p=0.20) while the 3-year overall survival (OS) rates were 44%±6% and 40%±6.1% respectively (p=0.10). In addition, deaths were higher in the ABMT group (15% versus 2.7%; p=0.005). As shown in the AIEOP trial [1], consolidation of remission with ABMT in children with AML did not offer any additional benefit when compared to postremission intensive chemotherapy.

In the AML 10 trial [3], following induction and consolidation therapy, children in complete remission (CR) who had a matched family donor were allocated to allogeneic bone marrow transplantation (allo-BMT). All other patients were randomized between ABMT and no further treatment. Children below the age of 15 years with previously untreated AML, including those with secondary AML or with myelodysplastic syndrome (MDS), were the subjects of this report. See Hann et al. [4] for details of the chemotherapy regimens and randomizations. One hundred children who were in CR at the end of four courses of chemotherapy were randomized between ABMT (n=50) and no further treatment (n=50). Disease-free survival (DFS) at 7 years in the ABMT group was 68% versus 46% in the stop arm (p=0.02) while relapse-free survival (RFS) at 7 years in the ABMT group was 69% versus 48% in the stop arm (p=0.03). Although the DFS and RFS rates were lower in patients in the stop arm, OS did not differ between the two treatment groups (70% versus 59%; p=0.2) and this appeared to be related to inferior salvage rate after relapse in the ABMT group. The report concluded that ABMT did not improve survival in children with AML in first remission.

In the CCG 2891 trial [5], patients who had completed four cycles of chemotherapy and had no matched family donor were randomized to either ABMT or intensive chemotherapy (IC) . All patients with previously untreated AML <21 years of age except those with Fanconi anemia, Down or Philadelphia-positive chronic myeloid leukemia in the blast phase were included in the study. Children with Down syndrome, secondary AML, isolated granulocytic sarcoma or MDS were also excluded from the analyses. There was one other randomization in this trial; the first randomization at diagnosis was between a standard induction regimen and intensively timed regimen (see Woods et al. [6] for more details). One hundred and seventy-seven patients were randomized to ABMT and 179 to IC. The 8-year OS and DFS for patients randomized to ABMT were 48%±8% and 42%±8% respectively compared to 53%±8% (ABMT versus IC; p=0.21) and 47%±8% (ABMT versus IC; p=0.31) respectively for patients who received IC. The report also concluded that ABMT did not offer any advantage over IC in children with AML.

References

1 Amadori S, Testi AM, Aricò M et al. Prospective comparative study of bone marrow transplantation and postremission chemotherapy for childhood acute myelogenous leukemia. The Associazione Italiana Ematologia ed Oncologia Pediatrica Cooperative Group. J Clin Oncol 1993;11:1046–5.

2 Ravindranath Y, Yeager AM, Chang MN et al. Autologous bone marrow transplantation versus intensive consolidation chemotherapy for acute myeloid leukemia in childhood. Pediatric Oncology Group. N Engl J Med 1996;334:1428–34.

3 Stevens RF, Hann IM, Wheatley K, Gray RG. Marked improvements in outcome with chemotherapy alone in paediatric acute myeloid leukemia: results of the United Kingdom Medical Research Council's 10th AML trial. MRC Childhood Leukaemia Working Party. Br J Haematol 1998;101:130–40.

4 Hann IM, Stevens RF, Goldstone AH et al. Randomized comparison of DAT versus ADE as induction chemotherapy in children and younger adults with acute myeloid leukemia. Results of the Medical Research Council's 10th AML trial (MRC AML10). Adult and Childhood Leukaemia Working Parties of the Medical Research Council. Blood 1997;89:2311–18.

5 Woods WG, Neudorf S, Gold S et al., for the Children's Cancer Group. A comparison of allogeneic bone marrow transplantation, autologous bone marrow transplantation, and aggressive chemotherapy in children with acute myeloid leukemia in remission. Blood 2001;97:56–62.

6 Woods WG, Kobrinsky N, Buckley JD et al. Timed-sequential induction therapy improves post remission outcome in acute myeloid leukemia: a report from the Children's Cancer Group. Blood 1996;87:4979–89.

New studies

The authors have been unable to identify any new randomized trials regarding autologous bone marrow transplantation in acute myeloid leukemia in children published since the previous edition of this book.

CHAPTER 17

Acute myeloid leukemia: miscellaneous

Ananth Shankar

University College London Hospitals NHS Foundation Trust, London, UK

New study

Study 1

Creutzig U, Zimmermann M, Bourquin JP *et al.* CNS irradiation in pediatric acute myeloid leukemia: equal results by 12 or 18 Gy in studies AML BFM 98 and 2004. *Pediatr Blood Cancer* 2011;**57**: 986–92.

Objectives

To evaluate whether a lower dose of prophylactic cranial irradiation in children with acute myeloid leukemia (AML) is sufficient to prevent central nervous system (CNS) relapse of leukemia.

Study design

AML BFM 98, 98 interim, and AML BFM 2004 were prospective multicenter randomized studies conducted between July 1998 and April 2009 and included patients aged between 0 and 18 years with *de novo* AML, therapy-related or myelodysplastic-related AML or mixed lineage leukemia. Patients with Down syndrome, CNS leukemia at diagnosis, not in complete remission after 140 days of treatment or those assigned to stem cell transplantation were excluded from trial enrollment. Details of the randomization methodology were not specified in the report. The main analysis was performed on actual treatment received rather than on an intention-to-treat principle. The median follow-up was 4.8 years.

Treatment regimens in all the trials were largely similar. AIE (cytosine arabinoside [ARAC], idarubicin and etoposide) or ADxE (ARAC, liposomal daunorubicin and etoposide) induction was followed by HAM (high-dose ARAC and mitoxantrone, in high-risk patients only) and two further cycles with intermediate- and high-dose ARAC and anthracyclines. Intensification and maintenance were similar in all three study periods. Patients with high-risk disease were offered allogeneic stem cell transplantation if a suitable family donor was available. All patients received 11 doses of intrathecal (IT) ARAC (12 for high-risk patients). On completion of the intensification block, eligible patients were randomized to receive either 12 Gy or 18 Gy cranial irradiation as prophylaxis against CNS relapse of leukemia.

Statistics

Survival outcomes were estimated using the Kaplan–Meier method with standard errors according to Greenwood, and were compared with the log-rank test. The cumulative incidences of relapse and second malignant neoplasms were estimated using the Kalbfleisch and Prentice methods.

Results

Out of 1206 patients enrolled on trials, 484 were not eligible for the CNS irradiation randomization because they met the exclusion criteria and a further 236 patients refused randomization. Of the remaining 486 patients,

---

Evidence-Based Pediatric Oncology, Third Edition. Edited by Ross Pinkerton, Ananth Shankar and Katherine K. Matthay.
© 2013 John Wiley & Sons, Ltd. Published 2013 by John Wiley & Sons, Ltd.

237 children were randomized to receive 18 Gy cranial irradiation (CRT) (15 Gy for children aged between 15–24 months) and 249 children to 12 Gy CRT. Sixteen patients randomized to 18 Gy CRT received 12 Gy CRT and five patients randomized to 12 Gy CRT actually received 18 Gy CRT. Additionally, 15 randomized patients did not receive CRT due to either an event after randomization (n=9), stem cell transplantation (n=2) or parent/physician choice (n=4). In summary, 252 children received 12 Gy and 219 received 18 Gy CRT.

One hundred and forty-five patients relapsed and there were no differences in the relapse rates between the two randomized groups. Of the six CNS relapses, five occurred in the 18 Gy CRT group and one in the 12 Gy group, which was not statistically significantly different (p=0.452).

The 5-year overall survival (OS) and event-free survival (EFS) as well as the cumulative incidence of relapse were similar in the randomized patients treated with 12 or 18 Gy CRT ($82\% \pm 3\%$ versus $79\% \pm 3\%$; $68\% \pm 3\%$ versus $63\% \pm 3\%$; $30\% \pm 3\%$ versus $34\% \pm 3\%$] respectively. An analysis on an intention-to-treat principle (12 Gy; n=236 and 18 Gy; n=214) also showed comparable results (5-year EFS $69\% \pm 3\%$ versus $62\% \pm 4\%$).

Four children developed secondary leukemia: one in the 12 Gy group and three in the 18 Gy arm.

Conclusions

It was concluded that 12 Gy cranial irradiation was as effective as 18 Gy in preventing CNS relapse in children with AML.

CHAPTER 18

Childhood lymphoblastic leukemia commentary

Vaskar Saha

The University of Manchester, Manchester Academic Health Science Centre, The Christie NHS Foundation Trust, Manchester, UK

It has been 6 years since the last edition of this book came out, which is a relatively short span of time for clinical trials in childhood acute lymphoblastic leukemia (ALL), but a reasonable time period for significant scientific advances. The interval between the last edition and this one has coincided with the increasing use of whole genome analysis and in particular, next generation sequencing. We have learnt that multiple clones are present at diagnosis and relapse and that the clones evolve as a process of Darwinian natural selection [1,2,3]. The ALL genome has fewer mutations compared to other cancers. Prosaically, none of these mutations offers an immediate explanation for therapeutic failure. While patients with IZKF and CRLF2 mutations [4,5] are associated with an inferior outcome in clinical protocols, they have better outcomes in other study group analyses [6]. This may reflect not only differences in therapeutic regimen but also the ethnic composition of the study population [7]. CRLF2 is associated with activated mutations of JAK2 in childhood ALL [5] and thus the role of JAK inhibitors is now being investigated. The recent discovery of CREBPP mutations suggests the possibility of histone deacetylase inhibitors as adjunctive therapy in relapsed ALL [8].

The mainstream of therapies in childhood ALL continues to be broad-spectrum and nonspecific chemotherapy. While this has been a highly successful strategy, it has been associated with considerable toxicity, particularly in older patients. Unlike epithelial cancers where aromatase, PARP and BRAF inhibition

have quickly found a place in the clinic, there are no obvious targets in childhood ALL. Only in the rare cytogenetic subset of Philadelphia-positive (Ph+) ALL has the targeted tyrosine kinase inhibitor imatinib entered mainline therapy. The high success rates in childhood ALL pose considerable difficulties for drug development. Fewer relapsed and refractory patients are available for early-phase clinical trials and clinicians are understandably anxious about introducing as yet unproven new agents into phase III trials.

Perhaps the most significant developments with regard to therapy lie in the now routine use of minimal residual disease (MRD) in risk stratification and the push towards decreasing toxicity. Both these topics will be examined in the next section. As mentioned earlier, the time span between the two editions is not long enough for some trial data to mature to publication, so when necessary abstracts from meeting are quoted proceedings are quoted so that this chapter is not out of date by the time it reaches print.

Remission induction

Steroid

The argument over whether to use prednisolone or dexamethasone continues. In the last edition, evidence that suggested a superior outcome of dexamethasone was reviewed, which is not fully explained by the purported 6:1 to 7:1 ratio of glucocorticoid activity compared to prednisolone. The superior penetration of dexamethasone into the cerebrospinal fluid (CSF) has also been

Evidence-Based Pediatric Oncology, Third Edition. Edited by Ross Pinkerton, Ananth Shankar and Katherine K. Matthay.
© 2013 John Wiley & Sons, Ltd. Published 2013 by John Wiley & Sons, Ltd.

quoted as an advantage. Three randomized studies now report a better event-free survival for patients who received dexamethasone over those who received prednisolone, with a decrease in both central nervous system (CNS) and bone marrow relapses [9,10,11]. Curiously, overall survival remains comparable, suggesting that postprednisolone relapses have a higher salvage potential. Of increasing concern has been the higher toxicity with dexamethasone, particularly in those aged over 10 years. In the IEOP BFM ALL 2000 trial, the steroid randomization was actually halted for those aged over 10 years due to increased toxicity. However, this trial used a dose of 10 mg/m² of dexamethasone, higher than that used by other groups. Evidence suggests that the dose, rather than the steroid, is key to outcome. A recent meta-analysis suggests that when the prednisolone dose is ≥7 times that of dexamethasone, they appear to be equally effective [12].

Clearly, steroids are still the mainstay of ALL therapy. In the context of intensive multiagent combination chemotherapy, groups are now investigating ways of maintaining efficacy and decreasing toxicity. These include using prednisolone for induction and dexamethasone for delayed intensification and shortening the duration of exposure to dexamethasone.

L-Asparaginase

This is another key drug, whose use is primarily during induction, intensification, and Capizzi-style blocks. A number of study groups are now using polyethylene glycol (PEG)-conjugated E.coli-derived L-asparaginase (ASNase) as the derivative of choice. PEG-ASNase has the advantage of a longer half-life, requiring less frequent dosage. The amount of enzyme required is also less, and thus there are fewer complications. Different formulations have different pharmacokinetics but most previous studies comparing formulations have not taken this into consideration, making interpretation of comparative efficacy difficult [13].

With the development of reliable pharmacokinetic assays, the evidence base for L-asparaginase is moving away from randomized studies to those based on enzyme activity, asparagine levels, and detection of antibodies. The dose, frequency, and route of administration of PEG-ASNase remain speculative. Given intramuscularly at 1000 u/m², fortnightly ASNase activity >100 u/L was achieved in the majority of patients treated in the UK [14]. Data suggest that a dose of 2500 u/m² may be

required to deplete asparaginase in the CSF. This is a reflection of the systemic asparagine depletion, as ASNase itself does not enter the CSF. Its therapeutic relevance remains unclear and intensifying the ASNase dose does not appear to correlate with an improved outcome [15]. Nevertheless, a number of groups use 2500 units/m² and the Dana-Farber group has reported that this can be administered safely intravenously [16].

Though L-asparaginase has been in use for over 40 years, we are still unclear about the mechanisms of its affect on lymphoblasts, resistance, and associated toxicity. Lymphoblasts are thought to be auxotrophic for asparagine. Depletion of asparagine by ASNase is cytotoxic. However, ASNase also has glutaminase activity and this appears to be necessary for its cytocidal effect [17]. As ASNase is a bacterial product, its antigenicity results in antibody formation in some patients. The presence of antibodies correlates with inactivation of ASNase and an inferior therapeutic outcome [18]. Inactivation also occurs in the absence of detectable antibodies. This raises the possibility that there are other mechanisms by which the enzyme is inactivated. Intrinsic resistance to asparaginase, i.e. absence of an effect in the presence of the drug, remains largely unexplored [19].

The importance of adequate ASNase activity and the scheduling lies in its synergy with steroids. Sustained ASNase activity is associated with decreased steroid clearance. Similarly, steroids presumably dampen the immune response to ASNase, leading to increased tolerance. Thus the two drugs potentiate each other and perhaps also increase respective toxicity [18,20].

Regulatory and financial pressures also pose hurdles. PEG-ASNase is not available as first-line treatment for patients in France and Japan. The cost of PEG-ASNase is prohibitive in less resourced countries. The activity of PEG-ASNase depends not only on the native enzyme but the degree and type of pegylation and the linker used for conjugation. Though PEG-ASNase is available in both the US and Europe and goes under the same trade name of Oncaspar™, the native E.coli products in these derivatives are different. The COG is trialing a new PEG-ASNase that uses urethane as a linker; this will have different properties from both the previous products as well as the one available in Europe. To enhance the purity of the enzyme, a new recombinant product has recently been evaluated [21] and this too will be subsequently pegylated, possibly with a different linker.

A recombinant pegylated Erwinia product is also expected to enter clinical trials.

Current evidence suggests that ASNase is a key drug in childhood ALL therapy and when used to provide optimal activity along with steroids, contributes significantly to outcome [13,22].

Postinduction therapy

Methotrexate

The folic acid antagonist methotrexate is a representative of the first class of drugs designed specifically for childhood ALL. Its wide pharmacotherapeutic window, oral availability ,and the ability to counter its effects with folinic acid have resulted in its wide use in childhood ALL. In comparison to steroids and ASNase, there is more extensive knowledge about its mode of action, pharmacokinetic variability, and pharmacogenomics. Key to its effectiveness is the conversion of methotrexate to methotrexate-polyglutamate and the retention of the active metabolites within the cell where it competes for nucleic acid synthesis. Certain subtypes of childhood ALL show an increased response to methotrexate, namely, T-cell ALL and high hyperdiploidy [23].

Oral methotrexate is universally used as part of continuation therapy. The role of intravenous methotrexate given at higher doses has also been investigated intensively. In this context a randomized study explored the benefit of intravenous methotrexate used in interim maintenance in standard-risk ALL[24]. This schedule had previously been shown to be of benefit in high-risk ALL [25]. The dose used here was 100 mg/m^2 every 10 days with dose escalation if tolerated. Intravenous methotrexate overall provided a survival advantage except in the good-risk cytogenetic subtype of ETV6-*RUNX1*.

The obvious question then is whether higher doses of methotrexate could provide additional benefit? There are a number of dosage schedules and infusion durations available. Unlike the former schedule which is relatively inexpensive and can be delivered as an outpatient therapeutic procedure, high-dose intravenous methotrexate is relatively expensive and an inpatient procedure. Thus we need to be clear about how best to use it and which patients are most likely to benefit from it. The second study demonstrates that more than the dose, it is the duration of infusion that is critical [23]. A longer duration of infusion results in a higher and more prolonged

accumulation of the active methotrexate metabolites intracellularly and this correlates with a better outcome. This study demonstrated that the longer duration of infusion increases the accumulation of methotrexate polyglutamates in all subsets of ALL except the ETV6-*RUNX1* subtype, providing an explanation for the previous study. These data also provide an explanation to an earlier randomized study which found similar benefit of 5 g/m^2 of methotrexate given intravenously over 24 h compared to 1 g/m^2 given over 36 h [26].

Central nervous system-directed therapy

In the previous edition, evidence that prophylactic cranial irradiation was no longer necessary for most patients treated on modern regimens was reviewed. With increasing systemic therapy, there has been a reduction in both systemic and CNS relapses and most study groups no longer irradiate prophylactically [27]. One ongoing debate has been the issue of those who have CNS3 (≥5 white blood cells [WBC]/mm^3 of CSF with blasts) in the CSF and those who have a traumatic lumbar puncture (TLP) associated with blasts. CNS3 does not appear to be of prognostic significance [28,29]. The incidence of TLP varies with practice, possibly due to the fact that some groups use prophylactic platelet infusions. While TLP is seen more frequently in high-risk patients, the increased risk of relapse is not entirely explained by this variable. Nevertheless, most study groups treat CNS3 and TLP with additional intrathecal therapy, avoiding cranial irradiation.

Intensifying therapy

In the 1970s the BFM introduced protocol Ib or what others term "consolidation." In addition to 6-mercaptopurine used by many groups, cyclophosphamide was added to cytarabine. This has proved to be a highly effective therapeutic block [30]. In the 1990s the Children's Cancer Group (now the Children's Oncology Group [COG]) introduced an augmented BFM regimen by adding vincristine and ASNase to consolidation and delayed intensification and replacing oral 6-mercaptopurine and methotrexate with intravenous methotrexate, ASNase and vincristine in interim maintenance [31]. Subsequently the same group examined the effect of a similar regimen in standard-risk patients and noted a survival advantage in this group as well, without an increase in toxicity

[24]. In the same study, the group also performed a randomization for 1 versus 2 interim maintenance and delayed intensification blocks, and found no benefit in any risk or age group [24,32]. This observation has now been confirmed by another study group [33].

Thus early intensification benefits all risk groups. Current evidence does not support a role for late intensification.

Continuation therapy

This is a phase of therapy peculiar to childhood ALL. Most groups continue therapy for 2 years, while some treat boys for 3 years. The mainstays of therapy are daily oral thiopurines and weekly methotrexate. Therapy is titrated to the white cell count to avoid severe neutropenia and this seems to produce the best results [34]. The key to this phase has been administering as much of the drugs as possible without large gaps in therapy. Thus intensification using intravenous therapy has not proven beneficial [35].

The degree of myelo- and immunosuppression during this period of therapy is not trivial and patients are frequently hospitalized with infection. The Brazilian co-operative group reported on the result of a randomization in maintenance where continuous therapy and intermittent therapy (with a higher dose of 6-mercaptopurine and intravenous methotrexate with leucovorin rescue) were compared. Overall, there was no difference in survival but a better outcome was noted with the intermittent schedule for boys. The intermittent schedule was also less toxic [36].

Similarly, the use of 6-thioguanine (6-TG) instead of its precursor 6-mercaptopurine has not been associated with an improved outcome. Though 6-TG appeared to have a beneficial effect on boys <10 years and decreased the incidence of CNS relapses, this was negated by a higher toxic death rate [37,38]. Moreover, late toxicity manifest as hepatic veno-occlusive disease was more frequent in those who received 6-TG [38,39].

A number of study groups use pulses of steroid and vincristine during the continuation phase of therapy. The BFM group investigated the benefit of vincristine and steroid pulses in those classified by them as intermediate risk, i.e. <1 year or ≥6 years of age; presenting WC ≥20 × 10^9/L and good early response to prednisolone. There was no significant difference in outcome in those who did or did not receive pulses [40]. Other study groups are now attempting to confirm this result.

To simplify continuation therapy in the era of intensive systemic regimens, oral 6-mercaptopurine and methotrexate continue to be the most suitable form of therapy, given the considerable therapeutic burden of intravenous vincristine and steroids, particularly in older children. Further evidence is now required to confirm that these are no longer required.

Adolescents and young adults

A number of study groups now recruit patients up to 21 and some up to 25 years of age. In general, older patients have benefited from a pediatric-type protocol similar to that seen in younger patients [32,41,42,43].

Nevertheless, outcomes in the ≥10-year age group do not quite match those achieved in younger children in many studies. This is in part due to the biology of the disease. Older patients are more likely to have unfavorable cytogenetic subtypes, e.g. Philadelphia chromosome positivity, MLL gene rearrangements and fewer favorable cytogenetic subtypes, e.g. ETV6-*RUNX1*. Older patients also have a higher molecular burden at the end of induction [44]. Another reason is increased toxicity, particularly sepsis, osteonecrosis, and hyperglycemia [32,45]. This likely relates to altered pharmacokinetics of the drugs in older patients [18,20,46]. A recent study in a small cohort shows that intensive pediatric-style therapy and appropriate management of complications can produce survival rates in those aged 15–18 years comparable with younger children. However, success was also associated with considerable morbidity with significantly increased rates of sepsis (including postremission deaths), osteonecrosis (requiring core decompression), thrombosis, and hyperglycemia [45].

Thus, arguably, we need a better understanding of the pharmacokinetics in the older age group to develop age-adapted protocols that maximize efficacy without increasing toxicity.

Minimal residual disease

Quantitative assessment of disease burden, using either flow cytometry or real-time quantitative polymerase chain reaction (RQ-PCR), is now routinely used in clinical trials. Sensitivity of current assays is able to detect disease at 10^{-4}–10^{-5} levels. The absence of detectable disease at all follow-up times from the first postinduction time points is associated with almost 95% survival. One recent report shows that minimal residual disease (MRD) is the most sensitive predictor of outcome, superior to all other risk factors [44]. Thus low/negative MRD can now be used to lessen the intensity of therapy in this low-risk group who show a >90% survival [33]. Intensification of therapy in those with postinduction MRD levels $\geq 10^{-3}$ appears to be beneficial [33]. However, the therapy of choice for those with persistent detectable MRD is unclear, as they tend to relapse early while still in therapy. In the UK, those with persistent MRD positivity beyond intensification are now eligible for experimental therapy.

As newer and cheaper techniques to monitor MRD become available, it is likely that MRD will be used universally to identify those who have low/negative MRD at the end of induction. These patients can be mostly cured with the least intensive therapy.

Relapsed acute lymphoblastic leukemia

Few new drugs have entered routine practice for over four decades. Thus current survival rates are the result of optimizing the use of available drugs. As is evident from the preceding sections, this has been achieved through a combination of risk stratifications and intensifications. What is also evident is that therapy-related toxicity prevents further intensification. Thus the focus has moved to the identification of potential cellular mechanisms amenable to targeted therapy, not only to decrease toxicity but also to treat those who relapse despite current therapy. What has become clear from a number of observations is that relapses on therapy do poorly even with allogenic transplantation [47,48,49]. Almost paradoxically, those who relapse off therapy remain curable with more or less similar chemotherapy, with or without an allogeneic stem cell transplant. In this context, opportunity still exists to explore novel contributions with existing drugs. A recent randomized trial reported the superiority of mitoxantrone over idarubicin in patients with first relapse, particularly in those risk stratified to receive a transplant [50]. Another important lesson was learnt from this trial. Survival in those who received mitoxantrone was significantly better than for those

who received idarubicin, but there was no difference in the postinduction MRD levels between the two groups. Although MRD at the end of induction is the most sensitive predictor of outcome, it cannot be used as a surrogate marker of survival.

This study suggests that while we wait for newer drugs, there is still mileage to be made from existing drugs and newer combinations. If MRD had been used as a surrogate marker, then clearly the most effective combination would not have received further evaluation.

Long-term effects

With the progressive improvement in outcome, it is also important to minimize long-term side-effects of therapy. Cranial irradiation is associated with an increased incidence of brain tumors but is now hardly used as a therapeutic modality. In theory, steroid-induced osteonecrosis could be prevented by bisphosphonates and a randomized trial would be logical. However, there remains uncertainty about the natural history of osteonecrosis and what if anything needs to be done for those with minor disabilities [51]. Thus, the endpoint of such a trial would be difficult to define. More headway has been made with the long-term cardiac effects of anthracyclines. Anthracycline and now anthracenediones (mitoxantrone) are intensively used in childhood ALL. Anthracycline-induced late cardiomyopathy is associated with female sex, young age of exposure, and cumulative dose. The cardiotoxic effects are due partially to the drug forming complexes with iron, leading to increased formation of reactive oxygen species in cardiomyocytes [52]. Dexrazoxane chelates iron, reducing this effect. In a small randomized cohort study, dexrazoxane given at the time of anthracycline infusion was shown to be cardioprotective without affecting survival at 5 years [53]. Thus in the future dexrazoxane should be considered as adjunctive cardioprotective therapy in ALL patients who are to receive high cumulative doses of anthracyclines.

New agents

This is an exciting time for drug discovery. Different biological mechanisms that appear to be crucial to cancer cell survival have been characterized and novel compounds that potentially target these pathways are also being identified [54]. The difficulties in evaluating these new drugs in a rare and highly curable disease have already been highlighted and as yet most remain in the study phase.

The one new drug that has entered routine practice is imatinib. This tyrosine kinase inhibitor has proven benefit in Ph+chronic myeloid leukemia (CML) and newer tyrosine kinase inhibitors are being tested. Dasatinib is now becoming routine in the clinical management of CML patients. Ph+ALL was one of the earliest recognized high-risk cytogenetic subtypes and most groups have transplanted such patients in first remission [55]. A COG nonrandomized study suggested that Ph+ALL patients not only tolerated imatinib when given in conjunction with standard combination chemotherapy but this improved outcome. Most significantly, their data suggested that such patients no longer required transplantation [56]. The European intergroup study (EsPhALL) has recently confirmed this observation in a randomized trial [57].

The experience with imatinib in this rare but high-risk cytogenetic subtype highlights the well-tested paradigm of ALL therapy. One needs to identify the drug combination(s) to which the cells are most sensitive and use them intensively and early to achieve the best outcome. With the advent of tyrosine kinase inhibitors, there is now a drug specific for this group of patients and fewer will be treated with ablative transplantation. Going forward, we now need to see if new-generation tyrosine kinase inhibitors will provide better outcomes, without adding to the burden of therapy. More poignantly, we need to maintain the faith that such targeted therapy will become available for other high-risk subgroups so that we may eventually close the chapter on curing all children with ALL, worldwide.

References

1 Anderson K, Lutz C, van Delft FW *et al.* Genetic variegation of clonal architecture and propagating cells in leukemia. *Nature* 2011;**469**(7330):356–61.

2 Greaves M, Maley CC. Clonal evolution in cancer. *Nature* 2012;**481**(7381):306–13.

3 Notta F, Mulligan CG, Wang JC *et al.* Evolution of human BCR-ABL1 lymphoblastic leukaemia-initiating cells. *Nature* 2011;**469**(7330):362–7.

4 Chen IM, Harvey RC, Mulligan CG *et al.* Outcome modeling with CRLF2, IKZF1, JAK and minimal residual disease in pediatric acute lymphoblastic leukemia: a Children's Oncology Group Study. *Blood* 2012;**119**(15)3512–22.

5 Mulligan CG, Collins-Underwood JR, Phillips LA *et al.* Rearrangement of CRLF2 in B-progenitor- and Down syndrome-associated acute lymphoblastic leukemia. *Nat Genet* 2009;**41**(11):1243–6.

6 Ensor HM, Schwab C, Russell LJ *et al.* Demographic, clinical, and outcome features of children with acute lymphoblastic leukemia and CRLF2 deregulation: results from the MRC ALL97 clinical trial. *Blood* 2011;**117**(7):2129–36.

7 Harvey RC, Mulligan CG, Chen IM *et al.* Rearrangement of CRLF2 is associated with mutation of JAK kinases, alteration of IKZF1, Hispanic/Latino ethnicity, and a poor outcome in pediatric B-progenitor acute lymphoblastic leukemia. *Blood* 2010;**115**(26):5312–21.

8 Mulligan CG, Zhang J, Kasper LH *et al.* CREBBP mutations in relapsed acute lymphoblastic leukaemia. *Nature* 2011;**471**(7337):235–9.

9 Bostrom BC, Sensel MR, Sather HN *et al.* Dexamethasone versus prednisone and daily oral versus weekly intravenous mercaptopurine for patients with standard-risk acute lymphoblastic leukemia: a report from the Children's Cancer Group. *Blood* 2003;**101**(10):3809–17.

10 Mitchell CD, Richards SM, Kinsey SE *et al.* Benefit of dexamethasone compared with prednisolone for childhood acute lymphoblastic leukaemia: results of the UK Medical Research Council ALL97 randomized trial. *Br J Haematol* 2005;**129**(6):734–45.

11 Schrappe M, Zimmermann M, Moricke A *et al.* Dexamethasone in induction can eliminate one third of all relapses in childhood acute lymphoblastic leukaemia (ALL): results of an international randomized trial in 3655 patients (trial AIEOP-BFM ALL 2000). *ASH Annual Meeting Abstracts* 2008;**112**(11):7.

12 Teuffel O, Kuster SP, Hunger SP *et al.* Dexamethasone versus prednisone for induction therapy in childhood acute lymphoblastic leukemia: a systematic review and meta-analysis. *Leukemia* 2011;**25**(8):1232–8.

13 Moghrabi A, Levy DE, Asselin B *et al.* Results of the Dana-Farber Cancer Institute ALL Consortium Protocol 95-01 for children with acute lymphoblastic leukemia. *Blood* 2007;**109**(3):896–904.

14 Fong CY, Parker CA, Hussain A *et al.* Intramuscular PEG-asparaginase at 1000 u/m^2 achieves adequate trough activity levels in the majority of patients treated on the UKALL 2003 Childhood Acute Lymphoblastic Leukemia (ALL) Protocol. *ASH Annual Meeting Abstracts* 2011;**118**(21):2573.

15 Pession A, Valsecchi MG, Masera G *et al.* Long-term results of a randomized trial on extended use of high dose L-asparaginase for standard risk childhood acute lymphoblastic leukemia. *J Clin Oncol* 2005;**23**(28):7161–7.

16 Silverman LB, Stevenson K, Vrooman LM *et al.* Randomized comparison of IV PEG and IM E. coli asparaginase in children and adolescents with acute lymphoblastic leukemia:

results of the DFCI ALL Consortium Protocol 05-01. *ASH Annual Meeting Abstracts* 2011;**118**(21):874.

17 Offman MN, Krol M, Patel N *et al.* Rational engineering of L-asparaginase reveals importance of dual activity for cancer cell toxicity. *Blood* 2011;**117**(5):1614–21.

18 Kawedia JD, Liu C, Pei D *et al.* Dexamethasone exposure and asparaginase antibodies affect relapse risk in acute lymphoblastic leukemia. *Blood* 2012;**119**(7):1658–64.

19 Patel N, Krishnan S, Offman MN *et al.* A dyad of lymphoblastic lysosomal cysteine proteases degrades the antileukemic drug L-asparaginase. *J Clin Invest* 2009;**119**(7):1964–73.

20 Yang L, Panetta JC, Cai X *et al.* Asparaginase may influence dexamethasone pharmacokinetics in acute lymphoblastic leukemia. *J Clin Oncol* 2008;**26**(12):1932–9.

21 Pieters R, Appel I, Kuehnel H-J *et al.* Pharmacokinetics, pharmacodynamics, efficacy, and safety of a new recombinant asparaginase preparation in children with previously untreated acute lymphoblastic leukemia: a randomized phase 2 clinical trial. *Blood* 2008;**112**(13):4832–8.

22 Wetzler M, Sanford BL, Kurtzberg J *et al.* Effective asparagine depletion with pegylated asparaginase results in improved outcomes in adult acute lymphoblastic leukemia: Cancer and Leukemia Group B Study 9511. *Blood* 2007; **109**(10):4164–7.

23 Mikkelsen TS, Sparreboom A, Cheng C *et al.* Shortening infusion time for high-dose methotrexate alters antileukemic effects: a randomized prospective clinical trial. *J Clin Oncol* 2011;**29**(13):1771–8.

24 Matloub Y, Bostrom BC, Hunger SP *et al.* Escalating intravenous methotrexate improves event-free survival in children with standard-risk acute lymphoblastic leukemia: a report from the Children's Oncology Group. *Blood* 2011;**118**(2): 243–51.

25 Nachman J, Sather HN, Cherlow JM *et al.* Response of children with high-risk acute lymphoblastic leukemia treated with and without cranial irradiation: a report from the Children's Cancer Group. *J Clin Oncol* 1998;**16**(3):920–30.

26 Von Stackelberg A, Hartmann R, Buehrer C *et al.* High-dose compared with intermediate-dose methotrexate in children with a first relapse of acute lymphoblastic leukemia. *Blood* 2008;**111**(5):2573–80.

27 Krishnan S, Wade R, Moorman AV *et al.* Temporal changes in the incidence and pattern of central nervous system relapses in children with acute lymphoblastic leukaemia treated on four consecutive Medical Research Council trials, 1985–2001. *Leukemia* 2010;**24**(2):450–9.

28 Sirvent N, Suciu S, Rialland X *et al.* Prognostic significance of the initial cerebro-spinal fluid (CSF) involvement of children with acute lymphoblastic leukaemia (ALL) treated without cranial irradiation: results of European Organization for Research and Treatment of Cancer (EORTC) Children Leukemia Group study 58881. *Eur J Cancer* 2011;**47**(2): 239–47.

29 Te Loo DM, Kamps WA, van der Does-van den Berg A, van Wering ER, de Graaf SS. Prognostic significance of blasts in the cerebrospinal fluid without pleiocytosis or a traumatic

lumbar puncture in children with acute lymphoblastic leukemia: experience of the Dutch Childhood Oncology Group. *J Clin Oncol* 2006;**24**(15):2332–6.

30 Moricke A, Schrauder A, Zimmermann M *et al.* Major improvement of outcome in pediatric high-risk acute lymphoblastic leukemia by addition of BFM chemotherapy element "phase IB": a comparative data analysis of trials ALL-BFM 95 and ALL-BFM 2000. *ASH Annual Meeting Abstracts* 2011; **118**(21):1504.

31 Nachman JB, Sather HN, Sensel MG *et al.* Augmented post-induction therapy for children with high-risk acute lymphoblastic leukemia and a slow response to initial therapy. *N Engl J Med* 1998;**338**(23):1663–71.

32 Nachman JB, La MK, Hunger SP *et al.* Young adults with acute lymphoblastic leukemia have an excellent outcome with chemotherapy alone and benefit from intensive postinduction treatment: a report from the Children's Oncology Group. *J Clin Oncol* 2009;**27**(31):5189–94.

33 Vora AJ, Mitchell C, Goulden N, Richards S. UKALL 2003, a randomised trial investigating treatment reduction for children and young adults with minimal residual disease defined low risk acute lymphoblastic leukaemia. *ASH Annual Meeting Abstracts* 2010;**116**(21):496.

34 Schmiegelow K, Bjork O, Glomstein A *et al.* Intensification of mercaptopurine/methotrexate maintenance chemotherapy may increase the risk of relapse for some children with acute lymphoblastic leukemia. *J Clin Oncol* 2003;**21**(7):1332–9.

35 Silverman LB, Stevenson KE, O'Brien JE *et al.* Long-term results of Dana-Farber Cancer Institute ALL Consortium protocols for children with newly diagnosed acute lymphoblastic leukemia (1985–2000). *Leukemia* 2010;**24**(2):320–34.

36 Brandalise SR, Pinheiro VR, Aguiar SS *et al.* Benefits of the intermittent use of 6-mercaptopurine and methotrexate in maintenance treatment for low-risk acute lymphoblastic leukemia in children: randomized trial from the Brazilian Childhood Cooperative Group Protocol ALL-99. *J Clin Oncol* 2010;**28**(11):1911–18.

37 Vora A, Mitchell CD, Lennard L *et al.* Toxicity and efficacy of 6-thioguanine versus 6-mercaptopurine in childhood lymphoblastic leukaemia: a randomised trial. *Lancet* 2006; **368**(9544):1339–48.

38 Stork LC, Matloub Y, Broxson E *et al.* Oral 6-mercaptopurine versus oral 6-thioguanine and veno-occlusive disease in children with standard-risk acute lymphoblastic leukemia: report of the Children's Oncology Group CCG-1952 clinical trial. *Blood* 2010;**115**(14):2740–8.

39 Escherich G, Richards S, Stork LC *et al.* Meta-analysis of randomised trials comparing thiopurines in childhood acute lymphoblastic leukaemia. *Leukemia* 2011;**25**(6):953–9.

40 Conter V, Valsecchi MG, Silvestri D *et al.* Pulses of vincristine and dexamethasone in addition to intensive chemotherapy for children with intermediate-risk acute lymphoblastic leukaemia: a multicentre randomised trial. *Lancet* 2007; **369**(9556):123–31.

41 Barry E, DeAngelo DJ, Neuberg D *et al.* Favorable outcome for adolescents with acute lymphoblastic leukemia treated on

Dana-Farber Cancer Institute Acute Lymphoblastic Leukemia Consortium Protocols. *J Clin Oncol* 2007;**25**(7):813–19.

42 Haiat S, Marjanovic Z, Lapusan S *et al*. Outcome of 40 adults aged from 18 to 55 years with acute lymphoblastic leukemia treated with double-delayed intensification pediatric protocol. *Leuk Res* 2011;**35**(1):66–72.

43 Ram R, Wolach O, Vidal L, Gafter-Gvili A, Shpilberg O, Raanani P. Adolescents and young adults with acute lymphoblastic leukemia have a better outcome when treated with pediatric-inspired regimens: systematic review and meta-analysis. *Am J Hematol* 2012;**87**(5):472–8.

44 Conter V, Bartram CR, Valsecchi MG *et al*. Molecular response to treatment redefines all prognostic factors in children and adolescents with B-cell precursor acute lymphoblastic leukemia: results in 3184 patients of the AIEOP-BFM ALL 2000 study. *Blood* 2010;**115**(16):3206–14.

45 Pui CH, Pei D, Campana D *et al*. Improved prognosis for older adolescents with acute lymphoblastic leukemia. *J Clin Oncol* 2011;**29**(4):386–91.

46 Donelli MG, Zucchetti M, Robatto L *et al*. Pharmacokinetics of HD-MTX in infants, children, and adolescents with non-B acute lymphoblastic leukemia. *Med Pediatr Oncol* 1995;**24**(3):154–9.

47 Nguyen K, Devidas M, Cheng SC *et al*. Factors influencing survival after relapse from acute lymphoblastic leukemia: a Children's Oncology Group study. *Leukemia* 2008;**22**(12): 2142–50.

48 Roy A, Cargill A, Love S *et al*. Outcome after first relapse in childhood acute lymphoblastic leukaemia – lessons from the United Kingdom R2 trial. *Br J Haematol* 2005;**130**(1):67–75.

49 Tallen G, Ratei R, Mann G *et al*. Long-term outcome in children with relapsed acute lymphoblastic leukemia after timepoint and site-of-relapse stratification and intensified short-course multidrug chemotherapy: results of trial ALL-REZ BFM 90. *J Clin Oncol* 2010;**28**(14):2339–47.

50 Parker C, Waters R, Leighton C *et al*. Effect of mitoxantrone on outcome of children with first relapse of acute lymphoblastic leukaemia (ALL R3): an open-label randomised trial. *Lancet* 2010;**376**(9757):2009–17.

51 Vora A. Management of osteonecrosis in children and young adults with acute lymphoblastic leukaemia. *Br J Haematol* 2011;**155**(5):549–60.

52 Lipshultz SE, Rifai N, Dalton VM *et al*. The effect of dexrazoxane on myocardial injury in doxorubicin-treated children with acute lymphoblastic leukemia. *N Engl J Med* 2004;**351**(2):145–53.

53 Lipshultz SE, Scully RE, Lipsitz SR *et al*. Assessment of dexrazoxane as a cardioprotectant in doxorubicin-treated children with high-risk acute lymphoblastic leukaemia: long-term follow-up of a prospective, randomised, multicentre trial. *Lancet Oncol* 2010;**11**(10):950–61.

54 Saha V, Kearns P (eds). *New Agents for the Treatment of Acute Lymphblastic Leukaemia*. London: Springer, 2011.

55 Arico M, Schrappe M, Hunger SP *et al*. Clinical outcome of children with newly diagnosed Philadelphia chromosome-positive acute lymphoblastic leukemia treated between 1995 and 2005. *J Clin Oncol* 2010;**28**(31):4755–61.

56 Schultz KR, Bowman WP, Aledo A *et al*. Improved early event-free survival with imatinib in Philadelphia chromosome-positive acute lymphoblastic leukemia: a Children's Oncology Group study. *J Clin Oncol* 2009;**27**(31):5175–81.

57 Biondi A, Schrappe M, di Lorenzo P *et al*. Efficacy and safety of imatinib on top of BFM-like chemotherapy in pediatric patients with Ph+/BCR-ABL+ acute lymphoblastic leukemia (Ph+ALL). The EsPhALL Study. *ASH Annual Meeting Abstracts* 2011;**118**(21):873.

CHAPTER 19

Remission induction in childhood lymphoblastic leukemia

Ananth Shankar

University College London Hospitals NHS Foundation Trust, London, UK

Summary of previous studies

Prednisolone was the main steroid used in early trials during the remission induction phase of treatment in childhood lymphoblastic leukemia. However, with the development of other forms of synthetic steroids with potent glucocorticoid activity, it became clear that some might be more potent, with greater antileukemic activity than prednisolone.

The randomized trial by Yetgin *et al.* [1] compared high-dose intravenous (IV) methylprednisolone (HDMP) against standard prednisolone (PDN) during remission induction in previously untreated children with common childhood acute lymphoblastic leukemia (cALL). Other than the type of steroid, both groups of randomized patients received IV vincristine, IV or intramuscular (IM) L-asparaginase, IV daunorubicin, IV cytosine arabinoside, IV cyclophosphamide, IV etoposide, and IV methotrexate during the induction of remission/consolidation phase of therapy. Central nervous system (CNS) prophylaxis consisted of intrathecal methotrexate (IT MTX), cytosine arabinoside, and prednisolone. High-risk patients also received cranial irradiation plus five additional IT injections immediately after the consolidation phase of treatment. If remission was not achieved by day 15, one additional dose of daunorubicin and three additional doses of L-asparaginase were given. Two hundred and five patients were randomized: 108 to

prednisolone (group A; n=108) and 97 to HDMP (group B; n=97). The 8-year event-free survival (EFS) rates for all 205 patients, group A patients alone and group B alone were 60%, 53% and 66% respectively (p=0.05 between group A and B). For high-risk patients, 8-year EFS was 39% for group A versus 63% for group B (p=0.002) but this difference in EFS was not seen for patients with low-risk disease. Additionally, the EFS rates were significantly better for children who were either ≥2 or ≤10 years of age who received HDMP (n=28; 74%) compared to PDN (n=42; 44%; p=0.05). During the 11-year follow-up period, a total of 64 relapses were seen, with higher rates of relapse in group A (39%) than in group B (23%) (p=0.05). There was a significant difference between the groups with regard to bone marrow (BM) relapses (33 versus 15) but CNS relapses were equal (8 versus 7). The toxicity profile was similar in both groups of patients.

The authors concluded that HDMP during remission induction chemotherapy improved the EFS rate significantly for high-risk patients and improved survival outcome.

The fact that dexamethasone (DEX) had better penetration into the cerebrospinal fluid (CSF) and probably superior cytotoxicity led to the next randomized trial by Lopez-Hernandez *et al.* [2] which evaluated the impact

---

Evidence-Based Pediatric Oncology, Third Edition. Edited by Ross Pinkerton, Ananth Shankar and Katherine K. Matthay.
© 2013 John Wiley & Sons, Ltd. Published 2013 by John Wiley & Sons, Ltd.

of 4 days of prephase IV DEX before commencement of definitive therapy. Only previously untreated children below the age of 20 years were included in this prospective randomized trial and chemotherapy was according to the Memorial Sloan-Kettering (MSK) New York protocol II regimen. The study population included 52 patients randomized to the prephase DEX arm and 43 to the no DEX arm. Although there were no significant differences in the mean age (p=0.66), presence of mediastinal disease (p=0.48), presenting white blood cell count (p=0.61) or B/T cell distribution (p=0.88) between the two groups of patients, the male: female ratio was significantly different between the two groups (17:35 DEX arm versus 26:17 no DEX arm; p=0.01). Relapses were lower in the DEX arm (n=2) compared to no DEX arm (n=10) and the distribution of relapses (bone marrow/central nervous system) was 1/1 in the DEX arm compared to 9/1 in the no DEX arm. The 5-year disease-free survival (DFS) was also better in the DEX arm with a trend towards significance (p=0.07). There were four deaths in the DEX arm compared to 11 deaths in the no DEX arm.

This trial showed that administration of DEX for a very short duration prior to commencement of remission induction improved early bone marrow disease clearance and probably improved DFS in children and adolescents with ALL.

The role of DEX in the treatment of childhood lymphoblastic leukemia was investigated by Bostrom et al. [3] in the Children's Cancer Group (CCG) 1922 trial which was a prospective randomized study conducted between March 1993 and August 1995. The objective of this trial was to determine whether DEX was superior to PDN in preventing CNS relapses and thereby improve EFS in children with standard-risk ALL. Only children with previously untreated ALL aged between 1 and 10 years with a white blood cell (WBC) count $<50\times10^9$/L were eligible for study entry. During the first 6 months of this trial, a subset of standard-risk (SR) patients (1 to <2 years of age with WBC counts $<50\times10^9$/L; 2 to <10 years with a WBC count of $10\times$ to $<50\times10^9$/L and boys between 2 and 10 years with a WBC count $<10\times10^9$/L and platelet counts $<100\times10^9$/L) were enrolled in the CCG 1891 study for intermediate-risk ALL. All patients were randomly assigned at diagnosis to one of four treatment arms (2×2 factorial design – oral PDN/oral mercaptopurine, oral PDN/IV mercaptopurine, oral DEX/oral mercaptopurine, and oral DEX/IV mercaptopurine). The total duration of treatment was 38 months for boys and 26 months for girls. Of the 1060 eligible patients enrolled on the trial, 530 patients each were randomized to DEX and PDN respectively.

Isolated CNS relapses were lower in the DEX arm compared to the PDN arm (6-year cumulative estimates: DEX 3.7%±0.8% versus PDN 7.1%±1.1%; p=0.01). Although there were no differences in either the day 7 or end of induction marrow status by randomized steroid, patients randomized to DEX showed a trend toward fewer bone marrow relapses, with a 6-year estimate of 7.9%±1.3% versus 11.1%±1.5% (p=0.08). The 6-year EFS for patients randomized to DEX was significantly better: 85%±2% versus 77%±2% for PDN (p=0.002). Patients randomized to DEX had more toxicity, especially myopathy (6.3% versus 1.5% for PDN, p<0.0001 by chi-square), symptomatic pancreatitis, grade 3–4 hyperglycemia (DEX 26/528, 5% versus PDN 8/529, 1.5%; p=0.001) and neuropsychiatric symptoms were almost entirely seen in the DEX group.

This trial showed that despite a greater toxicity profile, DEX reduced the incidence of isolated CNS relapses and improved EFS in children with SR ALL.

A later randomized study by the UK Medical Research Council [4] conducted between April 1997 and June 2002 also compared DEX with PDN in the treatment of childhood lymphoblastic leukemia. Randomization used minimization to balance treatments over gender, age, white blood cell count, and other treatment allocation groups. Previously untreated children with ALL between 1 and 18 years of age were included in the trial. Remission induction chemotherapy comprised weekly vincristine, daily oral steroid as randomized PDN or DEX and Erwinia asparaginase (E Asp). Two intensification blocks were given at weeks 5 and 20 and patients were randomized to receive or not a third intensification block at week 35. In April 1998, the number of E Asp doses was increased to 12 and they were given on alternate days. In May 1998, interim data analysis suggested that patients who received three intensification blocks had an improved survival outcome and hence all subsequently diagnosed patients with ALL and all patients who had not reached week 35 received three intensification blocks. In November 1999, the treatment protocol underwent a further revision and although the basic treatment template and randomization question were retained, the intensification modules were modified to resemble the intensification regime of the BFM Group. A further change took place in April 2001, when *E. coli* asparaginase (Elspar) replaced *Erwinia* asparaginase.

All patients received the same randomized steroid during remission induction, intensification, and the continuing phase of treatment. Presymptomatic CNS prophylaxis consisted of 16 doses of IT MTX with dosage based on age. Patients who had CNS leukemia at diagnosis received additional IT MTX during remission induction followed by 24 Gy cranial irradiation during the consolidation phase of treatment. The total duration of therapy was 3 years for boys and 2 years for girls.

In this trial, 805 patients were randomized to receive PDN and 798 to receive DEX. CNS relapses were significantly lower in patients who were randomized to DEX. The 5-year isolated CNS relapse rate was 2.5% (95% confidence interval [CI] 1.3–3.7%) compared to 5% (95% CI 3.4–6.6%) for children in the PDN arm (p=0.007). In addition, the overall CNS relapse rate was also significantly lower in the DEX arm (p=0.0004), as was the incidence of non-CNS relapses (p=0.002). The relative risk reduction for CNS relapses with DEX was highest for those aged 10 years or above (p=0.03) while for non-CNS relapse it was highest for those <10 years of age (p=0.05). Although the 5-year EFS was significantly better for the DEX group (84.2%, 95% CI 81.5–86.9%) compared to the PDN group (75.6%, 95% CI 72.3–78.9%), there were no differences in the 5-year overall survival (OS) rates between the two groups of patients. Overall toxicity was higher in the DEX group (11% versus 5% with PDN), with behavioral problems (6% versus 1%) and myopathy (2.8% versus 0.5%) being particularly high in patients who received DEX.

Clearly, DEX, despite its increased toxicity, significantly reduced the incidence of isolated and overall CNS relapses and improved EFS and the authors concluded that DEX should be considered as part of standard treatment in childhood ALL.

Another study that compared DEX with PDN was the Tokyo Children's Cancer Study Group (TCCSG) L95-14 trial [5] that was conducted between Mach 1995 and March 1999. Previously untreated children with SR (non-T phenotype ALL, age 1–6 years, WBC count at diagnosis <20×10⁹/L) or intermediate-risk ALL (IR) (age 1–6 years, WBC count between 20 and 100×10^9/L or a child between 7 and 9 years of age with a WBC count $<20 \times 10^9$ or a child who fulfilled the SR criteria but had a T-cell phenotype) were included in this trial. In each risk group, patients were randomized to receive DEX or PDN at diagnosis. IR patients with a WBC count $>50 \times 10^9$/L received 18 Gy prophylactic cranial radiotherapy (CRT) while all other IR and SR patients received IT MTX plus high-dose MTX for CNS prophylaxis.

Of the 359 entered on the TCCSG L95-14 trial, 231 were categorized as SR and 128 as IR. The complete remission rates in the four groups were 98.3% in the SR DEX arm, 99.1% in the SR PDN arm, 95.2% in the IR DEX arm, and 98.5% in the IR PDN arm. Two extramedullary relapses occurred in the DEX arm versus seven in the PDN arm. In addition, there were no differences either in the relapse sites or relapse rates in the DEX and PDN group of patients who received CRT. There were no differences in the EFS between the PDN and DEX arms; 8-year EFS in the DEX (n=117) and PDN (n=114) arms were 81.1% ± 3.9% versus 84.4% ± 5.2%; no differences were seen in EFS rates in either the SR ALL (p=0.217) or IR ALL (p=0.625). Complications including pancreatitis, osteonecrosis and neuropsychiatric symptoms were exclusively seen in patients randomized to DEX.

The investigators concluded that DEX did not offer any advantage over PDN in the treatment of SR or IR ALL in children.

Types of L-asparaginase have also been compared. Pharmacokinetic studies have shown that *E. coli* asparaginase (*E. coli* ASP) has a longer half-life than asparginase derived from *Erwinia* (Erw ASP). The European Organization for Research and Treatment of Cancer (EORTC) trial 58881 [6] compared the efficacy and toxicity of *E. coli* ASP with Erw ASP in previously untreated children (<18 years) with ALL (FAB L1 and L2) or lymphoblastic non-Hodgkin lymphoma (NHL) during remission induction (protocol 1A) and reinduction (protocol II). Patients were randomized at diagnosis to receive either *E. coli* ASP or Erw ASP: a total of 12 doses of 10,000 IU/m² IV twice weekly. Of the 700 eligible patients, 354 were assigned to *E. coli* ASP and 346 to the Erw ASP arm. Complete remission rate was higher with *E. coli* ASP: 94.5% (n=335) versus 91% (n=315) with Erw ASP. The relapse rate was 1.5 times higher in the Erw Asp arm and the EFS was shorter in the Erw Asp arm; the 6-year EFS in the Erw

ASP arm was 59.8% (standard error [SE] 2.6%) versus 73.5% (SE 2.4%) in the *E. coli* ASP arm (p=0004). The 6-year OS was also superior for patients who received *E. coli* ASP: (83.9%, SE 2.0%) versus 75.1% (SE 2.3%) (p=0.002). The estimated hazards ratio for remission failure, relapse or death for patients in the Erw ASP arm was 1.60 (95% CI 1.22–2.09). Coagulation abnormalities were, however, more common amongst patients who received *E. coli* ASP (30.2% versus 11.8%; odds ratio 3.20; p<0.0001).

The report concluded that E. coli ASP was superior to Erw ASP in the treatment of childhood lymphoid malignancies.

The study by Risseeuw-Appel *et al.* [7] focused on coagulation profile with the two different asparaginases – *E. coli* ASP and Erw Asp. Twenty children with previously untreated childhood lymphoblastic leukemia treated on the Dutch Leukaemia Study Group ALL VII protocol were included in this randomized study. Remission induction therapy consisted of 4 weeks of oral prednisone, IV vincristine, IV daunorubicin, asparaginase, and IT MTX. Patients were randomized just prior to the start of phase B (day 18) to receive either Erw ASP or *E. coli* ASP. The mean activated partial thromboplastin time (APTT) levels showed a significant fall after the start of asparaginase treatment (p<0.001), and there were no significant differences in the APTT profiles between the two treatment groups. Although fibrinogen levels also declined significantly (p<0.001) after the start of asparaginase treatment in both treatment groups, the levels recovered more rapidly during phase B in the Erw ASP group and the difference in the change from baseline values was statistically significant at day 25 and at most time points thereafter. While protein C levels also demonstrated a significant decline in both treatment groups (p<0.001), the decreases in protein C levels were nonsignificantly higher in the *E. coli* ASP group.

The report concluded that the overall effect of ASP, either E. coli or Erwinia, on the coagulation system showed a tendency towards thrombosis, mainly because of a gradual decrease in protein C activity. This was less pronounced with Erwinia asparaginase.

As with corticosteroids, the choice of L-asparaginase has been shown to have a significant impact on survival outcome in children with ALL. The report by Avramis *et al.* [8] compared polyethylene glycol conjugated asparaginase (PEG ASP) against native *E. coli* asparaginase (*E. coli* ASP). Children with previously untreated SR ALL (WBC count $\leq 50 \times 10^9$/L) between 1 and 9 years of age enrolled in the CCG 1962 trial were included in the study. Treatment consisted of 4 weeks each of remission induction (RI) and consolidation blocks, two 8-week interim maintenance phases (IM), two 8-week delayed intensification blocks (DI) and a continuing treatment phase. The total duration of treatment from the first IM phase was 2 and 3 years for girls and boys, respectively. Randomization was at diagnosis and all patients received either 2500 IU/m^2 of PEG ASP during RI and two DI phases or 6000 IU/m^2 of *E. coli* ASP×3 /week for nine doses during RI and six doses during each DI block. Patients who received PEG ASP had a more rapid bone marrow leukemic blast clearance on days 7 and 14 as well as more prolonged asparaginase activity than those treated with native ASP. Additionally, the mean asparaginase antibody level during DI was lower in those who received PEG ASP (1.9 ± 0.8) compared to 3 ± 0.7 for those treated with native ASP (p=0.001). Moreover, 26% of native asparaginase patients had high-titer antibodies versus 2% for PEG ASP patients. High-titer antibodies were associated with low asparaginase activity in the native arm but not in the PEG asparaginase arm. Half-lives of asparaginase were 5.5 days and 26 hours for PEG ASP and native asparaginase, respectively. There was correlation between asparaginase enzymatic activity and depletion of asparagine or glutamine in serum. However, no significant differences in the CSF asapargine levels were seen between the two groups of patients. The 3-year EFS rates for PEG ASP and *E. coli* ASP patients were 85% and 78% respectively (p NS). Adverse events, infections, and hospitalizations were similar in both groups.

The report concluded that in view of the fact that PEG ASP had a more prolonged asparaginase activity, lower incidence of silent antibodies and similar safety profile, it should replace native asparaginase in the treatment of children with SR ALL.

References

1 Yetgin S, Tuncer MA, Cetin M *et al.* Benefit of high-dose methylprednisolone in comparison with conventional-dose prednisolone during remission induction therapy in childhood acute lymphoblastic leukemia for long-term follow-up. *Leukemia* 2003;**17**:328–33.

2 López-Hernández MA, Alvarado M, de Diego J, Borbolla-Escoboza JR, Jiménez RM, Trueba E. A randomized trial of dexamethasone before remission induction, in de novo childhood acute lymphoblastic leukemia. *Haematologica* 2004;**89**:365–6.

3 Bostrom BC, Sensel MR, Sather HN *et al.*, for the Children's Cancer Group. Dexamethasone versus prednisone and daily oral versus weekly intravenous mercaptopurine for patients with standard-risk acute lymphoblastic leukemia: a report from the Children's Cancer Group. *Blood* 2003;**101**:3809–17.

4 Mitchell CD, Richards SM, Kinsey SE *et al.*, for the Medical Research Council Childhood Leukaemia Working Party. Benefit of dexamethasone compared with prednisolone for childhood acute lymphoblastic leukaemia: results of the UK Medical Research Council ALL97 randomized trial. *Br J Haematol* 2005;**129**:734–45.

5 Igarashi S, Manabe A, Ohara A *et al.* No advantage of dexamethasone over prednisolone for the outcome of standard- and intermediate-risk childhood acute lymphoblastic leukemia in the Tokyo Children's Cancer Study Group L95-14 protocol. *J Clin Oncol* 2005;**23**:6489–98.

6 Duval M, Suciu S, Ferster A *et al.* Comparison of Escherichia coli-asparaginase with Erwinia-asparaginase in the treatment of childhood lymphoid malignancies: results of a randomized European Organisation for Research and Treatment of Cancer-Children's Leukemia Group phase 3 trial. *Blood* 2002;**99**:2734–9.

7 Risseeuw-Appel IM, Dekker I, Hop WC, Hählen K. Minimal effects of E. coli and Erwinia asparaginase on the coagulation system in childhood acute lymphoblastic leukemia: a randomized study. *Med Pediatr Oncol* 1994;**23**:335–43.

8 Avramis VI, Sencer S, Periclou AP *et al.* A randomized comparison of native Escherichia coli asparaginase and polyethylene glycol conjugated asparaginase for treatment of children with newly diagnosed standard-risk acute lymphoblastic leukemia: a Children's Cancer Group study. *Blood* 2002;**99**:1986–94.

New studies

Study 1

Teuffel O, Kuster SP, Hunger SP *et al*. Dexamethasone versus prednisone for induction therapy in childhood acute lymphoblastic leukemia: a systematic review and meta-analysis. *Leukemia* 2011;**25**:1232–8.

Objectives

This systematic review compared the efficacy and toxicity of DEX versus PDN during RI therapy in childhood ALL.

Study design

Electronic searches of OVID MEDLINE (from 1950 to September 2010), EMBASE (from 1980 to September 2010), and the Cochrane Central Register of Controlled Trials (CENTRAL) until the third quarter of 2010, as well as relevant references and conference proceedings from 2007 to 2010 using the Web of Science and Scopus databases of all randomized controlled trials comparing DEX with PDN during RI therapy in childhood ALL, were performed to extract the relevant data. Data collection was not restricted by dose, frequency or method of drug administration or by length of RI therapy and/or concurrent chemotherapy. There was also no restriction by study site/country, quality of the study or follow-up period. Final inclusion of studies was determined by agreement between two reviewers with the involvement of a third author in cases of discrepancy.

The primary outcome measures included event rate (death from any cause, relapsed or refractory leukemia, second malignancy), relapse rate (specifically any CNS relapse or extramedullary relapse, isolated bone marrow relapse, isolated testicular relapse, combined relapse), and mortality rate.

Secondary outcome measures were death during RI (i.e. death within 60 days of initiation of therapy), osteonecrosis, numbers of patients coming off study following steroid randomization, sepsis (including fungal infection), diabetes, neuropsychiatric events, pancreatitis, and myopathy.

Statistics

To assess methodological quality and risk of bias, included articles were assessed for sequence generation, allocation concealment, blinding, incomplete outcome data, and intention-to-treat analysis. The report was based on an intention-to-treat analysis and determined risk ratios (RR) with 95% CI for dichotomous data (Mantel–Haenszel method). P-values < 0.05 were considered significant. A subgroup analysis was performed for all outcomes to investigate the effect of PDN/DEX dose ratio (< 7 versus ≥ 7). The cut-off of 7 was chosen because this was the typical conversion between DEX and PDN as reported in the literature (i.e. 1 mg DEX is equivalent to 7 mg PDN). Statistical heterogeneity was inspected graphically (forest plot) and assessed by calculating tests of heterogeneity using the Cochran Q-test (χ^2test). The degree of heterogeneity was quantified using the I^2 statistic. Publication bias was investigated using a funnel plot in which the standard error of the effect estimate of each study was plotted against the estimate. An asymmetrical plot suggested possible publication bias.

Results

Of the 23 full articles retrieved and reviewed, only eight studies which satisfied the eligibility criteria were included in the meta-analysis. While blinding status was not reported in any of the studies, withdrawal information could only be retrieved from four of the eight selected studies and intention-to-treat analyses were reported for three trials. When weighted data from five studies were studied, DEX was associated with a significantly lower event rate compared to PDN (RR 0.8; 95% CI 0.68–0.94; p=0.005). As there was significant heterogeneity between the five studies ($I^2 = 60\%$; p=0.04) a stratified analysis (PDN/DEX dose ratios < 7 versus ≥ 7) was performed to explore the heterogeneity. This showed that the superiority of DEX was confined only to studies where PDN/DEX dose ratio was < 7

(RR 0.73; 95% CI 0.66–0.81; p < 0.001) in contrast to studies where the dose ratio was ≥ 7 (RR 1.01; 95% CI 0.84–1.22; p = 0.88).

Corticosteroid choice (prednisone or prednisolone), intensity of RI (three- versus four-drug RI therapy), length of randomization (corticosteroid randomization restricted to RI versus corticosteroid randomization in RI plus other treatment phases) did not significantly affect the results of the report.

Central nervous system and bone marrow relapses

Six studies (8873 patients) provided information related to CNS and bone marrow relapse rates. Whereas DEX compared to PDN significantly reduced CNS relapse in children with ALL (RR 0.53; 95% CI 0.44–0.65; p < 0.001), DEX did not have any significant impact on bone marrow relapse rates (RR 0.9; 95% CI 0.69–1.18; p = 0.45). Qualitatively, DEX appeared superior to PDN in studies where the PDN/DEX ratio was < 7 while PDN appeared superior to DEX in studies where the PDN/DEX ratio was ≥ 7 (both were nonsignificant). No significant differences were observed between DEX and PDN with regard to testicular relapse rates (two studies) or overall mortality (three studies). Only one study provided data on combined relapse.

Adverse events

Dexamethasone compared to PDN was significantly associated with higher deaths during RI (RR 2.31; 95% CI 1.46–3.66; p < 0.001), neuropsychiatric adverse effects (RR 4.55; 95% CI 2.45–8.46; p < 0.001) and myopathy (RR 7.05; 95% CI 3.00–16.58; p < 0.001). In addition, more patients randomized to DEX compared to PDN were likely to have come off study due to adverse treatment effects (RR 121.7; 95% CI 16.34–906.64; p < 0.001). There were no significant differences between DEX and PDN in the incidence of osteonecrosis, sepsis, fungal infections, diabetes or pancreatitis.

Overall survival

No significant differences were identified between DEX and PDN in terms of overall survival (three studies).

Conclusions

The report concluded that while dexamethasone appeared to be more effective during remission induction therapy for children with ALL, it did not alter the incidence of bone marrow relapse or improve overall survival and was significantly more toxic, with higher treatment-related adverse events.

Study 2

Liang DC, Yang CP, Lin DT *et al.* Long-term results of Taiwan Pediatric Oncology Group studies 1997 and 2002 for childhood acute lymphoblastic leukemia. *Leukemia* 2010;24:397–405.

Objectives

In the TPOG-ALL-97 trial, the primary aim was to determine whether epirubicin can replace *E. coli* asparaginase during the remission induction phase of treatment with compromising efficacy in children with SR ALL.

In trial TPOG-ALL-2002, the main aims were to determine whether a single intensification block was as effective as two intensification blocks in the treatment of children with SR ALL and whether replacing cranial irradiation with triple intrathecal (TIT) chemotherapy was safe and effective

This review focuses only on the randomization between *E. coli* asparaginase and epirubicin during the remission induction treatment phase in trial TPOC-ALL-97.

Study design

Although the detailed treatment protocol for trial TPOG-ALL-97 was not described in the publication, the treatment phases for patients with SR ALL were similar to the treatment protocol in TPOG-ALL-2002 and consisted of a 5-week induction phase with four drugs (vincristine, prednisolone, asparaginase or epirubicin [R] and TIT), 8 weeks of consolidation with two drugs (moderate-dose IV methotrexate, oral 6-mercaptopurine and TIT), 2-week reinduction (dexamethasone, vincristine, epirubicin, *E. coli* asparaginase and TIT) followed by the maintenance phase (oral 6-mercaptopurine, oral methotrexate, cyclophosphamide, cytarabine with 8-week pulses of vincristine, dexamethasone, and TIT).

The definition of SR ALL was 1 to 10 years old with a presenting white blood cell count $<10\times10^9/L$.

Statistics

Event-free survival and OS were estimated by the Kaplan–Meier method and compared by the Mantel–Haenszel test. Details of the randomization methodology were not specified in the publication.

Results

Six hundred and fourteen patients were enrolled on the TPOG-ALL-97 trial. The 5- and 10-year EFS (± standard error [SE]) rates were 69.3%±1.9% and 68.0%±2.0% respectively. There was no statistically significant difference in the 10-year EFS rates between the two treatment arms: (E. coli asparaginase arm [SRL] (n=114), 82.8%±3.6% versus epirubicin arm [SRE] (n=153), 78.0%±3.5%; p=0.353.

Conclusions

It was concluded that asparaginase and epirubicin were of comparable efficacy during remission induction phase treatment that included prednisolone, vincristine, and TIT in children with SR ALL.

Study 3

Mikkelsen TS, Sparreboom A, Cheng C et al. Shortening infusion time for high-dose methotrexate alters antileukemic effects: a randomized prospective clinical trial. J Clin Oncol 2011;29:1771–8.

Objectives

To determine whether shortening infusion time of high-dose methotrexate (HDMTX) affects in vivo accumulation of active methotrexate (MTX) polyglutamates (MTXPG) in leukemic cells and whether this alters the antileukemic effects of MTX.

Study design

This was a prospective randomized trial in which HDMTX was given as a single agent before the start of conventional chemotherapy to patients with newly diagnosed ALL. All children between the ages of 1 and 18 years with a newly diagnosed ALL treated at either St Jude Children's Research Hospital or Cook Children's Medical Center between 2000 and 2007

were the subjects of this report. All patients were divided into five major subtypes based on cytogenetic and immunophenotypic analysis: T- or B-lineage ALL with hyperdiploidy (B-hyperdiploid), with t(12;21)/ETV6-RUNX1 translocation, t(1;19) translocation or with none of these chromosomal translocations (B-other). Because allopurinol (ALPN) inhibits de novo purine synthesis, patients who received ALPN before or during HDMTX infusion were excluded from analysis of the antileukemia effects of MTX.

Randomization

Patients were randomly assigned to receive in an open-label manner preinduction chemotherapy with IV HDMTX ($1\,g/m^2$) either as a 4-h constant infusion or 24-h infusion ($200\,mg/m^2$ over 5 min and then 800 mg/m^2 over the next 23 h and 55 min). The randomization was stratified according to ALL lineage (T versus B) and ploidy (hyperdiploid versus nonhyperdiploid B-lineage ALL). A computer software system generated a block randomization scheme with a block size of 6. The random assignment was stratified according to ALL lineage and ploidy. Standard remission induction therapy was not started until 3 days after HDMTX infusion.

Plasma pharmacokinetics of methotrexate

Peripheral blood was drawn at 1, 4, 24, and 42 h after the start of HDMTX infusion and concentrations of MTX in plasma were measured by a fluorescence polarization immunoassay.

Assessment of methotrexate polyglutamates in leukemia cells

Intracellular concentrations of MTXPG (pmol/10^9 cells) were measured in leukemia cells from the 42-h bone marrow sample and peripheral blood.

Measurement of de novo purine synthesis

De novo purine synthesis (DNPS) was measured in bone marrow lymphoblasts and percentage change from pretreatment to 42 h after start of HDMTX infusion was calculated as $DNPS_{42H} - DNPS_{PRE}/DNPS_{PRE}$.

Measurement of antileukemic effects

Circulating leukemia cells were measured in peripheral blood immediately before MTX infusion and at 3 days after start of infusion and the percentage change in pretreatment to day 3 was calculated.

Statistics

Sample size for MTXPG accumulation was estimated on the basis of pharmacokinetic data from the Total Therapy Study XIIIA in which children with ALL received HDMTX 1 g/m² infused over 24 h. All values were expressed as medians and normally distributed variables were compared by t test. Nonrandomly distributed variables were compared using the Wilcoxon rank sum or Kruskal Wallis test. Multivariable linear regression was performed to assess the association between log ($MTXPG_{1-7}$) and covariates.

Results

Three hundred and fifty-six children were randomized to IV HDMTX to either a 24-h infusion or 4-h infusion before start of conventional remission induction treatment. There were no demographic or biological differences between the 24-h infusion patient group (n = 180) and the 4- infusion patient group (n = 176).

Accumulation of methotrexate polyglutamates in leukemia cells

Patients randomized to the 24-h HDMTX infusion (1695 pmol/10⁹ cells) had significantly higher amounts of MTXPG in the leukemic cells compared to patients on the 4-h HDMTX infusion (1150 pmol/10⁹ cells; p = 0.0059). This difference remained significant after adjusting for cell lineage and ploidy. Within specific B-cell lineage genetic subtypes, the 24-h infusion resulted in significantly higher intracellular $MTXPG_{1-7}$ in hyperdiploid ALL (3919 versus 2417 pmol/10⁹ cells; p = 0.0038) and in the B-other ALL subtype (2210 versus 1576 pmol/10⁹ cells; p = 0.048). With either infusion rate, intracellular MTXPG accumulation was significantly higher in hyperdiploid ALL than in any other ALL subtype and was lowest in B-cell lineage ALL with t(1;19) and T-cell lineage ALL.

De novo purine synthesis inhibition

De novo purine synthesis inhibition was higher in patients who received the 24-h HDMTX infusion compared to patients who received the 4-h infusion (p = 0.021) and this remained significant after adjusting for ploidy and cell lineage (p = 0.044). In a multivariable model analysis, duration of MTX infusion and ALL subtype were the only factors significantly related to percentage inhibition of DNPS.

Antileukemia effects

The 24-h HDMTX infusion produced a significantly greater antileukemia effect in patients compared to the 4-h infusion and this was reflected in the mean day 3 WBC (p = 0.038). Among the ALL subtypes, T-cell ALL patients had a better response to the 24-h HDMTX infusion when measured as either day 3 WBC or percentage change in circulating leukemia cells. This better antileukemia effect with the 24-h HDMTX infusion remained when adjusted for ALL subtypes and white cell count at presentation in a multivariable model.

Methotrexate polyglutamates as a predictor of relapse

Low accumulation of MTXPG in ALL cells was significantly associated with a higher risk of relapse when compared to intermediate (hazard ratio 3.3; 95% CI 1.2–9.1; p = 0.018) or high accumulation of MTXPG (hazard ratio 3.6; 95% CI 1.0–12.5; p = 0.047) and this risk remained after adjusting for disease risk group and treatment arm.

Conclusions

It was concluded that shortening the duration of HDMTX infusion reduced MTXPG accumulation in leukemia cells and, consequently, the antileukemia effects, which varied among ALL subtypes.

Study 4

Matloub Y, Bostrom BC, Hunger SP *et al.* Escalating intravenous methotrexate improves event-free survival in children with standard-risk acute lymphoblastic leukemia: a report from the Children's Oncology Group. *Blood* 2011;118:243–52.

Objectives

The main aims of the trial were to:
• compare the survival outcome of children with SR ALL treated with escalating doses of intravenous methotrexate without leucovorin rescue and

vincristine versus standard oral MTX, oral 6-mercaptopurine (6-MP), dexamethasone and vincristine during the interim maintenance phases of treatment
• determine whether the addition of a second delayed intensification block improves survival outcome.

This report presents the outcome of randomized children with B precursor ALL who achieved a rapid early response to remission induction therapy.

Study design

CCG 1991 was a prospective multicenter randomized trial conducted between June 2000 and February 2005 and included children between 1 and 10 years of age who had a presenting white cell count $<50 \times 10^9$/L. Children who had an L3 morphology, poor-risk cytogenetics such as t(9;22), t(4;11), or t(2;8) or who had treatment with systemic corticosteroids >48 h during the preceding month were excluded from trial enrollment. Children with SR T-cell ALL were initially included in the trial but were excluded from trial enrollment after March 2004 when an interim analysis showed inferior outcome for children with T-cell ALL.

All children received a three-drug induction therapy that included IT ARAC $\times$ 1, IV vincristine (VCR), oral dexamethasone (DEX) and IM pegylated asparaginase (PEG ASP) and IT MTX $\times$ 2 doses. Marrow status was determined on days 7 and 14 and to be eligible for randomization, patients must have achieved an M1 or M2 status on day 7 (<25% blasts) and should have achieved morphological remission by day 28 (<5% blasts) and no unfavorable cytogenetics such as hypodiploidy, balanced t(1;19) (q23;p13).

Randomization occurred between days 21 and 28 and eligible patients were randomly assigned in a 2×2 factorial design to one of four treatment regimens: regimen OS – oral MTX, 6MP, VCR and DEX during IM phases and single delayed intensification (SDI); regimen OD – oral MTX, 6MP, VCR and DEX during IM phases and two intensification courses (DDI); regimen IS – IV MTX and VCR during IM phases and SDI; regimen ID – IV MTX and VCR during IM phases and DDI. All patients received two interim maintenance courses regardless of the number of courses of delayed intensification. The total duration of treatment for girls and boys was 2 and 3 years respectively from the start of the first interim maintenance course.

Bone marrow relapse was defined as an M3 marrow (>25% blasts) after achieving initial CR and CNS relapse was diagnosed when the CSF contained at least 5 WBC/µL with morphologically identifiable blasts on a cyto-spin sample.

Statistics

The primary endpoints were EFS and OS from the time of randomization. The Kaplan–Meier method was used to calculate EFS and OS and standard errors were calculated by the Peto method. The log-rank test was used to compare survival curves between groups. The χ^2 test of homogeneity of proportions was used to compare baseline patient clinical characteristics.

Results

Although a total of 3054 patients was entered on the trial, only 2078 eligible patients were randomized as a significant number were excluded because of trial ineligibility (n=28), refusal of trial enrollment or withdrawn from trial by parent/guardian (n=456), had high-risk ALL (n=283), had CNS disease at diagnosis (n=35) or were ineligible for randomization (n=26). Hence among the eligible patients (n=2078), 512 were randomized to the OS arm, 524 to the OD arm, 525 to the IS arm, and 517 to the ID arm.

The overall 5-year EFS and OS for the eligible B precursor randomized patients were 90.7% ± 0.9% and 96% ± 0.6% respectively. Comparing the randomized treatment arms, the 5- year EFS was significantly better for patients randomized to the IV MTX-based interim maintenance arms (92.6% ± 1.2% versus 88.7% ± 1.4%; p=0.009) compared to the oral MTX-based arms (OS and OD). The 5-year OS rates were comparable for the IV and oral-based regimens. The addition of a second DI provided no benefit, with the 5-year EFS and OS of 90.9% ± 1.3% and 97.1% ± 0.8% respectively for the single DI regimen compared to 90.5% ± 1.3% and 95.4% ± 1.0% respectively for the two-course DI regimen (p=0.71; 0.12).

Eighty-two relapses were observed among the 1037 patients randomized to the single DI arms (OS+IS) compared to 86 among 1041 children randomized to the DDI arms (IS+ID). Ninety-six relapses (n=1036) occurred in children randomized to the oral MTX-based IM arm compared to 72 relapses (n=1042) in the IV-based IM treatment arm. Patients randomized to the IV MTX-based IM treatment arm had a significantly lower extramedullary relapse rate compared to the oral MTX-based IM arm (CNS: 11 [1%] versus 26 [2.5%]; testicular: 0 [0%] versus 7 [0.7%]). While IV MTX eliminated CNS relapses in girls and testicular relapses in boys, IV MTX-based IM treatment had no effect on the incidence of bone marrow relapse. While the advantage of IV MTX was seen in both girls (5-year EFS 93.1% ± 1.7% versus 88.8% ± 2.1%; p=0.02, relative hazard rate [RHR] 1.7) and boys (92% ± 1.6% versus 88.6% ± 2.0%; p=0.13), it was statistically significant in girls alone.

Toxicity

Children randomized to the oral MTX arms had greater elevations in their hepatic transaminases and while seizure rates were very low in all four treatment arms, they were relatively higher in the IV MTX arms.

Conclusions

It was concluded that while there was no advantage for a second delayed intensification course, the use of escalating IV MTX along with vincristine during interim maintenance improved EFS in children with SR ALL.

Study 5

Pieters R, Appel I, Kuehnel HJ *et al.* Pharmacokinetics, pharmacodynamics, efficacy, and safety of a new recombinant asparaginase preparation in children with previously untreated acute lymphoblastic leukemia: a randomized phase 2 clinical trial. *Blood* 2008;**112**:4832–8.

Objectives

The main aim of this prospective randomized trial was to evaluate the safety, tolerability, and efficacy of recombinant asparaginase (R-ASP) in the treatment of children with newly diagnosed *de novo* ALL and whether it can safely replace native asparaginase (MEDAC).

Study design

Thirty-two children with previously untreated ALL were enrolled on this study that was conducted between January 2005 and October 2006. All were treated according to the DCOG ALL-10 trial protocol and received remission induction that comprised prednisolone (60 mg/m²/day, days 1–36), vincristine

(1.5 mg/ m², days 8, 15, 22, 29), daunorubicin (30 mg/ m², days 8, 15, 22, 29), asparaginase (5000 U/m², days 12, 15, 18, 21, 24, 27, 30, 33) and intrathecal chemotherapy (IT CT) with methotrexate, cytarabine, and prednisolone (days 15 and 33).

Children were randomized to receive either R-ASP or asparaginase MEDAC (M-ASP) in a double-blind manner. Asparaginase serum levels were measured within 72 h of administration of the first dose of ASP. Additionally, prior to IT CT on days 1, 15, and 33 (45 and 59 during treatment phase B), CSF was sampled for amino acid levels. Serum levels of asparaginase were determined by a sensitive microplate reader-based method. Serum and CSF levels of asparagine, glutamine, aspartic acid, and glutamic acid were analyzed by reverse-phase high-performance liquid chromatography (HPLC). The lower limit of quantification for asparagine in serum and CSF was 0.5 μM.

Treatment efficacy was determined according to complete remission (CR) rate and minimal residual disease (MRD) status at the end of remission induction (day 33). MRD negativity was defined as MRD $< 10^{-4}$ with two MRD PCR targets. MRD status was assessed by determination of clonal immunoglobulin H (IgH), T-cell receptor (TCR) rearrangements (TCR-δ and TCR-λ) with polymerase chain reaction (PCR) on day 33. The primary endpoint of the study was a comparison of the area under the curve (AUC) of asparaginase in serum after the first dose.

Statistics

A total of 32 patients were randomized in a 1:1 ratio to show equivalence with a power of 80% using two one-sided *t*-tests at 5% significance level on the log transformed data. This sample size assumed treatment-specific coefficient of variations of 25%.

Results

Thirty-two children were included in the study. Two patients were excluded (both received R-ASP) from the pharmacokinetic analysis because of missing serum samples although both were included for efficacy and safety analysis. The median age of the cohort was 4.5 years. Patients who were randomized to R-ASP had a higher mean white blood cell count and leukemic blasts in the peripheral blood at diagnosis.

Asparaginase pharmacokinetics after first dose

Maximum serum activity (C_{MAX}), half-life, total clearance, and volume of distribution were not significantly different in the treatment groups. C_{MAX} was reached immediately after infusion for most patients. The point estimate of AUC_{0-72h} for the treatment ratio recombinant asparaginase/asparaginase MEDAC was 86.01 (95% CI 77.52–95.43) and was contained within the predefined acceptance range of equivalence of 75–133%. Although the AUC_{0-72h} value was statistically significantly (p=0.02) different between R-ASP and M-ASP, it was too small to be considered clinically relevant.

Asparaginase trough levels during acute lymphoblastic leukemia remission induction

While the observed trough activities (measured just before asparaginase administration) were above the desired threshold of >100 U/L in both treatment groups, the R-ASP treatment group had slightly lower values than those who received M-ASP.

Pharmacodynamic results

Mean asaparagine concentrations in serum dropped from the predose concentrations of 45.83 μM R-ASP and 42.52 μM M-ASP to below the lower limit of quantification (<0.5 μM.) in both treatment groups. Mean serum asaparagine depletion was >99% (immediately after the first dose on day 12 until last day of ASP treatment on day 33) in both treatment groups and serum asparagine levels correlated to asparaginase activity in both treatment groups (i.e. the higher the serum concentrations of asparaginase, the lower the asparagine concentrations). The mean duration of depletion after the end of ASP treatment was 7.6 days (standard deviation [SD] 3.2) with R-ASP and 9.0 (SD 3.5) days with M-ASP treatment. Similarly, mean CSF asparagine levels dropped below the level of quantification (days 15 and 33) in both treatment groups. Whereas both ASP preparations completely depleted serum and CSF of asparagine, glutamine levels were only moderately affected with a very high interindividual variability.

Remission status and safety

A high percentage of patients had MRD levels < 10^{-4} on day 33 of remission induction with both asparaginase preparations. Both preparations were well tolerated and no differences in the severity or

frequency of adverse reactions were observed. No differences in hepatic and kidney function parameters or abnormalities of coagulation profile were observed between the two asparaginase preparations. Two patients in each treatment arm experienced a serious adverse reaction (deep vein thrombosis×2, severe neutropenia (M-ASP) and severe hyperglycemia (R-ASP)).

Conclusions

It was concluded that the recombinant asparaginase was bioequivalent to native asparaginase with a good safety profile when used in children during ALL remission induction.

Study 6

Moghrabi A, Levy DE, Asselin B *et al*. Results of the Dana-Farber Cancer Institute ALL Consortium Protocol 95-01 for children with acute lymphoblastic leukemia. *Blood* 2007;**109**:896–904.

Objectives

The aims of this study were to:

• determine whether cardiac toxicity could be prevented by the use of the cardioprotectant dexrazoxane in children with high-risk ALL without compromising efficacy

• compare and evaluate the safety and efficacy of two different asparaginase preparations (*E. coli* ASP and *Erwinia chrysanthemi* [Erwinase] asparaginase) when administered during remission induction and consolidation phases of therapy in children with ALL

• compare the efficacy of 18 Gy cranial irradiation with intensive intrathecal chemotherapy as presymptomatic CNS treatment

• compare two dosing schedules of cranial irradiation (once-daily versus twice-daily fractions).

This review focuses only on the asparaginase question.

Study design

The DFCI Protocol 95-01 was a multicenter randomized trial conducted between January 1996 and September 2000 and children (0–18 years of age) with previously untreated ALL were eligible for study enrollment. All patients were categorized as SR or high-risk (HR) ALL according to DFCI risk group criteria that incorporated the National Cancer Institute (NCI) age and WBC count criteria.

Standard-risk and HR patients were randomized to receive 20 weekly doses of either Erwinase or *E. coli* ASP (both 25,000 IU/m^2 intramuscularly) until December 1998 when the randomization target accrual was met. Thereafter, all patients received *E. coli* ASP only.

The asparaginase preparation was switched after an allergic event; patients allergic to *E. coli* ASP were switched to twice-weekly Erwinase (25,000 IU/m^2/dose) while those allergic to Erwinase switched to weekly *E. coli* ASP (25,000 IU/m^2/dose) to complete 20 weeks of treatment. All patients were switched to weekly polyethylene glycol (PEG) asparaginase (2500 IU/m^2/dose) if they experienced a subsequent allergic reaction.

Statistics

Overall survival, EFS, and leukemia-free survival (LFS; time from complete remission to relapse) were estimated by the Kaplan–Meier method and the Greenwood formula was used to calculate standard errors. Univariate analyses of differences in LFS, OS, and EFS were conducted with log-rank tests. Multiple regression was conducted using Cox proportional hazards model to assess prognostic factors for EFS, OS, and LFS. P-values ≤ 0.05 were deemed statistically significant.

Results

A total of 286 patients were involved in the randomized comparison between Erwinase and *E. coli* ASP; patients received a single dose during remission induction followed by 20 weekly injections during postremission consolidation. Although asparaginase-related toxicity was lower in the Erwinase group compared to those randomized to *E. coli* ASP (10% versus 24%; p < 0.01), more patients in the Erwinase treatment arm relapsed at any site (19% versus 10%; p = 0.02), including CNS relapses (6% versus 1%; p < 0.01). At a median follow-up of 6.5 years for randomized patients, the 5-year EFS for Erwinase patients was 78% ± 4% versus 89% ± 3% for *E. coli* patients (p = 0.01). The difference in EFS remained significant when stratified by risk group (p = 0.02).

Toxicity

Asparaginase toxicity was observed in 21% of patients. While patients between 10 and 18 years had higher probability of an asparaginase-related toxicity compared to those < 10 years of age (29% versus 19%; p = 0.03), this difference was not observed for allergic events (8% versus 14%).

Conclusions

It was concluded that while once-weekly Erwinase was less toxic than *E. coli* ASP, it was also significantly less efficacious.

Study 7

Silverman LB, Stevenson KE, O'Brien JE *et al.* Long-term results of Dana-Farber Cancer Institute ALL Consortium protocols for children with newly diagnosed acute lymphoblastic leukemia (1985–2000). *Leukemia* 2010;24:320–34.

Objectives

This publication reported the long-term results of four consecutive Dana-Farber Cancer Institute (DFCI) pediatric clinical trials conducted between 1985 and 2000. It focuses on the randomization results between *E. coli* asparaginase, polyethylene glycol asparaginase (protocol 91-01), and *Erwinia* asparaginase (protocol 95-01).

Study design

The DFCI Protocol 91-01 and 95-01 were multicenter prospective trials. Treatment was assigned based on risk group classification determined at diagnosis. There were four phases of therapy: remission induction, CNS-directed treatment, intensification, and continuation.

Randomizations

• Eligible patients treated on protocol 91-01 received 30 weeks of asparaginase during the intensification phase and were randomized to receive either *E. coli* asparaginase 25,000 IU/m^2/week or polyethylene glycol (PEG) asparaginase 2500 IU/m^2 every 2 weeks.
• Eligible patients in protocol 95-01 were randomized to receive either *E. coli* asparaginase or *Erwinia*

asparaginase 25,000 IU/m²/week for 20 weeks during the intensification phase.

- Eligible patients on protocol 91-01 were randomized to receive standard oral 6-MP (50 mg/m²/day on days 1–14 every 3 weeks or high-dose IV 6-MP (1000 mg/m²/dose over 20 hours weekly×2 every 3 weeks for 1 year after completion of remission induction phase; thereafter all patients receive standard oral 6-MP.

This review focuses on the first and second randomization questions: native *E. coli* asparaginase versus PEG asparginase and *E. coli* asparaginase versus *Erwinia* asparaginase alone.

Statistics

Event-free failure and OS was estimated by the Kaplan–Meier method and compared with the log-rank test. Multivariable regression was performed using the Cox proportional hazards model to assess prognostic factors for EFS and OS for each protocol.

Results

Protocol 91-01

One hundred and ninety-eight patients (SR/HR/very high risk [VHR]) were randomized to receive either *E. coli* asparaginase (25,000 IU/m² IM weekly) or PEG asparaginase (2500 IU/m² IM every 2 weeks) for a total of 30 weeks during the postinduction consolidation. There was no significant difference in either the EFS (p=0.29) or OS (p=0.29) based on the type of asparaginase.

Protocol 95-01

Two hundred and eighty-six patients (SR.HR/VHR) were randomized to either *E. coli* asparaginase or *Erwinia* asparaginase for 20 weeks during postinduction consolidation. Patients randomized to *Erwinia* asparaginase had significantly inferior 10-year EFS (75.2% ± 3.8% versus 84.6% ± 3.4%; p=0.02) and OS (85.3% ± 3.1% versus 93.1% ± 2.1%; p=0.04). More patients randomized to *Erwinia* asparaginase experienced a relapse involving the CNS (7% versus 1%; p<0.01).

Conclusions

It was concluded that fortnightly IM PEG asparaginase was similar in efficacy to weekly IM native *E. coli* asparaginase but was associated with reduced risk of hypersensitivity reactions. As previously reported, *E. coli* asparaginase was superior to *Erwinia* asparaginase in improving survival outcomes in children with ALL.

CHAPTER 20

Central nervous system-directed therapy in childhood lymphoblastic leukemia

Ananth Shankar

University College London Hospitals NHS Foundation Trust, London, UK

Summary of previous studies

Prior to 1960, when there was no presymptomatic central nervous system (CNS)-directed therapy, > 50% of children relapsed in the CNS. Radiotherapy had been shown to be effective in controlling overt CNS disease after the first demonstration that craniospinal irradiation (CSRT) given to children without detectable CNS disease (but invariably subclinical involvement). Subsequently, many collaborative study groups conducted randomized trials of pre-symptomatic or prophylactic cranial radiotherapy (CRT) or CSRT aimed at optimizing the effect of chemo-radiation in this setting but minimizing toxicity, particularly late sequelae.

Dose of irradiation

In the Children's Cancer Group (CCG) trials CCG-101 and CCG 143 [1], patients were randomized to either craniospinal radiotherapy (CSRT) (24 Gy or 18 Gy) or cranial radiotherapy (CRT) (24 Gy or 18 Gy) plus intrathecal (IT) methotrexate (MTX). All patients received identical induction and continuing treatment therapy. At 2 years after randomization, the proportion of patients who experienced a CNS relapse was: CSRT 18 Gy 0.05, 24 Gy 0.07; 18 Gy CRT + IT MTX

0.08, 24 Gy CRT + IT MTX 0.06. There were no statistically significant differences in the CNS relapse rate in poor-risk acute lymphoblastic leukemia (ALL) patients (presenting white blood cell count > 50×10^9/L) who received either 24 Gy or 18 Gy CSRT (p=0.84) or 24 Gy CRT + IT MTX or 18 Gy CRT + IT MTX (p=0.45). In fact, patients who received 18 Gy CRT + IT MTX had fewer events than any other combination of treatment. The report concluded that the reduction of CNS irradiation to 18 Gy did not result in any significant increase in the frequency of CNS relapse, bone marrow or death among any prognostic group of patients.

The UK ALL VII trial [2] also focused on reducing the dose of presymptomatic cranial irradiation and randomized previously untreated children (< 14 years old) with ALL to either 18 Gy or 24 Gy cranial irradiation. Black children as well as those with T-ALL or B-ALL were excluded from the trial. In addition, it had a second randomization: whether the extra doses of IT MTX at 6-weekly intervals during the first year of continuing therapy reduced subsequent CNS relapse. There was no difference in the CNS relapse rates between the two CRT schedules or the differing IT MTX schedules when analyzed by both intention to treat and actual treatment

Evidence-Based Pediatric Oncology, Third Edition. Edited by Ross Pinkerton, Ananth Shankar and Katherine K. Matthay.
© 2013 John Wiley & Sons, Ltd. Published 2013 by John Wiley & Sons, Ltd.

received. The authors concluded that the reduction in the dose of presymptomatic cranial RT was not detrimental for children with ALL.

The Brazilian ALL Study Group trial GBTLI-80 [3] compared and evaluated the efficacy of 18 Gy CRT against 24 Gy CRT as presymptomatic CNS-directed therapy in the treatment of children with low-risk ALL. Patients with low-risk ALL who had achieved complete remission after the remission induction phase of treatment were randomized to either 18 Gy or 24 Gy CRT CNS prophylactic treatment. The incidence of combined and isolated CNS relapse was 6.7%. Similar to the UK ALL VII trial, there was no statistically significant difference in CNS relapse rates between patients who received 18 Gy and 24 Gy CRT (p=0.61). It was concluded that 18 Gy CRT was adequate irradiation for CNS prophylaxis in children with low-risk ALL.

The three previous reports showed that the reduction of presymptomatic CNS irradiation to 18 Gy had no adverse impact on either CNS relapse rates or survival outcome. The Berlin-Frankfurt-Münster (BFM) ALL-83 trial [4] went a step further in reducing the dose of CRT to 12 Gy and conducted a randomized trial in high standard-risk (SR) ALL patients (n=143): 12 Gy versus 18 Gy as presymptomatic CNS-directed therapy. The cumulative incidences of CNS relapses were not significantly different between the two groups of patients. The 8-year disease-free survival (DFS) rate for the 12 Gy CRT group (n=72) was 62.7%±5.6% compared to 68.1%±5.6% for the 18 Gy group (p=0.68). Clearly, 12 Gy CRT was as effective as 18 Gy in preventing CNS relapse of leukemia and did not adversely impact on DFS in patients with high SR ALL.

Another study that compared 18 Gy against 24 Gy CRT as CNS prophylaxis for SR ALL patients was the Tokyo Children's Cancer Group L81-10 trial [5]. SR ALL patients were randomized to 18 Gy CRT plus IT MTX (n=46) and hydrocortisone (IT MH) or 24 Gy CRT plus IT MH (n=40) after the completion of remission induction phase. There were three CNS relapses in each group and the 5-year event-free survival (EFS) in the 18 Gy group was 81.7%±5.8% compared to 62.3%±8% in the 24 Gy group (p=0.14). The authors concluded that 18 Gy CRT with IT MH was adequate in preventing CNS relapses in children with SR ALL.

The need for irradiation in central nervous system-directed therapy

The CCG-123 trial [6] was a randomized prospective multicenter trial that evaluated the need for cranial radiotherapy as CNS prophylaxis in the treatment of children with high-risk ALL (bulky extramedullary disease and T-cell phenotype or other poor prognostic features). Patients were randomized to one of four treatment regimens.

- **Regimen A** was the CCG modified version of the BFM-76/79 study. Treatment included intensive induction/consolidation, a reinduction/reintensification phase after a period of interim maintenance and 18 Gy cranial radiotherapy plus IT MTX for CNS prophylaxis.
- **Regimens B and C** were the CCG modified versions of the Memorial Sloan-Kettering LSA2-L2 protocol. Regimen B included 18 Gy CRT plus IT MTX while regimen C was without cranial radiotherapy. Patients with CNS disease at diagnosis were not eligible for regimen C. Patients in both regimens B and C received 15 Gy irradiation to extra-abdominal bulky disease.
- **Regimen D** (New York regimen) was based on a five-drug induction therapy combined with 15 Gy irradiation to bulky extra-abdominal and 18 Gy CRT plus IT MTX given during the consolidation phase of treatment.

Outcome measures included EFS and overall survival (OS). The final randomization tally when the study was closed was regimen A 261, B 163, C 84, and D 170.

Results

The EFS at 6 years from diagnosis for the entire cohort was 60%±4% and OS was 67%±4%. The EFS rates were similar for regimens A (67%±6%) and D (67%±7%) and this was significantly better than either of the two LSA2-L2 regimens (regimen B 53%±8% and regimen C 42%±0%). The difference in the EFS rates between the two LSA2-L2 arms was small (relative hazard rate [RHR] was 1.3 for regimen C; p=0.34). The comparison of CNS remission duration for regimen B versus regimen C was significant (p=0.02); the CNS recurrence rate for regimen B was 6% versus 18% for regimen C. Bone marrow (BM) relapse rates were 32%±8% and 39%±12% for regimen B and C patients respectively. The report concluded that the LSA2-L2 chemotherapy regimen with cranial radiotherapy as CNS prophylaxis resulted in lower CNS relapse rates compared to the same treatment regimen without cranial irradiation.

The Alin C-9 trial [7] aimed to evaluate whether triple intrathecal (TIT) chemotherapy alone was an effective form of presymptomatic CNS therapy. Children < 15 years of age were randomized at diagnosis to either TIT alone or to TIT plus 24 Gy CRT. Briefly, systemic therapy consisted of vincristine and prednisolone or cyclophosphamide, asparaginase, vincristine, and prednisolone. Continuing therapy consisted of 6-mercaptopurine (6-MP) plus vincristine with prednisolone ± daunorubicin reinforcement. TIT consisted of IT MTX 15 mg/m^2, IT cytosine arabinoside (ARAC) 30 mg/m^2 and IT hydrocortisone (IT HC) 15 mg/m^2 given weekly during the first month of CT and thereafter once every 2 months. No significant difference was noted in the duration of CNS remission or in the CNS relapse rate between the two groups of patients (p=0.44) irrespective of the presenting white blood cell count. In addition, there were no differences in the duration of disease-free remission (p=0.84) or OS (p=0.85) between the two treatment groups. Furthermore, hematological toxicity was greater in the CRT group (P=0.05). The report concluded that the addition of cranial irradiation to TIT for presymptomatic CNS therapy was unnecessary in children with ALL.

The Alin C-11 trial [8] was similar to the Alin C-9 study and compared the efficacy of IT chemotherapy alone against 24 Gy CRT plus IT MTX as CNS prophylaxis for children with ALL. All patients received induction therapy with vincristine and prednisolone and continuing therapy consisted of oral MTX and oral 6-MP. Patients were randomized at diagnosis to one of four treatment regimens. Allocation to regimens 1 and 4 (conventional CNS regimens) was weighted 2:1 with the other two regimens. Total duration of treatment was 3 years. The number of CNS relapses including those combined with a bone marrow relapse in the IT alone regimens (regimens 1–3) was 10/234 (4.3%) compared to 7/105 (6.1%) in the CRT plus IT MTX (p=NS) group. It was, therefore, concluded that IT chemotherapy alone was as effective as CRT plus IT MTX in preventing CNS relapse of leukemia when used with effective systemic regimens.

The CALGB trial 7111 [9] was similar to the previous Alin C-11 trial as its aim was to determine the effectiveness of IT MTX as presymptomatic CNS treatment for children with ALL. All previously untreated children below the age of 20 years with ALL were entered on the trial. Remission induction consisted of vincristine (VCR), prednisolone (PDN) or dexamethasone (DEX) with or without L-asparaginase (L-ASP) (prior to, simultaneously or subsequent to a 3-week course of VCR and steroids). Patients in CR after 2 months of treatment were randomized to weekly IT MTX (12 mg/m^2) alone or to weekly IT MTX plus 24 Gy CRT. Of the 493 randomized patients, 255 were randomized to IT MTX alone while 238 were assigned to CRT plus IT MTX. With the CNS prophylaxis regimens, CNS relapse occurred in 30 of 238 (12.6%) patients who received CRT plus IT MTX compared to 70/255 (27.5%) who received IT MTX alone. Additionally, patients who received CRT had a longer duration of CR (p=0.037). It was concluded that CNS prophylaxis with CRT plus IT MTX offered greater protection against CNS relapse compared to IT MTX alone.

The Alin C-12 trial [10] compared the efficacy of TIT CT versus CRT plus IT MTX as CNS prophylaxis in children with high-risk ALL. Previously untreated children and adolescents with high-risk ALL below 21 years were included in this trial. All patients were randomized at diagnosis to one of two treatment arms.

• Arm 1: induction consisted of VCR, PDN, and L-ASP with 2 additional weeks of VCR and PDN given to those who had not achieved a CR after 4 weeks of treatment. CNS prophylaxis consisted of 15–24 Gy CRT that was age dependent along with five doses of IT MTX during CRT.

• Arm 3: remission induction was identical to arm 1 with the exception that L-ASP was given during the consolidation block along with cyclophosphamide. CNS prophylaxis in this arm was with TIT CT along with intravenous MTX every 2 weeks for six courses and also during the entire continuing therapy phase of treatment in 8-weekly cycles.

Continuing therapy consisted of oral 6-MP and oral MTX with pulses of VCR and PDN and treatment ended at 3 years from date of remission. Two hundred and seven patients were randomized to treatment arm 1 and 223 patients to treatment arm 3. There were in total 37 CNS relapses in treatment arm 1 patients compared to 26 in treatment arm 3 (relative risk 0.59;

95% confidence interval [CI] 0.36–0.98; p=0.04). Additionally, relapses at other extramedullary sites were higher in arm 1 patients compared to arm 3 patients (n=54 versus n=39; p=0.013) although there was no significant difference in bone marrow relapses between the two treatment arms (p=0.13). The report concluded that TIT CT provided adequate protection against CNS relapse of leukemia in patients with high-risk ALL.

The efficacy of IT MTX as CNS prophylaxis treatment in children with low-risk ALL was addressed by the CCSG 161 trial [11]. All children with previously untreated ALL who achieved complete remission or M2 marrow (<25 blasts) at the end of remission induction (day 28) with vincristine, prednisolone, asparaginase and two doses of IT MTX were randomized to one of four treatment groups.

• Group 1: CRT (18 Gy/10 fractions) as CNS prophylaxis plus continuing treatment with oral 6-MP and oral MTX.
• Group 2: as above with additional pulses of VCR and PDN every 12 weeks during continuing therapy.
• Group 3: IT MTX as CNS prophylaxis plus oral 6-MP, oral MTX and IT MTX at 12-weekly intervals during continuing therapy.
• Group 4: similar to Group 3 with regard to CNS prophylaxis but with the additional pulses of VCR and PDN to standard continuing therapy of oral 6-MP and oral MTX.

Of the 504 patients who were randomized to the CNS prophylaxis regimens, 250 were assigned to CRT and 254 patients to IT MTX. The CNS relapse rate was 6.1% in the CRT group compared to 8.4% in the IT MTX group that was not statistically significant (p=0.48). The incidence of bone marrow relapses was also comparable between the two groups (CRT 21% versus IT MTX group 22%; p=0.88). As the DFS and OS rates were not significantly different between the two groups of patients (p=0.82), it was concluded that IT MTX could be safely substituted for CRT in children with low-risk ALL without compromising efficacy or DFS.

Intensified IT chemotherapy without cranial radiation therapy prevents CNS relapse in children with low-risk and intermediate-risk ALL. The CCG 1882 trial [12] had a similar objective of determining whether cranial irradiation could be avoided in children with high-risk ALL without compromising survival. In this report, high-risk ALL patients who achieved a rapid early response to induction chemotherapy were randomized to receive intensive systemic chemotherapy and presymptomatic CNS therapy that consisted of either IT MTX and CRT (regimen A, n=317) or intensified IT MTX alone (regimen B, n=319). Randomization for the CNS prophylactic therapy was at the end of the remission induction phase of therapy. Rapid early response was defined as ≤25% blasts on day 7 bone marrow examination. Outcome measures were CNS relapse rate and EFS.

Central nervous system relapses were more frequent in regimen B patients: 11 (isolated 10) compared to 8 in regimen A patients (isolated 5). The temporal sequence of events differed in the two groups of patients: in the first 2 years of follow-up, the number of bone marrow relapses was similar in both groups of patients (regimen A 31 versus regimen B 33) but between 2 and 6 years of follow-up, regimen A patients had more bone marrow relapses (26 versus 10). Eight out of 10 CNS relapses in regimen B patients occurred within the first 2 years of follow-up. Analysis on an intention-to-treat principle showed that at 5 years follow-up the probability of an isolated CNS relapse was 2.3%±1.1% and 3.6%±1.1% for regimens A and B respectively (p=0.72). Survival after an isolated CNS relapse was better in patients on regimen B (p=0.009); all 10 regimen B patients who had an isolated CNS relapse were alive compared to only two of five regimen A patients. Two patients treated in each regimen developed leukoencephalopathy. The report concluded that IT MTX was a satisfactory form of presymptomatic treatment in high-risk children who achieved a rapid early response to remission induction therapy and furthermore, IT MTX afforded protection against late bone marrow relapse.

The study by Ortega et al. [13] was slightly different from the previous study (CCSG trial 161) as it aimed to compare the efficacy of IT chemotherapy (MTX and ARAC) alone versus CRT plus IT MTX in the prevention of CNS relapse of leukemia. The two CNS prophylaxis regimens were regimen A – CRT 24 Gy in 12 fractions plus six doses of IT MTX, and regimen B – six doses of IT MTX and IT ARAC with four additional monthly doses during year 1 of continuing therapy. Of the 243 patients who achieved a CR, 114 patients were randomized to regimen A while 129 patients were assigned to regimen B. There was a total of 108 relapses, of which 19 were within the CNS. As there were no significant differences in the CNS relapse rates between the two groups, the report concluded that CNS prophylaxis with IT chemotherapy with MTX and ARAC alone was an effective form of CNS prophylaxis in children with ALL.

Similar to the previous report, the CCG 105 trial [14] also compared the efficacy of 18 Gy CRT plus IT MTX in the first 6 months of treatment against IT MTX alone throughout the duration of treatment as presymptomatic CNS treatment. This trial was based on a 2×4 factorial design in which the first factor refers to the two types of CNS prophylaxis regimens and the second factor refers to the four systemic regimens. The 7-year survival outcomes were:
• CRT arm (n=697): CNS relapse-free survival (RFS) 93%, DFS 69%, EFS 68%
• IT MTX arm (n=691): CNS RFS 91%, DFS 67%, EFS 64%.
When survival rates were analyzed by age, outcomes were as follows.
• CRT arm 1–9 years: CNS RFS 94%, DFS 72%, EFS 70%; 10–21years: CNS RFS 91%, DFS 61%, EFS 60%
• IT MTX arm 1–9 years: CNS RFS 91%, DFS 71%, EFS 68%; 10–21 years: CNS RFS 90%, DFS 54%, EFS 53%.
The trial showed that IT MTX during the whole duration of treatment afforded comparable protection against CNS relapse of leukemia as CRT but in patients aged > 10 years, CRT provided better CNS protection. In addition, CNS relapse rate was higher in those patients who had received standard systemic treatment in both CNS regimens, especially so in the IT MTX arm (p< 0.0001).

The CCG 101 trial [15] evaluated the effectiveness of four different CNS prophylaxis regimens in previously untreated children < 18 years with ALL. All children who achieved a CR after remission induction with vincristine, prednisone, and asparaginase were randomized to one of four arms: (1) 24 Gy CSRT with 12 Gy to liver, spleen, kidneys, and gonads; (2) 24 Gy CSRT alone; (3) 24 Gy CRT with IT MTX 12 mg/m^2 twice a week×6 doses; or (4) IT MTX 12 mg/m^2 twice a week×6 doses. Continuing therapy consisted of daily oral 6-MP, weekly oral MTX plus monthly pulses of VCR and PDN. For outcome analysis, patients were categorized into two groups: cranial irradiation group (regimens 1, 2, 3) and IT MTX group (regimen 4). Although isolated CNS relapses were higher in the IT

MTX group (n=55 versus n=29; p< 0.0001), isolated bone marrow relapses as first event were higher in the CRT group. Overall survival was not significantly different (p=0.16) between the CRT (regimens 1, 2, 3) and IT MTX groups (regimen 4). The report concluded that although short-term IT MTX alone was ineffective as CNS prophylaxis, this did not significantly affect OS due to a higher incidence of bone marrow relapses in the CRT group.

The CLCG-EORTC report [16] provided long-term results of three randomized trials (58831, 58832, and 58881). Trial 58832 randomized all eligible children with intermediate- and high-risk ALL after the completion of reinduction phase (protocol II) therapy to receive 24 Gy prophylactic cranial irradiation or not. All patients received five doses of IT MTX during the first 8 weeks of induction/consolidation treatment. Following induction/consolidation was the interim maintenance phase that consisted of an 8-week course of oral 6-MP 25 mg/m^2/day, high-dose IV MTX 2.5 g/m^2/dose×4 plus IT MTX×4. Maintenance therapy consisted of daily oral 6-MP 50 mg/m^2/day and weekly oral MTX 20 mg/m^2. The total duration of treatment for all patients was 2 years.

Outcome measures were CNS relapse rate and DFS. The CNS relapse rate in patients randomized to cranial RT was 15%±4% compared to 9%±3.2% in patients who did not receive cranial RT (hazard ratio [HR] 0.57, 95% CI 0.24–1.35). Isolated CNS relapse rate for patients who did not receive cranial RT was 7%±2.8% versus 7%±2.9% for those who received CNS prophylaxis with cranial RT. Six-year DFS was 66%±5% and 68%±4.8% for patients with and without cranial RT. The report concluded that in medium- and high-risk patients, the omission of radiotherapy did not increase the risk of CNS or systemic relapse (trial 58832).

Schedule of irradiation

Hyperfractionated radiotherapy, with delivery of larger numbers of smaller fractions of radiotherapy, is a possible way to increase tumor control without increasing neurological toxicity. In an attempt to reduce the neuropsychological effects of cranial radiotherapy, Waber et al. [17] randomized patients with high-risk ALL to either conventional fractionated radiotherapy (CFRT) or hyperfractionated radiotherapy (HYFRT). All patients were treated on one of two

Dana-Farber Cancer Institute ALL consortium protocols – 87-01 and 91-01. Patients randomized to CFRT received 18 Gy in 10 fractions of 1.8 Gy/fraction/day over 12–14 days while those randomized to HYFRT received the same total dose in 20 fractions of 900 cGy: 2 fractions/day at least 6 h apart over 12–14 days. Both groups of patients received IT ARAC and IT MTX along with cranial radiotherapy. Infants with ALL had CRT delayed until they reached 1 year of age. All high-risk patients with CNS disease at diagnosis were excluded from the study. Of the 467 eligible patients, only 369 were randomized to either CFRT (n=180) or HYFRT (n=189). The 8-year EFS and OS for patients who received CFRT were 80%±3% and 85%±3% respectively compared to 72%±3% and 78%±3% respectively for the HYFRT group (p=0.06 amd 0.06). CNS relapses occurred in five patients in each treatment group (p=0.99) and remission death rates were also equal in both treatment groups (p=0.99). Children randomized to HYFRT achieved higher scores for visual learning than those assigned to CFRT (p=0.03), the Rey–Osterrieth Complex Figure Organization Recall (p=0.04) and structural accuracy (p=0.06) but there were no significant differences in any of the other variables. Repeating the analysis for children below 3 years of age at diagnosis showed there were no cognitive late sequelae for children randomized to either arm. Achievement testing scores for English-speaking children were similar for the two treatment groups. It was concluded that hyperfractionated cranial radiotherapy provided no benefits in terms of cognitive late effects and should not be substituted for conventional fractionated radiotherapy in children with ALL who require cranial irradiation.

Type of intrathecal therapy and duration of treatment

The report by Matloub et al. [18] of the CCG 1952 trial compared the efficacy of presymptomatic TIT consisting of IT ARAC, IT MTX and IT hydrocortisone against IT MTX alone in reducing the incidence of CNS relapses in children with SR ALL. Children between 1 and 10 years of age with previously untreated SR ALL (WBC count <50×10^9/L) were eligible for trial enrollment. Children with FAB L3 morphology or who had received treatment with corticosteroids for more than 48 h were ineligible for

the study. Only patients who achieved M1 (<5% blasts) or M2 (5–25% blasts) bone marrow status by day 14, complete remission at the end of induction on day 28 and had no unfavorable cytogenetics such as hypodiploidy t(9;22) or t(4;11) were eligible for the randomization. Outcome endpoints included isolated CNS relapse rate, EFS, and OS. The median follow-up from randomization was 6 years for patients alive in continuous remission at the time of the report.

Isolated CNS relapse rates were significantly higher in the IT MTX group (n=58) than in the TIT group (n=31; p=0.004; RHR=0.53). The 6-year cumulative estimates of isolated CNS relapses were 5.9%±1.2% and 3.4%±1.0% in the IT MTX and TIT groups respectively. Children randomized to TIT had a higher BM relapse rate (n=117) compared to those who received IT MTX (n=79). The 6-year EFS rates for the TIT and IT MTX groups were 80.7%±1.9% and 82.5%±1.8% respectively (p=0.3). Because more patients died of BM relapse than from isolated CNS relapse, the OS was in favor of IT MTX; 6-year OS was 90.3%±1.5% and 94.4%±1.1% for the TIT and MTX groups (p=0.01) respectively with a relative death rate 1.5 times higher for TIT compared to IT MTX. CNS toxicity (seizures, severe ataxia, facial nerve palsy, hemiplegia, GB syndrome) occurred in 6.7% of patients randomized to TIT compared to 5.8% for the IT MTX group. The report concluded that while presymptomatic CNS treatment with TIT chemotherapy significantly reduced the isolated CNS relapse rate, it did not improve overall survival outcome because of a higher incidence of bone marrow relapses in this group.

The report by Bleyer et al. [19] evaluated the influence of maintenance IT MTX on CNS relapse rates in children with average-risk ALL who were treated on the CCG 160 series of trials. Previously untreated children and adolescents under the age of 18 years were eligible for enrollment. Average risk was defined as age <3 years or >6 years with a white blood cell (WBC) count <50×10^9/L or 3–6 years of age with a WBC count of 10–50×10^9/L or low–risk patients with FAB L2 morphology. Remission induction therapy consisted of VCR, PDN, and L-ASP. A third of the average-risk patients received standard maintenance therapy, a third received periodic pulses of VCR, PDN, and L-ASP in addition to standard maintenance therapy and a third received pulses of ARAC, doxorubicin or cyclophosphamide added at monthly intervals to standard maintenance therapy. All patients also received 18 Gy cranial radiotherapy. Patients randomized to maintenance IT were given IT MTX at 12-weekly intervals during the maintenance program; 1024 patients were randomized to receive maintenance IT MTX or not. Although the CNS relapse rates were lower in the IT MTX group, especially in children >10 years of age, this was marginal and not statistically significant (p=0.06). However, bone marrow relapses, remission deaths, and deaths following relapse were higher in the maintenance IT MTX group. Moreover, patients under 10 years of age did not benefit from maintenance IT MTX. It was concluded that while maintenance IT MTX marginally improved CNS relapse rates, it did not improve 3-year continuous hematological remission or overall survival outcome in children with average-risk ALL.

Role of intermediate- and high-dose methotrexate

The strategy of using moderate- to high-dose intravenous (IV) MTX to decrease the occurrence of CNS relapse was investigated in the ALL BFM 81 trial [20]. Children and adolescents below 18 years with SR ALL (excluding B-ALL) were included in the study. Risk categorization was based on the BFM risk factor assessment with SR patients randomized to receive either CRT (n=180) or intermediate-dose IV MTX (ID MTX) (n=177). Comparing the ID MTX and CRT arms, isolated CNS relapses in the ID MTX arm were higher (n=12; 6.8%) than in the CRT arm (n=4; 2.2%). Similarly, combined CNS relapses were also higher in the ID MTX arm (n=13; 7.3%) compared to the CRT arm (n=3; 1.7%). The report concluded that ID MTX was not an adequate substitute for CRT in preventing CNS relapse in patients with SR ALL.

The CALGB 7611 trial [21] also evaluated the effectiveness of ID MTX as CNS prophylaxis in previously untreated children and adolescents <20 years of age with ALL. Patients in complete remission at the end of remission induction were randomized to 24 Gy CRT plus IT MTX or ID MTX plus IT MTX. The 12-year CNS relapse rates for the ID MTX and CRT arms were 28%±3% and 8%±2% respectively (p< 0.0001). However, the ID MTX regimen afforded greater protection against bone marrow relapse (p< 0.0006) and testicular relapse (p=0.002) compared to CRT.

The report concluded that ID MTX was inferior to CRT in preventing CNS relapse in children and adolescents with ALL but offered better systemic and testicular protection.

The study by Zintl et al. [22] compared the efficacy of moderate-dose IV MTX plus IT MTX against CRT plus IT MTX as presymptomatic CNS treatment in children with SR ALL. All previously untreated children with ALL excluding those with B-ALL were included in the trial. SR children were randomized to either 18 Gy CRT and IT MTX (SR-A) or moderate-dose IV MTX and IT MTX (SR-B) as CNS prophylaxis treatment. Of the 23 children who relapsed within the CNS, only six were in the SR-A treatment arm (3%). Interestingly, nine patients in the SR-A treatment arm developed testicular recurrence while none in the SR-B arm did. The 5-year EFS rates were 62% and 57% in the SR-A and SR-B treatment arms respectively. Clearly, moderate-dose IV MTX was less effective than CRT in preventing CNS relapse of leukemia in SR ALL patients.

The main objective of a Japanese study [23] was to determine whether the omission of presymptomatic CNS irradiation (CRT) in children with low-risk (LR) or intermediate-risk (IR) ALL adversely affected CNS relapse rate or survival outcome. Previously untreated children with LR or IR ALL who were in remission after remission induction therapy (vincristine 2.0 mg/m²/week, prednisone 60 mg/m-/day and L-asparaginase 2000 IU/m²) were randomized to either 18 Gy CRT plus IT CT or high-dose IV MTX (2–4.5 g/m²) plus IT CT. IT CT consisted of IT MTX (12 mg/m²) and IT hydrocortisone (50 mg/m²). Risk factor calculation was based on age and white blood cell count at diagnosis. Continuing therapy comprised IV intermediate-dose MTX (225 mg/m²) and alternating bi-weekly oral 6-MP (175 mg/m²). While all patients also received vincristine/prednisolone pulses, children with intermediate-risk ALL also received doxorubicin and L-asparaginase during continuing therapy. Outcome endpoints included CNS relapse rate and EFS. Of the 189 children with LR and IR ALL enrolled on the study, 97 (LR ALL 42 and IR ALL 55) were randomized to receive CRT plus IT CT while the remaining 92 were assigned to receive high-dose intravenous MTX plus IT CT.

While CNS relapse rates were lower in patients randomized to CRT plus IT CT (3/97; 3%) compared to those assigned to HD MTX plus IT CT (9/92; 9.7%), this did not result in statistically significant differences in the EFS rates between the two groups. Five-year EFS rates were 75.6%±5.7% and 70.5%±6.1% for LR and IR ALL patients who received CRT plus IT CT compared to 69.2%±5.5% and 67.5%±5.9% for the same risk group of patients who received HD MTX plus IT CT. It was concluded that the omission of CRT in LR and IR ALL patients had no significant impact on EFS despite a slightly higher rate of CNS relapse in this group.

Schrappe et al. [24] reported the updated results of the BFM trials BFM-81 and BFM-83 in 1998. The objectives of the BFM-81 trial were to examine whether CRT could be omitted as CNS prophylaxis in SR children with ALL without adversely affecting the CNS relapse rate, while the BFM-83 trial evaluated the efficacy of a reduction in the dose of CRT and its impact on the treatment outcome in children with high SR ALL. Children and adolescents up to the age of 18 with previously untreated disease were eligible for study enrollment. In the BFM-81 trial, the score for SR ALL was <1.2 while the risk score index for high SR ALL in the BFM-83 trial was between 0.8 ≤1.2. SR ALL patients in the BFM-81 trial (BFM RF <1.2) were randomized to 18 Gy CRT plus oral MTX ($0.02 g/m^2 \times 8$) and IT MTX×6 (SR-A) or to IV ID MTX) (SR-B) as CNS prophylaxis treatment. In the BFM-83 trial, high SR ALL (BFM RF 0.8–1.2) patients were randomized to 18 Gy CRT plus ID MTX ($0.5 g/m^2 \times 4$) and IT MTX×8 or to 12 Gy CRT plus ID MTX ($0.5 g/m^2 \times 4$) and IT MTX×8. Outcome endpoint in both trials was CNS relapse rate.

In the BFM-81 trial, a higher incidence of CNS relapses was observed in those who did not receive CRT (19 versus 3). However, subcategorizing this group, in those with LR ALL (BFM RF <0.8) the incidence of CNS relapses was small treated with ID MTX without CRT (n=137; 1.6% isolated CNS relapse and 3.2% combined CNS relapse). However, even in this good-risk group, long-term results showed that CRT was superior to ID MTX (all relapses 12.9% versus 22.2%). In the BFM-83 trial, 72 patients were randomly assigned to 12 Gy CRT while 71 children were assigned to 18 Gy CRT. Both CRT regimens were equally effective in preventing CNS relapses (12 Gy, isolated CNS relapse 2.8% and combined CNS relapse 2.8%; 18 Gy, isolated CNS relapse 2.8% and combined CNS relapse 1.4%).

The BFM-81 trial report concluded that in LR ALL patients CNS relapse can effectively be prevented with intensive systemic and IT chemotherapy without CRT but in high SR ALL (BFM RF 0.8 <1.2) patients, CNS prophylaxis without CRT was unsafe as it resulted in a significantly increased rate of CNS relapse. The BFM-83 trial demonstrated that the dose of cranial irradiation could be safely reduced to 12 Gy in high SR ALL patients (RF 0.8 ≤1.2) without increasing the incidence of CNS relapses when combined with IV ID MTX and IT MTX.

Role of high-dose cytarabine

The addition of high-dose IV ARAC to high-dose IV MTX to improve CNS and systemic protection against relapse of leukemia was examined by Millot et al. [25] in the EORTC 58881 trial for children with intermediate-risk ALL. In this trial, children and adolescents below the age of 18 with previously untreated ALL or lymphoblastic lymphoma who were in complete hematological remission after the consolidation course were randomized to IV HD MTX alone (arm A) or IV HD MTX plus IV HD ARAC (arm B) for presymptomatic CNS therapy. The total duration of therapy was 2 years. Outcome endpoints were DFS, OS, and CNS relapse rate. The median follow-up at the time of the report was 6.5 years.

Of the 656 children randomized to presymptomatic CNS therapy, 323 were randomized to arm A and 330 children to arm B (two were excluded due to ineligibility). The duration of the CNS prophylactic phase was statistically longer for patients randomized to arm B compared to arm A (Wilcoxon test, p=0.000). Isolated and combined CNS relapse rates for patients randomized to arm A were 5.6% and 5.3% compared to 3.3% and 4.6% respectively in patients assigned to arm B (HD ARAC plus HD MTX). There were no differences in the incidence of isolated bone marrow relapses in patients of both treatment arms.

The 6-year DFS was 70.4% (standard error [SE] 2.6%) and 71% (SE 2.5%) for patients randomized to arm A and arm B respectively (log-rank test, p=0.67). There was no difference in the OS of patients in both arms (83.5% versus 84%; p=0.55). Three patients (09%) in arm A and 10 in arm B died in CR as a result of treatment toxicity (mainly infection). The report concluded that the addition of high-dose ARAC to HD MTX during the presymptomatic CNS treatment phase did not significantly reduce the CNS relapse rate, decrease isolated bone marrow relapse or improve DFS in patients with intermediate-risk ALL.

Overview

Clarke et al. [26] performed a meta-analysis of 43 randomized trials in childhood lymphoblastic leukaemia (ALL) carried out worldwide before or during 1993. Individual patient data of more than 9000 children were retrieved for analysis and were compared according to the type of CNS-directed therapy. The various CNS-directed therapies were categorized into (1) intrathecal chemotherapy (IT CT), (2) intravenous methotrexate (IV MTX), (3) intravenous mercaptopurine (IV 6-MP), (4) cranial irradiation (CRT), and (5) craniospinal irradiation (CSRT). IT CT was further subdivided into short IT CT (2–8 doses) given early during treatment and long IT CT (10–26 doses). Variables included for subgroup analyses were age <10 or ≥10 years, white blood cell count at diagnosis (<50 or $≥50×10^9$/L) and ALL immunophenotype (B- or T-cell lineage). Primary outcome measures were EFS and OS from date of randomization. Secondary endpoints included CNS relapse (any relapse with CNS involvement), non-CNS relapse, isolated CNS relapse, and death in remission. All data were censored at first relapse.

All analyses were from time of randomization to event within the trial with observed minus expected (O-E) number of events and its variance (V) obtained by the log-rank survival analyses using the exact date of the event. Information from different trials was combined by summing up the separate O-E to calculate the odds ratio (OR) for annual event rates, their confidence intervals, and survival figures. Heterogeneity between trials was tested using χ^2 statistics.

The results can be summarized as follows.

• **Radiotherapy (RT) plus IT CT versus extra IT CT.** Seven trials that included a total of 2848 children were analyzed. Although the overall event rate was similar in both groups (CRT+IT CT 34.3% versus extra IT CT 36%), isolated CNS relapses were lower in the CRT group (4.9% compared to 6% in the IT CT group; p=0.03). There was no difference in the 10-year overall survival (CRT 73.5% versus IT CT 75.3%) or in the EFS (CRT 64% versus IT CT 62.8%) between the two groups of patients.

• **Addition of IV MTX to long-term IT CT versus CRT plus IT CT.** Eight trials were reviewed and included 3189 patients. All treatment arms included CRT plus nine or more IT CT or at least 12 IT CT. The IV MTX dose ranged from 0.5 to 8.0 g/m². Patients randomized to IV MTX plus IT CT had a 19% and 17% lower incidence of CNS (p=0.08) and non-CNS (p=0.02) relapses respectively. While there was a significant reduction in the annual event rate (17%; p=0.03) reflected by a 6.2% improved 10-year EFS, there were no significant differences in the OS rates (80.1% IV MTX versus 76.8% without IV MTX).

• **CRT plus short-term IT CT versus IV MTX plus short-term IT CT.** Three trials that included 958 children were analyzed. All patients received some IT therapy. While CRT reduced CNS relapse rate by 62% (p< 0.00001), this was counterbalanced by a 67% increase in non-CNS relapse rate (p=0.00005). Thus no differences were observed in the 10-year OS (CRT 65% versus IV MTX 64.2%) or EFS (RT 53% versus IV MTX 50.6%) between the two treatment arms.

• **Dose of CRT.** Seven trials were analyzed and in all the trials, short-term IT CT was used in all the treatment arms. Most trials compared 24 Gy with either 18 or 21 Gy but one (ALL-BFM-83) compared 18 Gy with 12 Gy. There was no significant difference between the various CRT doses with respect to CNS relapses (isolated or combined), non-CNS relapse or death in remission. The 10-year OS was nonsignificantly higher (59.1%) with lower doses than higher doses (55.9%) and the difference in the 10-year EFS was <1%.

• **CRT plus short-term IT CT versus IV MTX plus long-term IT CT.** Three randomized trials that included 512 patients were analyzed. There were no significant differences in CNS relapses, non-CNS relapses or deaths in remission between the two treatment arms. The 10-year EFS (CRT+IT CT 51.2% versus IV MTX+IT CT 49.6%) and OS (CRT+IT CT 66.7% versus IV MTX+IT CT 64.7%) were similar with both treatments.

• **Addition of IV MTX plus IT CT to CRT plus IT CT and/or IV MTX.** Three trials addressed the addition of IV MTX and IT therapy to other CNS therapies, including CRT. All three trials used RT in both the randomized arms. No differences were observed in non-CNS relapses, CNS relapses, and deaths in remission or OS with additional therapy.

- **Other comparisons**. While 29 trials were identified that addressed questions not addressed by any of the above six comparisons, data were available from only 14 trials. The St Jude VI trial showed a significant benefit when CSRT was added to a treatment regimen without any IT CT. The CCG 101 trial showed CRT+CSRT was more effective than short-term IT CT. Both the CCG 162 trial and the MRC UK VII trial showed that the addition of extra IT CT to CRT plus short-term IT CT had no significant effect on overall outcome. The EORTC trial 58881 suggested that the addition of IV 6-MP to a regimen of IV MTX plus IT CT had an adverse effect on outcome. Four trials (two in relapsed patients and two that included extra IT CT in the arm that had lower IV MTX) that examined the efficacy of higher doses of IV MTX found no benefit with higher doses.

Conclusions of these trials included the following.

- 18 Gy or 21 Gy cranial irradiation was as effective as 24 Gy in preventing CNS relapses.
- Intravenous methotrexate gives some additional benefit by reducing non-CNS relapses.
- While radiotherapy reduced the incidence of CNS relapses when compared to long-term IT CT, there was no difference in either OS or EFS due to a higher incidence of non-CNS relapses. It was, therefore, concluded that radiotherapy could be replaced by long-term IT CT.

References

1 Nesbit ME Jr, Sather HN, Robison LL et al. Presymptomatic central nervous system therapy in previously untreated childhood acute lymphoblastic leukaemia: comparison of 1800 rad and 2400 rad. A report for Children's Cancer Study Group. Lancet 1981;1:461–6.

2 Lilleyman JS, Richards S, Rankin A, on behalf of the Medical Research Council Working Party on Childhood Leukaemia. Medical Research Council Leukaemia Trial, UKALL-VII: a report to the Council by the Working Party on Leukaemia in Childhood. Arch Dis Child 1985;60:1050–4.

3 Brandalise S, Odone V, Pereira W, Andrea M, Zanichelli M, Aranega V. Treatment results of three consecutive Brazilian cooperative childhood ALL protocols: GBTLI-80, GBTLI-82 and -85. ALL Brazilian Group. Leukemia 1993;7(Suppl 2):S142–5.

4 Schrappe M, Reiter A, Zimmermann M et al. Long-term results of four consecutive trials in childhood ALL performed by the ALL-BFM study group from 1981 to 1995. Berlin-Frankfurt-Münster. Leukemia 2000;14:2205–22.

5 Tsuchida M, Ikuta K, Hanada R et al. Long-term follow-up of childhood acute lymphoblastic leukemia in Tokyo Children's Cancer Study Group 1981–1995. Leukemia 2000;14:2295–306.

6 Steinherz PG, Gaynon PS, Breneman JC et al. Treatment of patients with acute lymphoblastic leukemia with bulky extramedullary disease and T-cell phenotype or other poor prognostic features: randomized controlled trial from the Children's Cancer Group. Cancer 1998;82:600–12.

7 Komp DM, Fernandez CH, Falletta JM et al. CNS prophylaxis in acute lymphoblastic leukemia: comparison of two methods a Southwest Oncology Group study. Cancer 1982;50:1031–6.

8 Sullivan MP, Chen T, Dyment PG, Hvizdala E, Steuber CP. Equivalence of intrathecal chemotherapy and radiotherapy as central nervous system prophylaxis in children with acute lymphatic leukemia: a Pediatric Oncology Group study. Blood 1982;60:948–58.

9 Jones B, Freeman AI, Shuster JJ et al. Lower incidence of meningeal leukemia when prednisone is replaced by dexamethasone in the treatment of acute lymphocytic leukemia. Med Pediatr Oncol 1991;19:269–75.

10 Van Eys J, Berry D, Crist W et al. A comparison of two regimens for high-risk acute lymphocytic leukemia in childhood. A Pediatric Oncology Group study. Cancer 1989;63:23–9.

11 Littman P, Coccia P, Bleyer WA et al. Central nervous system (CNS) prophylaxis in children with low risk acute lymphoblastic leukemia (ALL). Int J Radiat Oncol Biol Phys 1987;13:1443–9.

12 Nachman J, Sather HN, Cherlow JM et al. Response of children with high-risk acute lymphoblastic leukemia treated with and without cranial irradiation: a report from the Children's Cancer Group. J Clin Oncol 1998;16:920–30.

13 Ortega JJ, Javier G, Olive T. Treatment of standard- and high-risk childhood acute lymphoblastic leukaemia with two CNS prophylaxis regimens. Haematol Blood Transfus 1987;30:483–92.

14 Tubergen DG, Gilchrist GS, O'Brien RT et al. Prevention of CNS disease in intermediate-risk acute lymphoblastic leukemia: comparison of cranial radiation and intrathecal methotrexate and the importance of systemic therapy: a Children's Cancer Group report. J Clin Oncol 1993;11:520–6.

15 Ortega JA, Nesbit ME, Sather HN, d'Angio GJ, Hammond GD. Long-term evaluation of a CNS prophylaxis trial - treatment comparisons and outcome after CNS relapse in childhood ALL: a report from the Children's Cancer Study Group. J Clin Oncol 1987;5:1646–54.

16 Vilmer E, Suciu S, Ferster A et al. Long-term results of three randomized trials (58831, 58832, 58881) in childhood acute lymphoblastic leukemia: a CLCG-EORTC report. Children Leukemia Cooperative Group. Leukemia 2000;14:2257–66.

17 Waber DP, Silverman LB, Catania L et al. Outcomes of a randomized trial of hyperfractionated cranial radiation therapy for treatment of high-risk acute lymphoblastic leukemia: therapeutic efficacy and neurotoxicity. J Clin Oncol 2004;22:2701–7.

18 Matloub Y, Lindemulder S, Gaynon PS *et al.*, for the Children's Oncology Group. Intrathecal triple therapy decreases central nervous system relapse but fails to improve event-free survival when compared with intrathecal methotrexate: results of the Children's Cancer Group (CCG) 1952 study for standard-risk acute lymphoblastic leukemia, reported by the Children's Oncology Group. *Blood* 2006;**108**:1165–73.

19 Bleyer WA, Coccia PF, Sather HN *et al.* Reduction in central nervous system leukemia with a pharmacokinetically derived intrathecal methotrexate dosage regimen. *J Clin Oncol* 1983;**1**:317–25.

20 Niemeyer CM, Reiter A, Riehm H, Donnelly M, Gelber RD, Sallan SE. Comparative results of two intensive treatment programs for childhood acute lymphoblastic leukemia: the Berlin-Frankfurt-Münster and Dana-Farber Cancer Institute protocols. *Ann Oncol* 1991;**2**:745–9.

21 Freeman AI, Boyett JM, Glicksman AS *et al.* Intermediate-dose methotrexate versus cranial irradiation in childhood acute lymphoblastic leukemia: a ten-year follow-up. *Med Pediatr Oncol* 1997;**28**:98–107.

22 Zintl F, Malke H, Reimann M *et al.* Results of acute lymphoblastic leukemia therapy in childhood: GDR-experiences 1981–1987. *Haematol Blood Transfus* 1990;**33**:478–82.

23 Koizumi S, Fujimoto T. Improvement in treatment of childhood acute lymphoblastic leukemia: a 10-year study by the Children's Cancer and Leukemia Study Group. *Int J Hematol* 1994;**59**:99–112.

24 Schrappe M, Reiter A, Henze G *et al.* Prevention of CNS recurrence in childhood ALL: results with reduced radiotherapy combined with CNS-directed chemotherapy in four consecutive ALL-BFM trials. *Klin Padiatr* 1998;**210**:192–9.

25 Millot F, Suciu S, Philippe N *et al.*, for the Children's Leukemia Cooperative Group of the European Organization for Research and Treatment of Cancer. Value of high-dose cytarabine during interval therapy of a Berlin-Frankfurt-Munster-based protocol in increased-risk children with acute lymphoblastic leukemia and lymphoblastic lymphoma: results of the European Organization for Research and Treatment of Cancer 58881 randomized phase III trial. *J Clin Oncol* 2001;**19**:1935–42.

26 Clarke M, Gaynon P, Hann I *et al.*, for the Childhood ALL Collaborative Group. CNS-directed therapy for childhood acute lymphoblastic leukemia: Childhood ALL Collaborative Group overview of 43 randomized trials. *J Clin Oncol* 2003;**21**:1798–809.

New studies

The authors have been unable to identify any new randomized trials regarding central nervous system-directed therapy in childhood lymphoblastic leukemia in children published since the previous edition of this book.

CHAPTER 21

Maintenance treatment in childhood lymphoblastic leukemia

Ananth Shankar

University College London Hospitals NHS Foundation Trust, London, UK

Summary of previous studies

Extended low-dose oral chemotherapy with oral 6-mercaptopurine (6-MP) and oral methotrexate (MTX) has been a consistent element of therapy of childhood lymphoblastic leukemia for over 40 years. The nature and duration of continuing or maintenance therapy have been the subject of numerous randomized clinical trials.

Duration of therapy

The Medical Research Council's (MRC) Working Party on Leukaemia report [1] described the outcome of three UK ALL trials (I, II and III) in which the duration of continuing therapy (CT) was examined in a randomized manner. Analysis of allocated duration of therapy was restricted to patients who were in remission and on chemotherapy at 80 weeks (UK ALL I) or 104 weeks (UK ALL II and III). The report concluded that 18 months or 2 years of CT was as effective as 3 years for girls but for boys 18 months was inferior to 3 years of treatment, although there was little difference between 2 and 3 years of treatment. It was concluded that there was no significant difference between 2 or 3 years of treatment for either sex.

Comment: The authors also noted that in view of the rather different results for girls in a later trial and the high testicular and bone marrow relapse rates in boys, the results should be interpreted cautiously.

The next MRC trial, UK ALL V [2], evaluated duration of CT in children (1–14 years of age with a presenting white blood cell [WBC] count $<20\times10^9/L$) in continuous remission at 96 weeks (n=292) who were randomized to either stop treatment or continue till week 144. All patients with central nervous system (CNS) leukemia or mediastinal disease at diagnosis were excluded. A statistically significant higher hematological relapse rate was seen in girls who only received 2 years of treatment (28 versus 17; p=0.01) and although not statistically significant, a slightly increased rate of testicular and bone marrow relapse was observed in boys who only received 2 years of CT. Overall, there was an apparent benefit for patients who received 3 years of CT.

Although the MRC UK ALL VIII trial [3] ran from September 1980 to December 1984, the randomization for 2 versus 3 years of CT only happened from January 1983 in patients who were in 2 years continuous clinical remission (CCR). Of the 406 patients eligible for randomization for the duration CT, 203 patients each were assigned to 2 and 3 years of CT. Even though more relapses were seen after stopping treatment at 2 than 3 years (17% versus 25%; p=0.04), there was a 4% increase in remission deaths in patients

---

Evidence-Based Pediatric Oncology, Third Edition. Edited by Ross Pinkerton, Ananth Shankar and Katherine K. Matthay.
© 2013 John Wiley & Sons, Ltd. Published 2013 by John Wiley & Sons, Ltd.

in the 3-year CT arm. This trial concluded that there was no significant survival benefit for those receiving 3 years of CT.

The CCG 101 and CCG 143 trials [4] (June 1972 to February 1975) also evaluated the optimum duration of CT in children with previously untreated acute lymphoblastic leukemia (ALL). All patients who were in continuous remission for 3 years after start of therapy were randomized to either stop treatment (n=160) or continue treatment for a further 2 years (n=156). Relapse-free survival of patients treated for 5 years compared to those treated for 3 years was not significantly higher in males (81% versus 75%; p=0.14) or in females (89% versus 89%; p=0.95) and at 5 years after randomization, no significant differences were seen in survival between patients who received 3 years of therapy versus those treated for 5 years (93% versus 89%; p=0.27).

While the CCG 141 trial [5] that ran from February 1975 to February 1977 was similar to the earlier CCG 101 and CCG 143 trials in determining the most advantageous duration of CT (3 or 5 years), a fundamental distinction was that it included both previously untreated children who were in 3 years CCR as well those in 3 years of CCR after having had an isolated extramedullary relapse. Patients who were in 3 years of CCR were randomized to stop treatment (group A) or receive 4 weeks of reinduction with vincristine, prednisolone, and asparaginase and stop (group B) or to continue maintenance treatment for a further 2 years (group C). Disease-free survival at 6 years after randomization was not statistically significant between those who stopped treatment at 3 years (93%) and those with an additional 2 years of CT (89.1%). Girls randomized to 5 years CT had a significantly worse survival than those randomized to the combined regimens A and B (p=0.03). It was concluded that prolongation of CT beyond 3 years did not improve survival or decrease risk of relapse in both sexes.

CCG trials 161, 162, and 163 [6] assessed the optimal duration of CT in children with low-, intermediate-, and high-risk ALL respectively. Only children in continuous remission 2 years after diagnosis were randomized to either stop treatment or continue treatment for an additional year. Boys who had 3 years of therapy had a lower rate of testicular relapses but girls had no benefit in extending treatment beyond 2 years.

In the AIEOP 79 trial [7], children between the ages of 1 and 14 years with previously untreated low- and standard-risk (SR) ALL (n=177) were randomized to 2 versus 3 years of CT. The 5-year disease -free survival (DFS) for patients randomized to 3 years of treatment was 70% versus 68.3% for those who received only 2 years of treatment ($X^2t=0.55$). Plainly, the duration of total treatment did not affect final outcome.

Results of all randomized trials that began before 1987 of duration of CT (usually 3 years versus 2 years) were included in the Childhood ALL Collaborative Group report [8]. Although 17 trials were conducted between 1970 and 1983, data were available only from 16 trials (with the last patients randomized in 1990) and involved a total of 3861 patients. The median follow-up was >5 years for all but one trial. The risk of relapse or death was 27.6% (n=538/1946) for patients who had a shorter duration of CT (usually 2 years) compared to 23.3% (n=446/1915) with longer CT. Longer duration of CT halved the relapse rate but did not translate into improved survival as deaths during first remission were increased by longer CT (2.7% versus 1.2%).

The Berlin-Frankfurt-Münster (BFM) 81 and 83 trials [9] randomized patients in CCR at 18 months of CT to either stop treatment or continue maintenance treatment for an additional 6 months (18 versus 24 months). The 8-year DFS for patients randomized to 24 months (n=375) and 18 months (n=389) of therapy was 77.3%±2.3% and 71.2%±2.4% respectively (log-rank p=0.11). A significant difference in overall survival was observed at 10 years for patients who had 24 months of treatment (p=0.025). It was concluded that 2 years of treatment was superior to 18 months.

Pulses of steroids and vincristine

Oral 6-MP and oral MTX have been the core components of CT of childhood ALL for over four decades. Many co-operative study groups have added pulses of vincristine and corticosteroids as intensification of the CT phase to reduce the relapse rate after stopping treatment.

One such study was the Children's Cancer Group (CCG) 161 trial [10] that was conducted between April 1978 and May 1983 in children with low-risk ALL. A single randomization was performed with a

2×2 multifactorial design. One factor was the use of cranial radiotherapy (CRT) or intrathecal (IT) MTX and the second factor was the use of monthly vincristine (VCR) and prednisolone (PDN) pulses (n=302) or not (n=303) during CT. The 5-year DFS in the 6-MP/MTX/VCR/PDN arm was 76.7% versus 63.9% (p=0.003) in the 6-MP/MTX alone arm, regardless of the presymptomatic CNS therapy. This was due to increased bone marrow relapses and, in boys, also due to testicular relapses. The difference between VCR-PDN pulses and no pulses was most pronounced in the group who received IT MTX rather than CRT. Likewise, 5-year continuous hematological remission in the VCR/PDN/6-MP/MTX arm was 86.3% versus 74.5% in the 6-MP/MTX alone arm (p=0.0008). There were a total of 10 excess deaths in the group that received VCR/PDN pulses, most due to viral or *Pneumocystis carinii* infections. In this study, VCR-PDN pulses improved survival outcome in children with low-risk ALL.

A similar randomized study was the BFM 79/81 trial [11] that evaluated the efficacy of adding regular pulses of VCR and PDN to oral 6-MP and oral MTX during CT to improve DFS in standard-risk ALL patients. Unlike the results of the CCG 161 trial, there were no differences in the relapse-free survival (RFS) among children treated with regular pulses of VCR-PDN compared to those who did not receive VCR-PDN pulses (RFS 0.83, standard deviation [SD]=0.06) versus 0.83, SD=0.05).

Dose and route of methotrexate

During the CT phase both MTX and 6-MP are usually given orally in the evening. In an effort to improve overall and disease-free survival, the Children's Cancer Group randomized 164 children with intermediate-risk ALL to standard continuing treatment with or without additional moderate-dose intravenous (IV) MTX ($500 \, \text{mg/m}^2$) every 6 weeks [12]. All patients were randomized prior to commencement of remission induction. Patients randomized to the IV MTX group received IV MTX ($500 \, \text{mg/m}^2$) three times during consolidation and at 6-weekly intervals during CT in addition to standard-dose oral 6-MP and oral MTX (during the 5 weeks when there was no IV MTX). All patients also received 6-weekly pulses of VCR and PDN

during the CT. Patients in the non-IV MTX group received standard-dose oral 6-MP ($75 \, \text{mg/m}^2/\text{day}$) and weekly oral MTX ($20 \, \text{mg/m}^2/\text{week}$) with 4-weekly pulses of VCR and PDN. Duration of CT was 2 years for girls and 3 years for boys. Of 164 eligible patients, 80 were randomized to the IV MTX group and 84 to the non-IV MTX group. The 6-year event-free survival (EFS) was 58.4% ($\pm 5.6\%$) for patients in the IV MTX group compared to 57.4% ($\pm 5.6\%$) for the non-IV MTX group (p=0.92) while the 6-year overall survival (OS) was 76.9% ($\pm 5.0\%$) and 83.1% ($\pm 4.3\%$) for the IV MTX and non-IV MTX groups respectively (p=0.31). It was concluded that the addition of pulses of IV MTX in this dose and schedule during CT did not confer any advantage over standard CT.

The UK ALL VII trial explored the use of intramuscular (IM) MTX during CT to improve bioavailability and compliance and potentially the survival outcome in children with ALL [13]. Even though 40 patients were randomized to receive IM MTX and 39 to receive it orally, only 36 patients received IM MTX while 41 received MTX orally. When analysis was performed by actual treatment received, patients who received IM MTX had fewer relapses, 5 compared to 17 in the oral MTX group. In contrast, deaths in remission were higher in the IM MTX group (n=4) versus one in the oral MTX group (log-rank p<0.05). Of the 36 patients given IM MTX, 27 (75%) were alive compared to 23 of 41 (56%) given oral MTX. The authors concluded that when analyzed according to the actual treatment received, IM MTX was more effective than oral MTX during CT but associated with increased toxicity.

Drug schedule

Modifying CT by altering the schedule of the administration of 6-MP and MTX, the Japanese Children's Cancer and Leukaemia Study Group (JCCLSG) conducted a randomized trial (JCCLSG-S811) wherein all previously untreated children with standard-risk ALL who had completed the CNS prophylaxis phase of treatment were randomized to a CT of either oral 6-MP ($175 \, \text{mg/m}^2/\text{day} \times 5$ days) alternating with IV MTX ($225 \, \text{mg/m}^2$) at 2-weekly intervals combined with pulses of VCR and PDN (intermittent cycle/regimen A) or oral 6-MP ($50 \, mg/m^2/day$) plus oral MTX ($20 \, mg/m^2/week$) combined with pulses of VCR and PDN at 4-weekly intervals (regimen B) at the same dosage as regimen A [14]. Patients who remained in remission at 2 years were given five courses of IV high-dose MTX with folinic acid rescue (late intensification). Of the total of 115 patients who achieved CR and completed CNS prophylaxis, 60 were randomized to regimen A and 55 to regimen B. Patients on regimen B had a higher incidence of bone marrow, CNS and testicular relapses, especially after 3 years of CCR. The CCR rate at 5 years for patients in regimen A was $72.1\% \pm 6.3\%$ versus $49.7\% \pm 7.3\%$ for regimen B patients ($p < 0.05$). The late intensification did not have any impact on the duration of CCR in either group of patients. The report concluded that intermittent administration of MTX and 6-MP was superior to continuous administration of both drugs during CT phase treatment in childhood ALL.

The UK ALL V trial [2] was designed to investigate whether intermittent continuing treatment might be less immunosuppressive and more effective in the management of childhood ALL. In this study, 496 low-risk ALL patients were randomized to one of three CT regimens: a conventional continuous regimen C (n=161), semi-continuous regimen G (intermittent course with a 1-week gap in the 6-MP) (n=166) and an intermittent regimen I (intermittent 5-day course every 3 weeks) (n=169). The 7-year DFS was $48.4\% \pm 7.64\%$ for regimen C, $46.4\% \pm 7.64\%$ for regimen G and $35.1\% \pm 7.25\%$ for regimen I patients. The authors concluded that intermittent CT was less effective than conventional CT in the treatment of childhood ALL.

The European Organization for Research and Treatment of Cancer (EORTC) Children's Leukaemia Group trial 58881 included a randomization to replace oral 6-MP with IV 6-MP for 1 week every month during CT [15]. The 5-year DFS in the group that received IV 6-MP was $71.2\% \pm 2.3\%$ compared to $78.6\% \pm 2.1\%$ for the conventional CT group (log-rank $p < 0.027$). This difference was more marked in the group who were randomized to receive the less potent *Erwinia* asparaginase ($59.2\% \pm 4.8\%$ versus $74.5\% \pm 4.3\%$; hazard ratio [HR] 1.71) compared to the group who received *E. coli* asparaginase ($78.2\% \pm 3.9\%$ versus $78.4\% \pm 3.9\%$; HR 1.08). Clearly, the addition of IV 6-MP to standard therapy during CT was ineffective and increased the risk of relapse.

6-Mercaptopurine primarily exerts its antileukemic effect through its conversion into 6-thioguanine nucleotides (6-TGN) that are incorporated into the leukemic cell DNA, leading to cell death. The Nordic Society of Paediatric Haematology and Oncology (NOPHO) conducted a randomized trial (ALL 92) which explored whether dose adjustment of 6-MP and MTX by erythrocyte (E) levels of 6-TGN and MTX polyglutamates could improve survival outcome in children with ALL [16]. Patients were randomized within 2 weeks of start of CT and were randomized to have their antimetabolite doses adjusted by blood counts (control group) or by a combination of blood counts and ETGN×E MTX (the product of ETGN and E MTX; the pharmacology group). The number of relapses in the control group was 34/269 (13%) compared to 45/269 (17%) in the pharmacology group with the majority occurring after completion of therapy. The risk was 6.6-fold higher for girls in the pharmacology group compared with those in the control group (9-year cumulative risk of relapse $19\% \pm 5\%$ versus $5\% \pm 2\%$; $p = 0.001$). No significant differences in relapse rates were observed between the two groups for boys. The report concluded that pharmacologically guided dose adjustments of 6-MP and MTX significantly increased the risk of relapse in girls.

Type of thiopurine

Theoretically, 6-TG is a more effective drug than 6-MP because it is more directly activated to TGN. To explore whether the use of 6-TG during CT offered a therapeutic advantage over 6-MP, the Co-operative Study Group for Childhood Acute Lymphoblastic Leukaemia (COALL) conducted a randomized trial in which 474 patients were randomized to receive either 6-TG (n=236) or 6-MP (n=238) during the CT phase of ALL treatment [17]. The 5-year EFS for patients on 6-TG was $80.1\% \pm 2.9\%$ versus $82.8\% \pm 2.6\%$ for 6-MP patients. Analysis according to risk status (low or high risk) showed no significant differences. Hematological toxicity was greater in patients who received 6-TG. The report concluded that CT with 6-TG had no impact on survival outcome.

Addition of other drugs during continuing therapy

The use of asparaginase to further reduce leukemic cell burden without increasing myelosuppression during standard CT was the focus of the Dutch Leukaemia Study Group (DLSG) ALL-8 trial [18]. Children and adolescents <18 years with standard-risk ALL in continuous remission after the reinduction phase of treatment were randomized to receive or not 25,000 IU of high-dose asparaginase (HD L-ASP) during the first 20 weeks of CT. The total duration of therapy was 2 years. As there were no differences in the 5-year EFS rate between the two randomized groups of patients (88%, standard error [SE] 5% in the HD L-ASP group versus 82%, SE 6% in the non-HD L-ASP group; p=0.58), the study concluded that the addition of HD L-ASP during CT did not improve survival outcome in children with SR ALL.

A similar study to the previous one was the Associazione Italiana Ematologica Oncologia Pediatrica (AIEOP) ALL 91 trial [19]. Previously untreated children <15 years with intermediate-risk (IR) ALL were randomized to receive or not HD L-ASP during both the reinduction and early CT phases of ALL treatment. As the DFS rates for patients in the two treatment groups were not statistically different (7-year DFS from randomization was 72.4%, SE 3.1% in the standard arm versus 75.7%, SE 2.6% in the HD L-ASP arm; p=0.64), the report concluded that HD L-ASP during reinduction and early CT for children with IR ALL did not improve overall survival.

The IDH ALL 91 trial [20] was an intergroup (Italy, Holland and Hungary) multicenter trial in which children with SR ALL were randomized to receive or not HD L-ASP during early CT with the aim of improving survival outcome. Previously untreated children aged 1–15 years were randomized at the start of CT to receive or not 20 weekly doses of HD L-ASP. Shortly after the commencement of the trial, the study asparaginase (E. coli ASP) became unavailable and Erwinia ASP was used instead. The few patients who received E. coli ASP were evenly distributed between the two randomized groups. Patients who received HD L-ASP during the CT had significantly better 5- and 10-year DFS (88.1%, SE 2.4 and 87.5%, SE 2.5) respectively compared to 82.5% (SE 2.9) and 78.7% (SE 3.3) respectively for patients who did not receive

ASP during CT (p=0.03). Similarly, the 5- and 10-year OS was 94.4% (SE 1.7) and 93.7% (SE 1.9), respectively, in HD L-ASP group compared to 89.8% (SE 2.3) and 88.6% (SE 2.4), respectively, in the group that did not receive ASP (p=0.05). The study concluded that HD L-ASP administered during early CT improved survival outcome in children with SR ALL.

References

1 Medical Research Council Working Party on Leukaemia in Childhood. Duration of chemotherapy in childhood acute lymphoblastic leukaemia. *Med Pediatr Oncol* 1982;**10**:511–20.

2 Chessells JM, Durrant J, Hardy RM, Richards S. Medical Research Council leukaemia trial-UK ALL V: an attempt to reduce the immunosuppressive effects of therapy in childhood acute lymphoblastic leukemia. Report to the Council by the Working Party on Leukaemia in Childhood. *J Clin Oncol* 1986;**4**:1758–64.

3 Eden OB, Lilleyman JS, Richards S, Shaw MP, Peto J. Results of Medical Research Council Childhood Leukaemia Trial UK ALL VIII (report to the Medical Research Council on behalf of the Working Party on Leukaemia in Childhood). *Br J Haematol* 1991;**78**:187–96.

4 Nesbit ME Jr, Sather HN, Robison LL, Ortega JA, Hammond GD. Randomized study of 3 years versus 5 years of chemotherapy in childhood acute lymphoblastic leukemia. *J Clin Oncol* 1983;**1**:308–16.

5 Miller DR, Leikin SL, Albo VC, Sather H, Hammond GD. Three versus five years of maintenance therapy are equivalent in childhood acute lymphoblastic leukaemia: a report from the Children's Cancer Study Group. *J Clin Oncol* 1989;**7**:316–25.

6 Bleyer WA. Remaining problems in the staging and treatment of childhood lymphoblastic leukemia. *Am J Pediatr Hematol Oncol* 1989;**11**:371–9.

7 Paolucci G, Masera G, Vecchi V, Marsoni S, Pession A, Zurlo MG. Treating childhood acute lymphoblastic leukaemia (ALL): summary of ten years experience in Italy. ALL Steering Committee of the Associazione Italiana Ematologia Oncologia Pediatrica (AIEOP). *Med Pediatr Oncol* 1989;**17**:83–91.

8 Childhood ALL Collaborative Group. Duration and intensity of maintenance chemotherapy in acute lymphoblastic leukaemia: overview of 42 trials involving 12 000 randomized children. Childhood ALL Collaborative Group. *Lancet* 1996;**347**:1783–8.

9 Schrappe M, Reiter A, Zimmermann M *et al.* Long-term results of four consecutive trials in childhood ALL performed by the ALL-BFM study group from 1981 to 1995. Berlin-Frankfurt-Münster. *Leukemia* 2000;**14**:2205–22.

10 Bleyer WA, Sather HN, Nickerson HJ *et al.* Monthly pulses of vincristine and prednisone prevent bone marrow and testicular relapse in low-risk childhood acute lymphoblastic leukemia: a report of the CCG-161 study by the Children's Cancer Study Group. *J Clin Oncol* 1991;**9**:1012–21.

11 Henze G, Langermann HJ, Fengler R et al. (Acute lympho-blastic leukemia therapy study BFM 79/81 in children and adolescents: intensified reinduction therapy for patients with different risk for relapse). Klin Padiatr 1982;194:195–203.

12 Lange BJ, Blatt J, Sather HN, Meadows AT. Randomized comparison of moderate-dose methotrexate infusions to oral methotrexate in children with intermediate risk acute lymphoblastic leukemia: a Children's Cancer Group study. Med Pediatr Oncol 1996;27:15–20.

13 Lilleyman JS, Richards S, Rankin A, for the Medical Research Council Working Party on Childhood Leukaemia. Medical Research Council Leukaemia Trial, UK ALL VII: a report to the Council by the Working Party on Leukaemia in Childhood. Arch Dis Child 1985;60:1050–4.

14 Koizumi S, Fujimoto T, Takeda T et al. Comparison of inter-mittent or continuous methotrexate plus 6-mercaptopurine in regimens for standard-risk acute lymphoblastic leukemia in childhood (JCCLSG-S811). The Japanese Children's Cancer and Leukemia Study Group. Cancer 1988;61:1292–300.

15 Vilmer E, Suciu S, Ferster A et al. Long-term results of three randomized trials (58831, 58832, 58881) in childhood acute lymphoblastic leukemia: a CLCG-EORTC report. Children Leukemia Cooperative Group. Leukemia 2000;14:2257–66.

16 Schmiegelow K, Björk O, Glomstein A et al. Intensi-fication of mercaptopurine/methotrexate maintenance chemotherapy may increase the risk of relapse for some children with acute lymphoblastic leukemia. J Clin Oncol 2003;21:1332–9.

17 Harms DO, Janka-Schaub GE. Co-operative study group for childhood acute lymphoblastic leukemia (COALL): long-term follow-up of trials 82, 85, 89 and 92. Leukemia 2000;14: 2234–9.

18 Kamps WA, Bökkerink JP, Hakvoort-Cammel FG et al. BFM-oriented treatment for children with acute lymphoblastic leukemia without cranial irradiation and treatment reduction for standard risk patients: results of DCLSG protocol ALL-8 (1991–1996). Leukemia 2002; 16:1099–111.

19 Rizzari C, Valsecchi MG, Aricò M et al., for the Associazione Italiano Ematologia Oncologia Pediatrica. Effect of protracted high-dose L-asparaginase given as a second exposure in a Berlin-Frankfurt-Münster-based treatment: results of the randomized 9102 intermediate-risk childhood acute lymphoblastic leukemia study – a report from the Associazione Italiana Ematologia Oncologia Pediatrica. J Clin Oncol 2001;19:1297–303.

20 Pession A, Valsecchi MG, Masera G et al. Long-term results of a randomized trial on extended use of high dose L-asparaginase for standard risk childhood acute lympho-blastic leukemia. J Clin Oncol 2005;23:7161–7.

New studies

Pulses of vincristine and steroids

Study 1

Conter V, Valsecchi MG, Silvestri D *et al*. Pulses of vincristine and dexamethasone in addition to intensive chemotherapy for children with intermediate-risk acute lymphoblastic leukaemia: a multicentre randomised trial. Lancet 2007;**369**:123–31.

Objectives

The main aim of this study was to determine whether the addition of pulses of vincristine and dexamethasone to the standard continuing phase of treatment improved survival outcome in children with intermediate-risk acute lymphoblastic leukemia.

Study design

The I-BFM-SG ALL IR 95 intermediate-risk trial was a multicenter randomized trial conducted between April 1995 and December 2000 by eight co-operative groups in 11 countries and included children below the age of 18 years with IR ALL. Children were categorized as having IR ALL if they were <1 year or ≥6 years or had a white blood cell count at diagnosis $\geq 20 \times 10^9/L$, had a good prednisone response (absolute peripheral blood blast count $<1 \times 10^9/L$ on day 8 of induction phase), and had no cytogenetic abnormalities such as t(9;22) or t(4;11). Only children in complete remission (CR) at the end of phase IA induction block were eligible for study enrollment. To be eligible for randomization, patients had to be in CR at the end of the reinduction phase and before the start of the continuing phase of treatment. Participating centers stratified randomization; each data center used a computer-generated sequence of allocation based on random permuted blocks. There was no blinding of the randomized treatment allocations. Patients randomized to vincristine and dexamethasone pulses during the continuing phase received this in addition to 6-MP and MTX. Pulses were given at 10-weekly intervals during the first

60 weeks of continuing therapy and thereafter treatment was as for the control group, i.e. 6-MP and MTX alone for a total of 2 years from diagnosis. The total cumulative dose of steroids (prednisone equivalent dose) was 4500 mg/m² for the treatment group compared to 3000 mg/m² for the control group.

Statistics

It was estimated that a sample size of 1700 patients would provide a power of 84% to detect a 6% difference in 4-year DFS, with a 75% baseline in the control group. However, the trial recruitment was extended to 5.5 years to increase the sample size to 2600 patients which had a 90% power to detect a 5% difference in 4-year DFS with a 79% baseline. All analyses were done on an intention-to-treat principle and treatment effects were estimated by the Cox model in terms of hazard ratio for DFS stratified by participating organization. All tests were two-sided and the proportional hazard assumption was verified by graphical checks. The follow-up was last updated on 31st January 2004. Forty-four patients were lost to follow-up. Data were analyzed with SAS software (version 8.2).

Results

Of the 3109 patients who were in CR at the end of phase IA induction, only 2935 were eligible for randomization as 174 patients either relapsed or died in CR before the start of the continuing phase of treatment. However, 317 patients were not randomized and hence, only 2618 patients were randomized to either the treatment group (pulses of vincristine and dexamethasone plus 6-MP and MTX; n=1325) or the control arm (6-MP and MTX alone; n=1293). There was no difference between the two groups with respect to age, sex, presenting white blood cell count or immunophenotype of ALL. Each group had 27 patients with CNS leukemia.

Two hundred and fifty-five events were seen in each of the groups; 241 relapses in the control group versus 240 in the treatment group. In the second year after randomization, there were fewer events in the treatment group (n=76; relapses 71) compared to 97 events in the control group of which 93 were relapses. This was mainly because of a decrease in isolated testicular relapse (2 versus 10) and combined bone marrow and extramedullary relapses (13 versus 20). However, in subsequent years, this was offset by a higher number of events in the treatment group. This transient improvement was seen in males, those with T-cell disease or with a presenting WBC count $\geq 100 \times 10^9$/L. No effect was consistently seen in patients aged 10 years or older.

The 5- and 7-year DFS rates were 79.8% (SE 1.2) and 77.5% (SE 1.5) in the treatment group compared to 79.2% (SE 1.2) and 78.4% (SE 1.3) for the control group. The addition of dexamethasone and vincristine was associated with a nonsignificant 3% relative risk reduction (hazard ratio 0.97; 95% confidence interval [CI] 0.81–1.15; p=0.7).

The 7-year OS was 87.1% in the treatment group (SE 1.2) compared to 88.9% (SE 1.0) in the control group (log-rank p=0.70); number of deaths from any cause were 133 and 122, respectively (hazard ratio 1.06; 95% CI 0.83–1.36; p=0.63).

When analysis was performed according to actual treatment received (33 patients in the control group received vincristine and dexamethasone pulses and 175 patients from the treatment group did not receive the allocated vincristine and dexamethasone pulses), the results were similar; 7-year DFS was 77.4% (SE 1.5) and 78.9% (SE 1.3) in patients who did or did not receive the dexamethsone and vincristine pulses (hazard ratio 1.02; 95% CI 0.86–1.22; p=0.80).

Vincristine and dexamethasone pulses did not substantially affect the total cumulative doses of 6-MP and MTX when the treatment group was compared with the control group (treatment group, mean and cumulative dose of 6-MP 18003 mg/m^2 and 18752 mg/m^2; MTX 1049 mg/m^2 and 1112 mg/m^2 versus control group, 6-MP 16974 mg/m^2 and 18128 mg/m^2 and MTX 1002 mg/m^2 and 1057 mg/m^2).

Toxicity

There were no significant differences in hepatic or neurological toxicities between the two groups of patients during the continuing phase of treatment. In addition, there were no differences in the need for blood product support or hospitalization rates (treatment group median 7 days versus 6 days in the control group) during the continuation phase of treatment.

Conclusions

It was concluded that dexamethasone and vincristine pulses during the continuing phase of treatment did not improve either the disease-free or overall survival of children with IR ALL when treated on intensive chemotherapy regimens based on BFM protocols.

Study 2

De Moerloose B, Suciu S, Bertrand Y *et al.*, for the Children's Leukaemia Group of the European Organization for Research and Treatment of Cancer (EORTC). Improved outcome with pulses of vincristine and corticosteroids in continuation therapy of children with average risk acute lymphoblastic leukemia (ALL) and lymphoblastic non-Hodgkin lymphoma (NHL): report of the EORTC randomized phase 3 trial 58951. *Blood* 2010;**116**:36–44.

Objectives

The objectives of the EORTC 58951 trial were to:
• compare and evaluate the efficacy of dexamethsaone (DEX) versus prednisolone (PDN) during remission induction therapy of children with acute lymphoblastic leukemia (ALL)
• determine the value of prolonged courses of L-asparaginase throughout consolidation and late intensification phases in the non-very high-risk patients
• evaluate the efficacy of vincristine (VCR) and corticosteroid pulses during the continuation phase of treatment in children with intermediate/average-risk ALL.

This review focuses on the efficacy of vincristine and corticosteroid pulses during the continuing phase of treatment.

Study design

Patients younger than 18 years of age with previously untreated ALL or non-Hodgkin lymphoma (NHL) were eligible for enrollment onto this EORTC 58951 trial. Patients with ALL of L3 morphology, diffuse large cell B-cell NHL, or Burkitt lymphoma were excluded as were patients who had previously received

>7 days corticosteroid treatment. Patients were risk categorized into very low-risk (VLR), intermediate- or average-risk (AR) and very high-risk (VHR) groups. VLR was defined as presenting WBC count $<10 \times 10^9$/L, hyperdiploid karyotype, DNA index >1.16 and with no CNS or gonadal involvement. VHR children were those with peripheral blood blast count $\geq 1 \times 1$ on completion of prephase, those who had t(9;22), t(4;11) or mixed lineage leukemia chromosomal translocations, near haploidy (<34 chromosome), acute undifferentiated leukemia, failure to achieve complete remission or minimal residual disease $>10^{-2}$ at the time of completion of remission induction. AR patients were all children without VLR or VHR characteristics and were further subdivided into AR1 (B-cell lineage ALL and WBC count $<100 \times 10^9$/L) and AR2 (T-cell ALL, WBC count $>100 \times 10^9$/L, those who had gonadal or CNS involvement). In this trial the value of DEX versus PDN was evaluated both during remission induction and continuing treatment phases as well as the increased number of doses of L-asparaginase during consolidation and late intensification phase of treatment. Children with AR were eligible for the randomization between VCR+corticosteroid pulses or no pulses during the continuing treatment phase.

Definitions

Central nervous system disease was defined as CNS 1 (no detectable blasts in cerebrospinal fluid [CSF]), CNS 2 (<5 leukocytes/µL with detectable blasts in centrifuged CSF) and CNS 3 (≥5 leukocytes/µL with detectable blasts in CSF) or ALL-related cranial nerve palsies. Grading of toxicity was according to the WHO criteria.

Treatment

Average-risk patients who were in CR at the end of late intensification were randomized to receive or not six pulses of VCR and corticosteroids along with standard CT of daily oral 6-MP and weekly oral MTX. The pulses were at 10-weekly intervals during the first 60 weeks of continuing treatment and consisted of 7 days of corticosteroids (PDN or DEX depending on first randomization) and VCR 1.5 mg/m^2 on days 1 and 7. After 60 weeks, standard CT (6-MP and MTX) was continued for a further 14 weeks.

Statistics

The primary endpoint was DFS and this was calculated from date of randomization to date of relapse, death or last follow-up. Overall survival was the secondary endpoint and was calculated from date of randomization to date of death or last follow-up. An additional secondary endpoint was treatment toxicity. Survival curves were calculated by the Kaplan–Meier life table method and standard errors (SE) were obtained by the Greenwood formula. The differences between curves were tested for statistical significance by the two-tailed log-rank test. The hazard ratio (HR with 95% or 99% CI) was estimated by the Cox proportional hazard model. All analyses were according to the intention-to-treat principle. SAS 9.1 software was used for statistical analysis.

Results

Between June 1999 and November 2002, 411 AR patients (ALL 384, NHL 27) enrolled on the EORTC 58951 trial were randomly assigned to receive or not pulses of VCR and corticosteroids during the CT phase. Of the 205 patients in the no pulse group, 101 (49.3%) were initially randomized to PDN and 100 to DEX. In the pulsed group (n=206), 101 patients each were randomized to PDN and DEX respectively. Eight patients registered on the trial were assigned to PDN during remission induction. The distribution of patients and disease characteristics were balanced in the two treatment groups. The mean daily dose of oral 6-MP and weekly oral MTX was not influenced by the administration of pulses.

Of the 205 patients randomized to no pulses, only 191 completed the CT phase while in the pulsed group of 206 patients, seven did not receive the allocated pulses.

The 6-year DFS rate was 90.6% (SE 2.1%) in the pulsed group and 82.8% (SE 2.8%) in the no pulses group (HR 0.54, 95% CI 0.31–0.94; p=0.027). There were 19 versus 34 events in the pulsed versus no pulses group: bone marrow (BM) relapse (10 versus 16), CNS relapses (1 versus 4), other isolated relapse (2 versus 3), combined BM and CNS relapses (2 versus 5), combined BM and other sites (4 versus 4) and deaths in CR (0 versus 2).

Six-year OS rate was 94.3% (SE 1.7%) in the pulsed group versus 91.1% (SE 2.1%) in the no pulses group (HR 0.63; 95% CI 0.29–1.34; p=0.225).

The effect of pulses was similar in the PDN (HR 0.56; 99% CI 0.18–1.74; p=0.18) and the DEX group (HR 0.59; 99% CI 0.22–1.59; p=0.17).

The 6-year DFS rates in girls and boys were 92.6% and 81.2% respectively (HR 0.40; 95% CI 0.22–0.73; p=0.002) while the 6-year OS rates were 95.7% and 90% respectively (HR 0.43; 95% CI 0.19–0.97; p=0.035). The pulses effect was more pronounced in girls (HR 0.24; 99% CI 0.04–1.25; p=0.015) than in boys (HR 0.71; 99% CI 0.30–1.66; p=0.30). In girls this was due to a reduction in BM relapses and in boys, pulses reduced the incidence of combined and isolated CNS relapses although BM relapses were similar in both arms.

Two hundred and forty-seven patients in this study corresponded to the IR criteria used in the Intergroup trial (I-BFM-SG ALL 1R 95); 128 and 119 randomized to VCR+PDN and VCR+DEX respectively. When analyzed according to the Intergroup risk criteria, DFS was better in the pulsed group, both in the VCR+DEX (HR 0.51; 99% CI 0.16–1.69) and VCR+PDN (HR 0.28; 99% CI 0.06–1.22) groups.

Toxicity

While grade 3 and 4 hepatic toxicity was lower in the pulsed group of patients (30% versus 40%), grade 2 and 3 osteonecrosis (4.4% versus 2%) and grade 3 and 4 infections (14.1% versus 9.8%) were higher in the pulsed group.

Conclusions

It was concluded that using this EORTC protocol, vincristine and corticosteroid pulses during the continuing phase of treatment improved survival outcome in children with average/intermediate -risk ALL and NHL.

Drug schedule

Study 3

Salzer WL, Devidas M, Carroll WL *et al.* Long-term results of the Pediatric Oncology Group studies for childhood acute lymphoblastic leukemia 1984–2001: a report from the Children's Oncology Group. Leukemia 2010;24:355–70.

Objectives

This publication reported the long-term outcome results of the 12 Pediatric Oncology Group (POG) studies conducted between 1984 and 2001. In this review we focus on the continuing phase randomization of the POG 9605 trial of the ALinC 16 studies where the aim was to identify the regimen that provided the best survival outcome for children with SR ALL.

Study design

The 9605 POG trial was a multicenter prospective trial conducted between 1996 and 1999. There was a randomization on a 2×2 factorial design: IM MTX (regimens A and C) versus divided dose (DD) MTX (regimens B and D) and daily (regimens A and B) versus twice-daily (regimens C and D) of 6-MP. There was another randomization during the intensification phase of the treatment.

Statistics

Datasets were frozen in January 2009 for analysis. EFS and OS rates were computed by the method of Kaplan–Meier and were compared using the log-rank test.

Results

Two hundred and sixty-six, 266, 260, and 271 patients were randomly allocated to IM MTX/daily 6-MP (regimen A), DD MTX/daily 6-MP (regimen B), IM MTX/twice-daily 6-MP (regimen C), and DD MTX/twice-daily 6-MP (regimen D) respectively.

Although there were no significant differences in survival outcomes within the MTX and 6-MP question, when reviewed by regimen, significant differences were evident, with the IM MTX/twice-daily 6-MP and the DD MTX/daily 6-MP arms showing improved survivals (5-year EFS: regimen A 71.1%±2.8%, regimen B 82.4%±2.4%, regimen C 82.8%±2.4%, regimen D 78%±2.6%). However, because the trial was designed as a 2×2 factorial, it was not sufficiently powered to compare the four arms.

Conclusions

It was concluded that because of a significant interaction between the two randomizations in the study, it was not possible to identify the regimen with the superior survival outcome.

Study 4

Silverman LB, Stevenson KE, O'Brien JE*et al.* Long-term results of Dana-Farber Cancer Institute ALL Consortium protocols for children with newly diagnosed acute lymphoblastic leukemia (1985–2000). *Leukemia* 2010;**24**:320–34.

Objectives

This publication reported the long-term results of four consecutive Dana-Farber Cancer Institute (DFCI) pediatric clinical trials conducted between 1985 and 2000. In this review we focus on the randomization results between *E. coli* asparaginase and polyethylene glycol asparaginase and oral 6-MP versus high-dose IV 6-MP (protocol 91-01) where the aims were to identify the regimen that provided the best survival outcome for children with ALL.

Study design

The DFCI protocol 91-01 was a multicenter prospective trial. Treatment was assigned based on risk group classification determined at diagnosis. There were four phases of therapy: remission induction, CNS-directed treatment, intensification, and continuation.

Randomizations

- Eligible patients treated on protocol 91-01 received 30 weeks of asparaginase during the intensification phase and were randomized to receive either *E. coli* asparaginase 25,000 IU/m²/week or polyethylene glycol (PEG) asparaginase 2500 IU/m² every 2 weeks.
- Eligible patients in protocol 95-01 were randomized to receive either *E. coli* asparaginase or *Erwinia* asparaginase 25,000 IU/m²/week for 20 weeks during the intensification phase
- Eligible patients on protocol 91-01 were randomized to receive standard oral 6-MP (50 mg/m²/day on days 1–14 every 3 weeks or high-dose IV 6-MP (1000 mg/m²/dose over 20 hours weekly×2 every 3 weeks for 1 year after completion of remission induction phase; thereafter all patients received standard oral 6-MP.

This review focuses on the third randomization: standard oral 6-MP versus high-dose IV 6-MP.

Statistics

Event-free survival and OS were estimated by the Kaplan–Meier method and compared with the log-rank test. Multivariable regression was performed using the Cox proportional hazards model to assess prognostic factors for EFS and OS.

Results

Three hundred and twenty two patients were randomized (SR and HR/VHR) to either standard oral 6-MP or IV high-dose 6-MP during the first year of postinduction therapy. There was no difference in either the EFS (p=0.99) or OS (p=0.66) based on 6-MP dosing. There was no difference between the two asparaginases.

Conclusions

It was concluded that high-dose IV 6-MP during the first year of continuing therapy was not superior to standard-dose oral 6-MP in either SR or HR/VHR children with ALL and both forms of asparaginase were equivalent.

Study 5

Brandalise SR, Pinheiro VR, Aguiar SS *et al.* Benefits of the intermittent use of 6-mercaptopurine and methotrexate in maintenance treatment for low-risk acute lymphoblastic leukemia in children: randomized trial from the Brazilian Childhood Co-operative Group – protocol ALL-99. *J Clin Oncol* 2010;**28**:1911–18.

Objectives

To determine whether intermittent use of 6-MP with intermediate-dose methotrexate during the continuing phase of treatment in children with low-risk ALL will improve survival outcome and also reduce treatment-related toxicity.

Study design

Children with low-risk (LR) ALL were enrolled on to the Brazilian Childhood Co-operative Group for ALL Treatment (GBTLI) ALL 99 protocol and this randomized multicenter study was conducted between October 2000 and December 2007. Patients were considered to be low risk if they were between 1 and 9 years old, WBC $<50\times10^9$/L, had a rapid early response to induction (i.e. WBC $<5\times10^9$/L on day 7, no peripheral blasts and <25% blasts in bone marrow on day 14 and <5% blasts on day 28 bone marrow). Randomization was done centrally at week 22 of their treatment.

Systemic chemotherapy was identical for all patients regardless of immunphenotype or cytogenetic abnormalities and consisted of a two-phase induction block; phase 1 consisted of four drugs (dexamethasone 6 mg/m^2/day orally for 28 days, vincristine 1.5 mg/m^2 on days 0, 7, 14 and 21, daunonomycin 25 mg/m^2/dose IV on days 0, 7, 14 and 21. and L-asparaginase 5000 U/m IM on days 3, 5, 7, 9, 11, 13, 15, 17 and 19 along with triple intrathecal (TIT) chemotherapy on days 0, 14 and 28 plus days 7 and 21 if CNS+). Induction phase 2 comprised cyclophosphamide 1 g/m^2 IV, cytarabine 75 mg/m^2 subcutaneously on days 29–32 and 36–40 and 6-MP 50 mg/m^2/day orally on days 28–42. An amendment was made in the protocol in 2001 for the use of prednisone instead of dexamethasone during the induction phase. This was followed by an 8-week intensification phase (MTX 2 g/m^2 IV infusion × 4 at 2-weekly intervals and TIT 1 week after IV MTX × 4, oral 6-MP 50 mg/m^2/day × 8 weeks).

After intensification, all patients received a two-part late consolidation block that consisted of oral dexamethasone 6 mg/m^2/day × 7 days at weeks 14, 16 and 18, vincristine 1.5 mg/m_2 IV on week 14–18, doxorubicin 30 mg/m^2/dose IV on weeks 15 and 17, L-asparaginase 5000 U/m^2 IM every other day × 4 doses at week 15 and TIT on weeks 14 and 18. The second part of late consolidation consisted of three drugs: cyclophosphamide 1 g/m^2 IV, cytarabine 75 mg/m^2 subcutaneously × 4 doses weekly on weeks 19, 20 and 21 and oral 6-thioguanine 60 mg/m^2/day for 21 days from week 19 plus TIT on week 22.

At the start of the continuing phase of treatment (maintenance), children received either continuous 6-MP (50 mg/m^2/day) and MTX (25 mg/m^2/week IM – group 1) or intermittent IV MTX (200 mg/m^2 every 3 weeks) with folinic acid rescue followed 24 h later by oral 6-MP (100 mg/m^2/day × 10 days followed by a 11-day rest – group 2. Both groups also received vincristine and dexamethasone pulses every 8 weeks until week 72: oral dexamethsaone 4 mg/m^2 every other day for 3 days, vincristine 1.5 mg/m^2/dose IV on day 1 and TIT.

Statistics

It was assumed that if 272 patients were recruited to the study, there would be sufficient power to detect a 10% difference between the two randomized arms at a significance level of 5% by a two-sided significance test. Treatment-related toxic episodes between the two groups were compared by the Mann Whitney test and survival curves were constructed by the Kaplan–Meier life table method. Differences in survival curves were compared by the log-rank test. All analysis was based on an intention-to-treat principle.

Results

A total of 635 patients were classified as low risk, of whom 544 children were randomized to either the continuous regimen (n = 272, group 1) or the intermittent regimen (n = 272, group 2) during the maintenance phase of treatment. There were no differences between the two groups of patients with respect to age, WBC count at diagnosis, immunophenotype or cytogenetic abnormalities.

Patients randomized to the continuous regimen (group 1) had lower 5-year EFS compared to patients who received intermittent treatment (group 2) although this was not statistically significant (80.9% ± 3.2% versus 86.5% ± 2.8%; p = 0.089). There was no difference in the OS rates between the two groups of patients (group 1 91.4% ± 2.2% versus group 2 93.6% ± 2.1%; p = 0.28).

Boys (n = 288) randomized to the intermittent treatment arm had significantly higher 5-year EFS compared to those in the continuous treatment arm (85.7% ± 4.3% group 2 versus 74.9% ± 4.6% group 1; p = 0.027). Similarly, OS rates were better in boys in group 2 (99.1% ± 0.9% group 2 versus 89.8% ± 3.2% group 1; p = 0015). The type of maintenance therapy had no impact on either EFS or OS rates in girls (n = 256; p = 0.78).

Although patients with common ALL (n = 467) appeared to have a better EFS with the intermittent maintenance regimen (p = 0.038), when stratified by sex, a significant difference in favor of the intermittent regimen was only seen in boys (p = 0.008; p = 0.88 for girls).

Toxicity

Grade 3 and 4 hepatic and hematological toxicities were higher in group 1 patients (p = 0.002 and 0.005 respectively). However, grade 1 and 2 renal toxicities were more common in patients on the intermittent maintenance regimen (326 versus 175; p = 0.002).

Grade 3 and 4 infections were not significantly different between the two groups of patients.

Conclusions

It was concluded that the intermittent use of 6-MP and MTX during continuing treatment was the less toxic regimen and significantly improved EFS rates in boys.

Type of thiopurine

Study 6

Vora A, Mitchell CD, Lennard L *et al.*, for the Medical Research Council/National Cancer Research Network Childhood Leukaemia Working Party. Toxicity and efficacy of 6-thioguanine versus 6-mercatopurine in childhood lymphoblastic leukaemia: a randomized trial. *Lancet* 2006;**368**:1339–48.

Objectives

To compare and evaluate the efficacy of 6-TG versus 6-MP during interim maintenance and continuing treatment in childhood lymphoblastic leukemia.

Study design

ALL 97 was a multicenter randomized trial conducted between April 1997 and June 2002 and included all children between 1 and 18 years of age with newly diagnosed ALL. There were three randomizations initially on this trial: the first randomization was between prednisolone and dexamethasone, the second between 6-MP and 6-TG during both the interim maintenance and continuing phases of treatment, and the third was for an additional third intensification block. Although the background treatment regimes underwent several modifications, the first two randomizations were retained throughout. Between 1997 and 1999, children with high-risk ALL (based on the Oxford hazard score using age, sex, and presenting white cell count) or the presence of adverse cytogenetic features were not randomized but treated on a more intensive treatment protocol. Between 1997 and 1999, the treatment consisted of a four-drug induction followed by two short intensification blocks at weeks 5 and 20 and a randomization to a third intensification block. In November 1999, the treatment template was altered and the US Childhood Cancer Study Group (US

CCSG) protocol was adopted, as the UK treatment outcomes were 10% worse than either the German or US treatment protocols.

This phase of the trial was designated as ALL 97/99 and three treatment regimens were used based on the US National Cancer Institute (NCI) risk stratification criteria of patients (leukemia karyotype and early bone marrow response: slow early response = presence of >25% blasts in the bone marrow at day 8 or 15 of induction, rapid early response = <25% marrow blasts at day 8 or 15 of induction). All three regimens used similar treatments but differed in treatment intensity. Regimen A (for standard-risk patients) used a three-drug induction regimen followed by the US CCSG modified consolidation and CNS directed phase and two blocks of delayed intensification (DI) at weeks 17 and 32 with 8 weeks of standard interim maintenance therapy between them. Regimen B (for intermediate-risk ALL patients) was a four-drug induction protocol and included a more intensive consolidation block, similar to the BFM consolidation block between weeks 6 and 10, than regimen A but otherwise was similar. Regimen C (for high-risk patients) contained additional vincristine and pegylated asparaginase in the consolidation and DI courses and Capizzi maintenance replaced standard interim maintenance courses. The duration of continuing therapy was 3 years for boys and 2 years for girls. Presymptomatic CNS therapy consisted of an age-adjusted dose of IT MTX apart from patients who had CNS leukemia at diagnosis. These patients received additional IT MTX during induction and 24 Gy cranial radiotherapy during consolidation.

During the continuing phase of treatment, patients received either daily oral 6-MP and weekly oral MTX) or daily oral 6-TG and weekly oral MTX along with pulses of vincristine and steroids (dexamethasone or prednisolone according to the randomized assignment at diagnosis) and IT MTX. Randomization for the thiopurine allocation was between diagnosis and day 35 in ALL 97 and between day 15 and day 29 for regimen A patients and between day 8 and day 29 for regimen B patients in ALL 97/99. Randomization was with minimization to balance sex, age, white blood cell count, and steroid allocation and in ALL 97/99 also according to early response to treatment.

Statistics

All analysis was based on an intention-to-treat principle. It was assumed that recruitment of 1800 patients would provide >99% power to detect a 10% difference but only a 65% power to detect a 5% difference between 6-TG and 6-MP. The trial was closed in June 2002 as interim analysis revealed a significant benefit of dexamethasone over prednisolone and an excess of 6-TG-related hepatotoxicity without a survival benefit. Subsequently, all patients still being treated were switched to dexamethasone and 6-MP for the remainder of their treatment. The primary endpoint was EFS and secondary endpoints were deaths in remission, isolated CNS relapse, CNS relapse combined with a relapse at another site, and non-CNS relapse. Differences between the patient groups who did or did not have thioguanine-related toxicities were assessed by the X^2 test or the Mann Whitney test.

Results

Seven hundred and fifty patients were randomized to receive 6-TG while 748 were randomized to receive 6-MP. The 5-year risk of overall CNS or non-CNS relapses was similar in both groups of patients. However, isolated CNS relapses were significantly lower in the 6-TG group than in the 6-MP group (2.5% 6-TG versus 4.6% 6-MP; p=0.02) with an odds ratio (OR) of 0.53 (95% CI 0.30–0.92). A subgroup analysis (variables included background treatment, steroid allocation, and patient risk group) showed that isolated CNS relapses were much the same whether the patients were NCI standard risk or high risk or whether they received dexamethasone or prednisolone. In the 6-TG group, events were half that of the 6-MP group.

Event-free survival did not differ between the two groups of patients (6-TG 80% [591/748] versus 6-MP 81% [596/744]; p=0.6). Similarly, there was no difference for overall survival between the two groups (88% 6-TG versus 90% 6-MP; p=0.3). The 5-year EFS rate of the 6-TG patients who were transferred to 6-MP at closure of randomization (79.3%) was very close to those who had received 6-TG during the entire continuing therapy (79.8%).

Toxicity

Death rate in remission was significantly higher in the 6-TG group than in the 6-MP group and was related to bacterial or viral infections with excess in the continuing phase of treatment. The frequency of infection-related deaths in remission during consolidation, interim maintenance, and delayed intensification phases was similar in both groups. It appeared that 6-TG was more problematic when combined with dexamethasone (6-TG/DEX 22/352 versus 5/349 with 6-MP/DEX) than with prednisolone (6-TG/PDN 6/394 versus 7/392 with 6-MP/PDN). The odds ratio was 0.86 in the prednisolone group (95% CI 0.29–2.54) and 3.55 (1.67–7.55) in the dexamethasone group.

Ninety-five patients developed hepatic veno-occlusive disease (HVOD) and all were related to 6-TG exposure; 82 patients were randomly assigned to 6-TG, one patient was nonrandomly on 6-TG and 12 patients assigned to 6-MP developed HVOD whilst taking 6-TG during the delayed intensification course. In patients assigned to 6-TG, the HVOD episodes occurred mainly during the continuing (75%) or interim maintenance phase (10%) of treatment (68/82) while 14 (15%) occurred during the intensification phase. All patients were switched to 6-MP after developing HVOD.

Conclusions

It was concluded that although 6-TG significantly reduced the incidence of isolated CNS relapses, it did not improve survival outcome due to an excess of deaths in remission due to infections, especially during the continuing phase of treatment, In addition, 6-TG was also directly causal to the development of hepatic veno-occlusive disease.

Study 7

Stork LC, Matloub Y, Broxson E *et al*. Oral 6-mercaptopurine versus oral 6-thioguanine and veno-occlusive disease in children with standard-risk acute lymphoblastic leukemia: report of the Children's Oncology Group CCG-1952 clinical trial. *Blood* 2010;**115**:2740–8.

Objectives

The CCG 1952 trial had two main aims:

• compare and evaluate the efficacy of 6-TG versus 6-MP during the consolidation, interim maintenance, and continuing phases of treatment in children with standard-risk childhood ALL

• compare the efficacy of TIT with standard IT MTX for presymptomatic CNS treatment in children with standard-risk ALL.

This review focuses on the thiopurine comparison.

Study design

The CCG 1952 was a prospective multicenter trial that enrolled patients between May 1996 and February 2000. Children with precursor B- or T-cell ALL considered as standard risk on the National Cancer Institute criteria (1 to <10 years with a presenting white cell count of $<50 \times 10^9$/L) were the subjects of this report. Patients treated with systemic corticosteroids for >48 h during the preceding month were ineligible. All children who had unfavorable cytogenetics such as t(9;22), t(4;11) or hypodiploidy and those who had M3 marrow status (>25% blasts) on day 14 were not eligible for the postinduction randomization. All patients had to be in morphological remission on day 28 of remission induction to be eligible for randomization. Those who had overt CNS or testicular disease at diagnosis were included. Eligible patients were randomized post remission induction to one of four treatment regimens on a 2×2 factorial design: (6-MP/IT MTX; 6-MP/TIT; 6-TG/IT MTX or 6-TG/TIT). The main treatment protocol consisted of an induction phase followed by consolidation, two interim maintenance phases, two delayed intensification phases (DI) followed by continuing treatment. Prednisone was the steroid used during induction, interim maintenance, and continuing treatment while dexamethasone was used during both DI phases. Girls were treated for 2 years and boys for 3 years from the start of the first interim maintenance phase. The doses of thiopurines and oral methotrexate were adjusted during continuing treatment to keep the neutrophil and platelet counts between $1–2 \times 10^9$/L and $\geq 100 \times 10^9$/L respectively.

Due to reports of the occurrence of hepatic veno-occlusive disease (HVOD), the target dose of 6-TG was reduced to 50 mg/m² in January 1998 and in early 2001, due to reports of portal hypertension as a late complication of 6-TG, all patients on 6-TG were switched to 6-MP.

Statistics

All analysis was based on intention-to-treat principle. Outcome analysis initially compared the entire 6-TG and 6-MP cohorts but later patients were subdivided into two subgroups, those enrolled before and after December 26th 1997, to reflect the reduction in target 6-TG dose to 50 mg/m². EFS and OS estimates were determined by the Kaplan–Meier method. Relative hazard rates (RHRs) were estimated by the log-rank method of observed divided by expected events. Chi-square tests for homogeneity of distributions, two-tailed Fisher exact test, and Cox proportional hazards model were used in some analyses.

Results

Of the 2175 patients who were enrolled on the trial, only 2030 were randomized, of whom three were excluded because they did not meet the inclusion criteria. One thousand and seventeen patients were randomized to 6-TG (6-TG/IT-MTX 509 and 6-TG/TIT 508) and 1010 randomized to 6-MP (6-MP/IT MTX 509 and 6-MP/TIT 501). The presenting features were similar in the two thiopurine cohorts except for hepatomegaly (more common in the 6-TG group) and CNS 2 status that was higher in the 6-MP group of patients.

Patients randomized to 6-TG had better EFS than those randomized to 6-MP despite the cross-over of 581 patients to 6-MP due to either toxicity or protocol modifications; 7-year EFS for 6-TG 84.1% (± 1.8%) versus 79% (± 2.1%) (p=0.004). However, 7-year OS rates were not statistically different between the two groups: 6-TG 91.9% (± 1.4%) versus 6-MP 91.2% (± 1.5%) (p=0.6).

Seven-year EFS rates for 6-TG patients on 60 mg/m² (cohort 1) were superior to patients on 6-MP (84.8%±2.0% versus 75.9%±2.4%; RHR 0.61; p=0.002) while it was not significantly different for 6-TG patients on the lower target dose (cohort 2) of 50 mg/m² (6-TG 83.7%±4.3% versus 6-MP 81.6%±4.4%; RHR 0.84; p=0.23). There was no survival advantage for 6-TG over 6-MP in cohort 1 or cohort 2 when comparing all randomized patients (p=0.51) or subdividing by sex (p=0.95).

Event-free survival rates were similar among patients randomized to 6-TG irrespective of whether or not they developed 6-TG-induced toxicities (with veno-occlusive disease [VOD] or disproportionate thrombocytopenia [DT] 89.4% versus 83.6% without VOD or DT).

Seven-year EFS for boys on 6-TG was higher than for boys on 6-MP: 82.5% (± 2.5%) versus 75.3% (± 3.0%) (RHR 0.66; p=0.002) and this was clearly evident in cohort 1 patients who received 60 mg/m² of

6-TG. In contrast, this difference in EFS rates for 6-TG versus 6-MP was not seen in girls in either cohort.

Compared to 6-TG patients, 6-MP patients had a higher rate of isolated CNS relapses (56 versus 33; 7-year cumulative incidence 5.8% versus 3.4%; p=0.01). The 7-year cumulative incidence of isolated CNS relapses was significantly higher for boys than girls on 6-MP (8.9%±2.2% versus 2.0%±1.2%; RHR 3.87; p<0.001) but was not statistically different between boys and girls on 6-TG. Similarly, 6-MP patients also had a higher incidence of bone marrow relapses than those on 6-TG (114 versus 84; 7-year cumulative incidence 12.9% versus 0.92%; p=0.018). The cumulative incidence of marrow relapse was sex equivalent for 6-TG and 6-MP. There were no differences in testicular or other extramedullary site relapses (22 versus 25), remission deaths (9 versus 10) or second malignancies (5 versus 4) between the two randomized groups.

Toxicity

Two hundred and six (20%) children randomized to 6-TG developed reversible HVOD and were switched to 6-MP on clinical recovery. In addition, three patients who were randomized to 6-MP developed HVOD after completing 14 days of the DI phase when the oral thiopurine was 6-TG. No patients developed HVOD while on 6-MP.

Fifty-one patients (5%) developed ongoing thrombocytopenia over a minimum of 2 months while on 6-TG that was out of proportion to the degree of neutropenia or anemia. In addition, a further six patients who were on 6-TG throughout their treatment were deemed to have developed DT during the second year of maintenance

In summary, HVOD or DT developed in 28.5% (n=118/414) and 23% (n=139/503) who received 6-TG at 60 mg/m² or 50 mg/m² doses respectively (p=0.056). Boys were more likely to develop these toxicities by the end of maintenance cycle number 4. The incidence of HVOD did not differ by age, presenting WBC count or intrathecal regimen. In total, 262 (26%) patients randomized to 6-TG switched to 6-MP because of toxicity.

Conclusions

It was concluded that although the EFS rates were higher in boys with 6-TG at 60 mg/m² compared to 6-MP, there was no difference in OS rates and, importantly,

acute as well as late toxicities preclude its use in the treatment of childhood ALL.

Study 8

Escherich GM, Richards S, Stork LC, Vora AJ. Meta-analysis of randomised trials comparing thiopurines in childhood acute lymphoblastic leukaemia. Leukemia 2011;**25**:953–9.

This report is a meta-analysis of three trials – COALL-05-92, CCG-1952, and MRC ALL 97 – in which there was randomization between 6-TG and 6-MP, conducted in Germany, the US, and the UK.

Objectives and study design

Data from each patient entered on the three trials were checked for internal consistency, balance between the treatment groups by initial features, randomization dates and length of follow-up and consistency with publications.

Statistics

All analyses were from time of randomization to event within the trial with observed minus expected (O-E) number of events and its variance obtained by the log-rank test method added over the three trials, used to calculate the overall odds ratio and the 95% CI. Outcomes analyzed were CNS relapse rate, non-CNS relapse, second malignancy, deaths not in remission as well as deaths in remission. Heterogeneity between trials was tested using χ^2-statistics and the I^2-measure of consistency. Subgroup analyses were prespecified by gender, age group (<10, ≥10 years), white blood cell count (<10, 10–19, 20–49, 50–99, and ≥100) and immunophenotype (T or B lineage). In the reported analyses, the two highest WBC groups were combined because the numbers were small.

Results

The COALL and MRC trials included children of all risk groups while the CCG-1952 trial was only for the National Cancer Institute standard-risk patients (age <10 years and white blood cell count <50×10⁹/L).

The total number of children randomized between 6-TG and 6-MP was 4000. With the maximum follow-up year of 2005 in COALL-05-92, 2005 in CCG-1952 and 2008 in MRC ALL 97, the median follow-up of all patients alive or lost to follow-up for the three trials

(COALL-05-92, CCG-1952, MRC ALL 97) was 8.9, 6.4, and 8.9 years respectively. The main difference between the trial cohorts was the inclusion of NCI standard-risk patients in the CCG-1952 trial and thus there were no children ≥10 years at diagnosis compared with 21% and 15% respectively in the COALL and MRC trials. Similarly, for the same reason there were no patients with a WBC count ≥50×10^9/L in the CCG-1952 trial compared to 21% and 18% in the COALL and MRC trials respectively.

Overall, there was a small but not statistically significant reduction in the event rate with 6-TG (OR 0.89; 95% CI 0.78–1.03; p=0.10).

The CNS relapse rate was lower for patients who received 6-TG (OR 0.74; 95% CI 0.58–0.95; p=0.02). As thiopurine treatments were balanced between intrathecal treatments in the CCG-1952 trial and between steroid types in the MRC ALL 97 trial, there was no evidence of a different effect of 6-TG on CNS relapse rate between these treatment groups. The reduction in the CNS relapse rate was offset by an increase in the death rate in first remission in the MRC trial (OR 1.67; 95% CI 1.00–2.78; p=0.05). Moreover, in the MRC ALL 97 trial, patients randomized to dexamethasone pulses had a higher incidence of death in first remission (6-TG 20/354; 6-MP 5/353; OR 3.36; 99% CI 1.02–9.43) compared with those who received prednisolone (6-TG 5/396, 6-MP 7/395; OR 0.73; 99% CI 0.16–3.17; p for heterogeneity =0.03). The absolute reduction in the proportion with CNS relapses in the 6-TG group was 1.8% and this resulted in a nonsignificant reduction of 2.5% in the proportion with any event at 5 years.

There were lower non-CNS relapses and more second malignancies in patients who received 6-TG compared with those received 6-MP but this was not statistically significant (OR 1.87; 95% CI 0.87–4.04; p=0.11). There was no evidence that the second tumors were related to the use of CNS irradiation. There was no difference in OS between the two groups of patients with the 5-year OS being 0.9% higher in those who received 6-MP (OR 1.07; 95% CI 0.89–1.30; p=0.47). In addition to the increased deaths in first remission and second malignancies, patients who relapsed had a nonsignificantly poorer survival after relapse if they had received 6-TG.

Although there was no evidence of a treatment effect on the overall event rate in subgroups by WBC count or immunophenotype, there appeared to be a possible gender effect (heterogeneity p=0.01). This was due to 50% reduction in CNS relapses amongst boys who received 6-TG (OR 0.52; 95% CI 0.39–0.72; p=0.0001) but this benefit was not seen in girls. There was no difference in non-CNS relapses or deaths in first remission. The difference in the 5-year EFS for patients who received 6-TG versus 6-MP was 5.4% higher in boys and 1.1% lower in girls who received 6-TG. Due to better salvage rates amongst boys who relapsed in the 6-MP group compared to those who relapsed in the 6-TG group, there was no difference in the OS rates between the two groups of patients. There were also differences in the incidence of overall events according to age. Patients <10 years who received 6-TG had a lower non-CNS relapse rate (OR 0.81; 95% CI 0.66–0.98; p=0.03) compared to patients ≥10 years (OR 144; 95% CI 0.89–2.33; p=14). There was a better survival for children ≥10 years who received 6-MP because of better salvage after relapse (heterogeneity p=0.006). The heterogeneity of treatment effect on EFS between the age groups and between the sexes was confirmed when the COALL and MRC trials were analyzed together after excluding the CCG-1952 trial.

Toxicity

Toxicity was a significant problem in the CCG-1952 and MRC ALL 97 trials which included steroid and vincristine pulses. In the MRC trial 82 patients developed HVOD, 68 during the continuing phase and 14 during the intensification phase, while 12 patients in the 6-MP arm developed this complication during the intensification phase when 6-TG was used. Similarly, in the CCG-1952 trial, 20% of patients randomized to 6-TG developed HVOD with the majority (n=182) developing it during the continuing phase of treatment. Three patients in the 6-MP arm developed HVOD while receiving 6-TG during the intensification phase of treatment. In both trials patients who developed HVOD were switched to 6-MP. The estimated increase in HVOD between the randomized groups was sevenfold (OR 7.16; 95% CI 5.66–9.06).

Conclusions

It was concluded that although there was significant improvement in EFS for boys <10 years who received 6-TG, this did not result in improved OS benefit and additionally, the toxicity associated with 6-TG was also higher.

Addition of other drugs during continuing therapy: role of intermediate-/high-dose cytarabine

Study 9

Möricke A, Reiter A, Zimmermann M *et al.*, for the German-Austrian-Swiss ALL-BFM Study Group. Risk-adjusted therapy of acute lymphoblastic leukemia can decrease treatment burden and improve survival: treatment results of 2169 unselected pediatric and adolescent patients enrolled in the trial ALL-BFM 95. *Blood* 2008;**111**:4477–89.

Objectives

The main objective was whether the addition of intermediate-dose cytarabine (ID ARAC) to high-dose IV methotrexate (HD MTX) would reduce the incidence of CNS and systemic relapses in children with intermediate-risk ALL. The study also considered a number of other issues not reported, including whether:

- a reduction in the dose of daunorubicin by 50% during the induction phase in standard-risk patients is feasible without affecting therapeutic efficacy
- extending the duration of the continuing phase of treatment in boys with SR ALL by an additional year will prevent late relapses
- the omission of cranial irradiation in intermediate-risk non-T-cell ALL patients compromises survival outcome
- modification of the consolidation and reinduction phases of treatment by intensification in the block elements and reintroduction of protocol II in high-risk ALL patients improves survival outcome.

Study design

This randomized multicenter trial was conducted between April 1995 and June 2000. There were two randomizations for patients with intermediate-risk ALL. At the end of intensification protocol I, intermediate-risk patients were randomly assigned to either receive additional ID ARAC (protocol MCA) or not (protocol M) and the second randomization involved the addition of six pulses of vincristine and dexamethasone every 10 weeks to standard

continuing-phase treatment versus standard continuing-phase treatment.

Statistics

For analysis of randomized patients, the DFS was calculated from the time of randomization to the first event or the last follow-up date. The Kaplan–Meier method was used to estimate the survival rates and differences were compared with the two-sided log-rank test. Cox proportional hazards model was used for univariate and multivariate analyses. Differences in the distribution of individual parameters among patient subsets were analyzed using the χ^2 test for categorized variables and the Mann-Whitney U test for continuous variables. All analysis was based on an intention-to-treat principle. The median follow-up for the analyzed patients was 7.2 years.

Results

Of the 1032 patients who were randomized to receive either additional high dose ARA-C (protocol MCA) or not (protocol M), 518 were assigned to the standard treatment arm (protocol M) and 514 to the experimental arm (protocol MCA). Seven patients died prior to this treatment phase and two patients withdrew from the trial. In addition, 13 patients randomized to protocol M and 69 to protocol MCA were treated in the opposite arm. Treatment analysis could not be performed in a further 18 patients and reasons were not clarified in the publication.

The 6-year DFS rates for patients randomized to protocols M and MCA were 80%±2% and 80%±2% respectively (p=0.99). Deaths in continuous complete remission (CCR) were similar (protocol M 3 versus protocol MCA 5) and none of them occurred during the treatment phase (i.e. protocol M/MCA).

Patients randomized to protocol MCA needed a median of 72 days (range 53–139 days) before they could commence the reinduction phase versus 71 days (range 60–119 days) for patients randomized to protocol M.

Conclusions

It was concluded that the addition of IV ID ARAC to the standard arm of IV HD MTX and 6-MP did not improve disease survival outcome in patients with intermediate-risk ALL.

CHAPTER 22

Relapsed childhood lymphoblastic leukemia

Ananth Shankar

University College London Hospitals NHS Foundation Trust, London, UK

New studies

Study 1

Parker C, Waters R, Leighton C *et al.* Effect of mitoxantrone on outcome of children with first relapse of acute lymphoblastic leukaemia (ALL R3): an open-label randomized trial. *Lancet* 2010;**376**: 2009–17.

Objectives

The primary objective of this randomized trial was to compare the efficacy of mitoxantrone (MTXN) versus idarubicin (IDA) during the induction phase of treatment in children and adolescents with relapsed acute lymphoblastic leukaemia (ALL).

Study design

This was an open-label randomized trial opened in January 2003 and was conducted in 31 centers across the UK, Ireland, Australia, and New Zealand. All patients between the ages of 1 and 18 years with a first relapse of ALL who had not received allogeneic stem cell transplantation (allo-SCT) in first complete remission were eligible for trial enrollment and were randomly assigned by stratified concealed randomization to receive either idarubicin or mitoxantrone as part of multiagent induction therapy. Neither patients nor those giving interventions were masked. Patients were stratified into high risk, intermediate risk or low risk on the basis of duration of first complete remission, site of relapse, and immunophenotype of relapsed ALL. Time to relapse was classified as very

early if relapse occurred within 18 months of first diagnosis, early if after 18 months of first diagnosis but within 6 months of end of treatment, and late if relapse was detected after 6 months from the end of treatment. All patients received three consecutive blocks of chemotherapy and were allocated to allogeneic stem cell transplantation according to risk group and minimal residual disease. Patients were deemed to be in second complete remission if they had <5% blasts in the marrow and no blasts in the cerebrospinal fluid at the end of phase 1 block. Minimal residual disease (MRD) was measured from marrow samples at diagnosis, at the end of induction (first time point), and after phase 3 (second time point). At first time point, low MRD was defined as $<10^{-4}$ cells with two sensitive markers and high MRD was defined as at least one marker of $\geq 10^{-4}$ cells. All others were classified as indeterminate. MRD was not estimated in isolated extramedullary disease.

The primary endpoint was progression-free survival (PFS) defined as time from randomization to the first induction failure, relapse, death from any cause or a second malignancy. Secondary endpoints were overall survival (OS), defined as time from randomization to death from any cause, and proportion of intermediate-risk patients with low MRD at the first time point. Adverse events were graded according to the National Cancer Institute (NCI) Common Terminology Criteria (CTCAE) v 3.0.

Evidence-Based Pediatric Oncology, Third Edition. Edited by Ross Pinkerton, Ananth Shankar and Katherine K. Matthay.
© 2013 John Wiley & Sons, Ltd. Published 2013 by John Wiley & Sons, Ltd.

Statistics

Randomization was stopped in December 2007 because of a significant difference in the PFS between the two groups of patients. Final analysis of the randomized objectives was done in 2009 to allow for maturation of data and all analysis was based on an intention-to-treat principle. All patients were included in the analysis apart from three ineligible patients being excluded and one additional patient was censored due to a major protocol violation. PFS and OS were estimated by the Kaplan–Meier plot and the unstratified log-rank test. Multiple Cox regression was done to assess treatment effect after adjustment for prespecified prognostic covariates: study group, risk group, age group (1<6, 6–10 and ≥10 years), sex, and presence of *ETV6-RUNX1* translocation.

The number of toxic effects at grade 3 or higher per patient was modeled with Poisson regression. Comparison of the number of patients who had at least one serious adverse event between treatments was by the χ^2 test.

Results

Of the 239 eligible patients enrolled on the study, 216 were randomized to receive either mitoxantrone (n=105) or idarubicin (n=111), of whom 103 and 109 patients respectively were analyzed. Although the two groups were well balanced with respect to age at relapse, sex and immunophenotype of relapsed ALL, there were differences between the treatment groups with regard to site of relapse, time to relapse and cytogenetic subtypes, with the mitoxantrone group having a higher proportion of patients with late relapses, isolated marrow relapses and high hyperdiploidy. The median follow-up in both treatment groups was 41 months.

Of the 212 evaluable patients, 108 were in second complete remission (CR) (MTXN 63/103, 61%, versus 45/109, 41%, in the IDA group). Of the 56 patients who had a subsequent relapse, a third CR was achieved in 6/38 in the IDA group versus 3/18 in the MTXN group.

Forty-nine patients were transplanted (allo-SCT) in each group; 16 (33%) patients relapsed after allo-SCT in the IDA group versus two (4%) in the MTXN group.

Three-year PFS and OS were significantly better for the MTXN group than for the IDA group (64.6%; 95% confidence interval [CI] 54.2–73.2) versus 35.9% (95% CI 25.9–45.9; p=0.0004) and 69.0% (95% CI 58.5–77.3) versus 45.2% (95% CI 34.5–55.3; p=0.004) respectively. The adjusted hazard ratio (HR) for PFS

was 0.54 (95% CI 0.36–0.82; p=0.003) and for OS was 0.56 (95% CI 0.36–0.87; p=0.01). The results remained unchanged when analysis was restricted to UK patients. Sensitivity analysis corroborated these findings.

No patient with a low MRD at the first time point had a high MRD at the second time point in either the high- or intermediate-risk group. There was no apparent difference between the two drugs with regard to MRD levels at the first time point in the intermediate-risk group of patients. The decreased relapse rate in the MTXN group was unrelated to the kinetics of disease clearance (adjusted odds ratio for low MRD 1.06; 95% CI 0.42–2.67; p=0.9).

Toxicity

Patients randomized to receive MTXN had significantly lower grade 3 toxicities than those who received IDA (incidence rate ratio MTXN:IDA 0.86; 95% CI 0.75–0.98; p=0.02). Toxicities (hepatic or gastrointestinal) were significantly higher in the IDA group during early treatment phases. However, toxic effects were significantly worse in the MTXN group during later treatment phases, with a delay in hemopoietic recovery being most common. Differences in PFS between the two groups were mainly related to a decrease in disease events (progression, second relapse, disease-related deaths; HR 0.56; 95% CI 0.34–0.92; p=0.007) rather than an increase in adverse treatment effects (treatment death, second malignancy; HR 0.52; 95% CI 0.24–1.11; p=0.11).

Conclusions

It was concluded that mitoxantrone was superior to idarubicin and significantly improved PFS and OS in children and adolescents with relapsed ALL.

Study 2

Von Stackelberg A, Hartmann R, Bührer C *et al.*, for the ALL REZ BFM Study Group. High-dose compared with intermediate-dose methotrexate in children with a first relapse of acute lymphoblastic leukemia. *Blood* 2008;**111**:2573–80.

Objectives

To evaluate, in a randomized manner, the efficacy of high-dose versus intermediate-dose methotrexate in the treatment of children with relapsed ALL.

Study design

Children and adolescents up to 18 years of age with first relapse of precursor B ALL (R-ALL) were eligible for enrolment on the ALL REZ BFM 90 that ran between July 1990 and June 1995. Eighty centers across Germany, Austria, Switzerland, Holland, Denmark, and Russia participated in this study. Patients were categorized into three groups: very early relapse (relapse occurring within 18 months of initial diagnosis), early relapse (occurring 18 months after diagnosis and within 6 months of completion of treatment), and late relapse (occurring 6 months after completing treatment). Patients enrolled on the study comprised those who had an isolated extramedullary relapse irrespective of the time point of relapse as well as those who had an early combined or isolated bone marrow (BM) relapse. Combined relapse was defined as ≥5% blasts in the marrow with extramedullary ALL while isolated BM relapse was defined as >25% blasts in the marrow without extramedullary disease. Patients were risk stratified into three groups according to time point of relapse and site of relapse (group A early isolated or combined BM relapse; group B late isolated or combined BM relapse; and group C isolated extramedullary relapse).

Treatment at diagnosis of relapse commenced with 5 days of prednisolone ($100 \, mg/m^2$/day) followed by alternating courses of R1, R2 and R3 blocks. All children were centrally randomized at relapse to receive either $1 \, g/m^2$ (intermediate-dose) methotrexate (ID MTX) over 36 h or $5 \, g/m^2$ (high-dose) methotrexate (HD MTX) over 24 h during the R1 and R2 blocks. Ten percent of the MTX dose was given IV over 30 min and the remaining 90% was administered during the subsequent 35.5 and 23.5 h respectively. Folinic acid rescue at a dose of $15 \, mg/m^2$ over 6 h was commenced at 42 h after start in those randomized to HD MTX and at 48 h after start in those randomized to ID MTX. Children in group A and B received a total of nine courses (6 R1/R2 and 3×R3 blocks) while those in group C received six courses (4×R1/R2 blocks and 2×R3 blocks). Interval at the start between R1 and R2 was 2 weeks and all subsequent blocks were at 3-weekly intervals.

Central nervous system (CNS) prophylaxis consisted of triple intrathecal (IT) chemotherapy consisting of MTX (12 mg), cytarabine (30 mg), and prednisolone (10 mg) administered with each block. Children who had CNS leukemia at relapse had 1–3 additional triple IT therapy courses till the cerebrospinal fluid (CSF) cleared as well as additional IT treatment after each R2 block. Patients who had BM relapse received cranial radiotherapy (RT) (12 Gy) while those who had CNS leukemia received craniospinal irradiation (18 Gy). Those with testicular involvement either had an orchidectomy or 24 Gy testicular irradiation (contralateral uninvolved testis received 15–18 Gy RT). Continuing therapy consisted of daily oral 6-thioguanine ($50 \, mg/m^2$) and alternate weekly IV MTX ($50 \, mg/m^2$) for 1 year in patients with isolated extramedullary relapse and 2 years for those who had a BM relapse.

Stem cell transplantation after 3–5 courses of relapse chemotherapy was recommended for patients who had a HLA identical sibling donor for patients with isolated or combined BM relapse within 4 years of diagnosis.

Statistics

Randomization was blinded using a randomization list with equal probabilities for the two arms and stratified according to treatment risk group (A/B/C). The study design required 133 patients in each of the two randomized arms and at a significance level of 5%, the study provided an overall power of 80% for a two-sided test to detect a 15% superiority of the HD MTX arm, assuming patients in the ID MTX arm had an event-free survival (EFS) rate of 35%. The Kaplan–Meier life table method was used to estimate EFS. Patients not in remission after three courses were considered induction failures and were censored at time zero. Children lost to follow-up were censored at the date of last contact. All analysis was based on an intention-to-treat principle.

Results

Of the 374 eligible patients recruited to the study, 269 were randomized to receive either HD MTX (n=128) or ID MTX (n=141). Four children who were randomized to receive HD MTX received ID MTX due to parents' choice. There were no significant differences between the two groups of patients with regard to age at relapse, sex, time or site of relapse, blast count at relapse, immunophenotype, the presence of *BCL-ABR* translocation or front-line therapy.

Although there appeared to be a trend of higher subsequent isolated extramedullary relapses in patients in the ID MTX arm, this was not significant with respect to frequencies or cumulative incidences of subsequent CNS, testicular or any isolated or combined extramedullary relapses.

Ten-year EFS rates were almost identical in both groups of patients: ID MTX 36 ± standard error [SE] 4% versus HD MTX 38 ± 4%; p = 0.919. Although the 5-year OS rate was 10% higher amongst patients in the ID MTX arm, at 15 years, the OS rates were no different (ID MTX 47% ± 4% versus HD MTX 43% ± 4%; p = 0.633). When data were analyzed by treatment received, irrespective of randomization, there was again no difference in the EFS rates (p = 0.564) between patients in the two treatment arms.

Seventy-one patients in the ID MTX group and 58 in the HD MTX group had a subsequent relapse and only 11 and six patients, respectively, were alive in third complete remission (p = 0.455). The total dose of MTX had no impact on survival outcome after allo-SCT as both groups had comparable treatment-related deaths (ID MTX n = 4, HD MTX n = 3) or a subsequent relapses (ID MTX n = 15, HD MTX n = 12). Additionally, the cumulative doses of IV MTX during front-line therapy had no impact on the effectiveness of MTX at different doses (1 g/m² or 5 g/m²) at relapse.

Conclusions

It was concluded that 24-h IV infusion of high-dose methotrexate (5 g/m²) compared with the 36-h IV infusion of intermediate-dose methotrexate (1 g/m²) did not improve EFS or OS in children with relapsed ALL.

Study 3

Freyer DR, Devidas M, La M *et al.* Post-relapse survival in childhood acute lymphoblastic leukemia is independent of initial treatment intensity: a report from the Children's Oncology Group. *Blood* 2011;**117**:3010–15.

Objectives

To determine whether initial therapy on the CCG-1961 trial was predictive of postrelapse survival (PRS) in patients who relapsed after receiving either augmented or standard treatment for newly diagnosed ALL.

Study design

The subjects of this report are the rapid early response (RER) patients randomized in the CCG-1961 trial. CCG-1961 was a multicenter prospective randomized trial that ran from September 1996 till May 2002. Eligibility criteria were age 1–9 years with a presenting white blood cell (WBC) count >50 × 10⁹/L or age 10–21 years with any WBC count.[1] All patients underwent a bone marrow examination for response assessment on day 7 and patients who had <25% blasts were considered RER and were randomized in a 2 × 2 factorial design to receive intensified or standard-intensity PII and longer versus standard-duration PII. Briefly, patients randomized to augmented PII received additional vincristine (VCR) and pegylated asparaginase (PEG ASP) during consolidation and delayed intensification (DI) phases and VCR, IV methotrexate (MTX) without leucovorin rescue and PEG ASP during the interim maintenance (IM) phases. Patients randomized to longer duration PII received two IM and DI phases rather than one. Patients with overt CNS disease and or those with Philadelphia-positive ALL were excluded from the RER randomization.

The occurrence of relapse, relapse site and postrelapse survival status were based on the individual treatment center report. The primary outcome measure in this report was postrelapse survival as a function of having received either augmented or standard-intensity PII as initial therapy on the CCG-1961 trial. Augmented PII included all patients treated on the stronger intensity regimen of either standard or longer duration therapy. Similarly, standard PII referred to all patients treated on the lesser intensity regimen irrespective of treatment duration. No patient who achieved RER on the CCG-1961 study was excluded from analysis.

Statistics

The χ² test for homogeneity of proportions was used to compare the study cohort of relapsed patients for similarities with all RER patients on the CCG-1961 trial. The Kaplan–Meier method was used to calculate postrelapse survival and the standard errors of the estimate were obtained by the method of Peto.[1]

[1] For treatment details see Seibel NL, Steinherz PG, Sather HN *et al. Blood* 2008;**111**:2548–55; Chapter 23, Study 1 of this book.

The log-rank test was used to compare survival curves between the groups. The Wilcoxon test was used to compare the median times to relapse for the initial treatment regimens.

Results

Two hundred and seventy-two patients who underwent randomization subsequently relapsed. There were no statistically significant differences between the groups on any of the characteristics that were compared.

Of the 272 patients who relapsed, 109 children were in the augmented PII arm while 163 received the standard PII treatment. The median time to relapse for the whole cohort was 396 days; 190 had an early relapse (<36 months from diagnosis) and the remaining 82 children were categorized as late relapses. One hundred and eighty-six patients had either isolated or combined bone marrow relapse, 66 had isolated CNS relapse, and 20 had isolated relapse at other extramedullary sites.

Of the relapsed cohort, 162 patients died; 99/163 (60.7%) were initially treated on standard PII and 63/109 (57.8%) were treated with augmented PII.

Although factors such as early relapse, older age at diagnosis, and bone marrow relapse were associated with inferior postrelapse survival, the, initial treatment did not significantly impact on postrelapse survival. For patients initially treated with augmented (n=109) versus standard-intensity (n=163) PII, the 3-year PRS was 36.4%+5.7% versus 39.2%+4.1% respectively (relative hazard ratio 1.06; log-rank p=0.72). There was no difference by initial regimen in the median time to death post relapse, which was 10.5 months for augmented PII versus 16.2 months for standard-intensity PII (p=0.27). No difference was seen in postrelapse survival after adjusting for time to relapse, site of relapse, age at diagnosis, and immunophenotype of ALL. Interestingly, the 3-year PRS amongst patients aged 16–20 years (n=19) who received standard PII was 21.1%+8.4% versus 0% for those who received augmented PII (n=15; log rank p=0.38).

Conclusions

It was concluded that initial therapy on the CCG-1961 trial had minimal impact on postrelapse survival and the emergence of a resistant subclone that had acquired spontaneous mutations was independent of the initial therapy.

Study 4

Panetta JC, Gajjar A, Hijiya N *et al.* Comparison of native E. coli and PEG asparaginase pharmacokinetics and pharmacodynamics in pediatric acute lymphoblastic leukemia. *Clin Pharmacol Ther* 2009;**86**:651–8.

Objectives

The objectives of the study were to compare native (*Erwinia chrysanthemi* asparaginase (Erwinase) or *Escherichia coli* asparaginase (Elspar)) and polyethylene glycol asparaginase (PEG ASP) during remission induction therapy of children with relapsed ALL.

Efficacy of depletion of asparagine (ASN) levels, the differences in their pharmacokinetics and the effects of asparaginase antibodies on their respective pharmacokinetics and depletion of ASN were the main endpoints.

Study design

This was not specified. Details of treatment were not reported.

Results

Previous asparaginase treatment and antibody status

Of the 40 patients included in the study, 36 had had received asparaginase (ASP) in prior front-line treatment: Elspar 30, PEG ASP1, Erwinase and Elspar ASP4, and all three types of ASP 1. Thirty-six patients were randomly assigned to receive native or PEG ASP, of whom 35 had ASP antibodies measured. In addition, four patients were allocated to receive Erwinase during remission induction therapy because of previous hypersensitivity reaction during front-line ALL therapy and three of them had developed antibodies to Elspar and *Erwinia* ASP. Of the randomized patients with evaluable antibody status at relapse, 13 were antibody positive to Elspar; of those, six patients were also antibody positive to PEG

ASP and another four of the 13 were antibody positive to Erwinase. All but one who were antibody positive to Elspar at relapse had received it during front-line ALL treatment. Twenty-eight patients randomized to either Elspar or PEG ASP received all their ASP treatment without being switched to Erwinase because of a clinical allergic reaction. Of these, 14 developed antibodies to either Elspar or PEG ASP prior to or during therapy. This group was considered to have silent hypersensitivity because they did not have clinical allergy.

Asparaginase pharmacokinetics

This was evaluable in only 33/40 patients (four non-randomly allocated to Erwinase and three patients had no samples taken) on day 8 (first pharmacokinetic course) and in 26 patients for the second pharmacokinetic course (four patients switched to Erwinase due to hypersensitivity reaction and three had no samples available). Clearance of ASP was significantly higher at both time points for patients on Elspar than for patients on PEG ASP. Additionally, ASP clearance increased for both formulations from day 8 to day 29 (Elspar, $p = 0.004$; PEG ASP, $p = 0.002$). PEG ASP clearance was significantly higher ($p = 0.004$) and the time PEG ASP was above the threshold of 1 IU/L was significantly shorter ($p = 0.03$) in those who were positive for PEG ASP antibodies. Although Elspar clearance was not significantly affected by Elspar antibody status, the trends were in the expected directions (higher median clearance on day 29 and shorter time of Elspar above the threshold level in antibody-positive patients).

Asparagine pharmacodynamics

Plasma and CSF ASN levels were available in 32 and 24 patients respectively. Specifically, patients who were ASP antibody positive at any time during the reinduction treatment had attenuated depletion of plasma ASN ($p = 0.01$) and CSF ASN ($p = 0.04$) levels compared to those who were negative for ASP antibodies. In addition, the time ASN was depleted below the threshold level of 3 µmol/L in plasma or 1 µmol/L in CSF was shorter in patients with antibodies ($p < 0.05$) than in those who remained antibody negative during reinduction therapy. A trend towards greater depletion of CSF ASN ($p = 0.1$) was seen in those who received Elspar compared to those who received PEG ASP.

The four patients who were switched to Erwinase (developed hypersensitivity reactions to Elspar or PEG ASP during remission induction therapy) had no significant reduction in their plasma or CSF ASN levels from day 8 to day 29.

Status at the end of remission induction

While no significant association was observed between remission induction rate and ASP treatment arm, the study was not powered to detect such a difference.

Conclusions

It was concluded that the presence of antibodies to asparaginase in children with relapsed ALL (native or PEG ASP) had an effect on both asparaginase clearance and asparagine depletion (plasma and CSF) during remission induction and there exist significant pharmacokinetic and pharmacodynamic differences attributable to asparaginase preparation and antibody status in these children.

CHAPTER 23

Postinduction therapy in adolescents and young adults with acute lymphoblastic leukemia

Ananth Shankar

University College London Hospitals NHS Foundation Trust, London, UK

New studies

Study 1

Seibel NL, Steinherz PG, Sather HN *et al*. Early post induction intensification therapy improves survival for children and adolescents with high-risk acute lymphoblastic leukemia: a report from the Children's Oncology Group. *Blood* 2008;**111**:2548–55.

Objectives

The purpose of the study was to determine whether a longer and more intensive postinduction intensification treatment improved survival in children and adolescents with high-risk acute lymphoblastic leukemia (ALL) who had a rapid early response to remission induction therapy.

Study design

CCG-1961 was a prospective multicenter randomized trial in children and adolescents with high-risk ALL that ran from September 1996 to May 2002. Previously untreated children and adolescents aged between 10 and 21 years or aged ≥1 year with a presenting white blood cell (WBC) count $\geq 50 \times 10^9$/L were eligible for study enrollment. Patients who had central nervous system (CNS) leukemia (CNS-3) or Philadelphia-positive (Ph+) ALL at diagnosis were excluded.

Remission induction consisted of IV vincristine 1.5 mg/m²/week×4, daunorubicin 25 mg m²/week×4,

oral prednisone 60 mg/m²/day×4 weeks, intramuscular L-asparaginase 6000 units/m² thrice weekly×9 doses, intrathecal (IT) cytosine arabinoside (ARAC) on day 0 and IT methotrexate (MTX) on days 7 and 28. All patients had a bone marrow assessment on day 7 and those who had ≤25% blasts on day 7 were considered rapid early responders (RER).

Rapid early responders who achieved a remission were randomized to standard (SPII) or increased-intensity (IPII) postinduction intensification and one or two delayed interim maintenance/intensification treatment blocks. Patients were assigned in a 2×2 factorial design to one of four regimens: regimen A, standard-intensity and one delayed intensification (DI) block; regimen B, standard intensification plus two DI blocks; regimen C, increased-intensity intensification plus one DI course; and regimen D, increased-intensity intensification plus two DI courses.

Statistics

The primary endpoints were event-free survival (EFS) and overall survival (OS) from the time of randomization. The target recruitment was 1052 randomized patients, which would have resulted in a statistical power of 96% at the final analysis to detect a relative hazard rate (RHR) of 0.626 (37% reduction in the EFS failure rate) for either of the main regimen comparisons in the 2×2 factorial design. Life table estimates

Evidence-Based Pediatric Oncology, Third Edition. Edited by Ross Pinkerton, Ananth Shankar and Katherine K. Matthay.
© 2013 John Wiley & Sons, Ltd. Published 2013 by John Wiley & Sons, Ltd.

were calculated by the Kaplan–Meier method and the standard deviation (SD) of the life table estimate was obtained with Peto's method. The log-rank test was used to compare outcome in treatment or prognostic groups and estimates of the RHR used observed and expected event rates from the log-rank tests. Tests for interaction effects of the treatment components were performed with Cox regression methods.

Results

Of the 2078 patients enrolled on the study, 21 patients were considered ineligible, 28 died during remission induction, and 24 did not achieve remission. In addition, 65 patients who achieved RER were excluded from randomization because they had CNS leukemia, Ph+ALL, parental or physician choice. Hence, 1299 eligible patient who had a RER were randomized in the 2×2 design: 649 and 650 patients were assigned to SPII and IPII; 651 and 648 patients to standard or longer duration PII respectively. There were no significant differences in patient characteristics between the standard and the stronger intensity groups.

For all RER, the 5-year EFS and OS rates post remission induction were 75.5% (SD 1.8%) and 84.7% (SD 1.5%) respectively. The median follow-up for the randomized continuously disease-free RER patients who had not had an event at the time of the analysis was 3.5 years.

Five-year EFS rates for patients randomized to IPII and SPII were 81.2% (SD 2.4%) and 71.7% (SD 2.7%) (p<0.001) and the corresponding 5-year OS rates were 88.7% (SD 1.9%) and 83.4% (SD 2.2%) (p=0.005) respectively. The RHR for EFS events and death were 1.61 and 1.56 times higher for the standard-intensity regimen. Bone marrow relapses were more common in the standard-intensity regimen patients (n=84) compared to the stronger intensity group (n=50; p=0.001; RHR 1.77). Isolated CNS relapses were similar in both groups of patients (32 and 29; p=0.61; RHR 1.14). Among the subgroups such as precursor B-cell ALL, T-cell ALL, age 1–9 or >10 years of age, the 5-year EFS rates were better for patients who received the stronger intensity PII.

No significant differences were seen in outcome for patients randomized to one IM/DI course (5-year EFS 76%; SD 2.6%) or two IM/DI courses (5-year EFS 76.8%; SD 2.6%) (p=0.94; RHR 1.00). Similarly, no differences were seen after subgroup analysis.

Toxicity

The incidence of avascular necrosis was higher in patients assigned to the standard duration treatment (n=67 events; 10.8%) compared to 5.5% (n=36 events) for patients treated on the increased duration arm (p=0.001). The number of days of hospitalization was not different between the increased-intensity and standard regimens except during consolidation (33.2% versus 23.1% for >8 days; p=0.001) and interim maintenance 1 (11.4% versus 3.9% for >8 days; p<0.001). The only difference between IPII and SPII during DI 1 was in the blood product use: 65.2% versus 59.2% (p=0.03).

Conclusions

It was concluded that, post induction, stronger early intensification but not prolonged duration delayed intensification improved outcome for children and young adults with high-risk ALL.

Study 2

Nachman JB, La MK, Hunger SP *et al.* Young adults with acute lymphoblastic leukemia have an excellent outcome with chemotherapy alone and benefit from intensive post induction treatment: a report from the Children's Oncology Group. *J Clin Oncol* 2009;27:5189–94.

Objectives

The main objective of the study was to examine the clinical outcome and prognostic factors of a subgroup of young adults treated on CCG-1961.

Study design and statistics

See previous study for details of CCG-1961. Primary outcome endpoints included OS and EFS in young adults from the time of randomization. A secondary endpoint was the evaluation of prognostic factors in young adults that predicted clinical outcome.

Results

Two hundred and sixty-two patients with newly diagnosed ALL between the ages of 16 and 21 were enrolled on the CCG-1961 trial. One hundred and seventy-seven achieved a RER, 75 a slow early response (SER) while 10 patients had no day 7 bone marrow evaluation performed. The ratio of RER:SER was similar to that seen among all patients entered on the CCG-1961 trial (70:30 versus 71:29 respectively). Of the patients who achieved a complete remission at the end of induction, 164 of the RER patients and 53 of the SER patients were randomized.

The 5-year EFS and OS rates for young adult patients were 71.5% (standard error [SE] 3.6%) and 77.5% (SE 3.3%) respectively.

Five-year EFS for the young adults who achieved RER was 81.8% (SE 5.4%) on the augmented-intensity arms (n=88) compared with 66.9% (SE 6.7%) for patients on the standard-intensity arm (n=76; p=0.07). There was no statistically significant difference in the EFS for young adult RER patients who were randomly assigned to one or two DI phases (71.8% versus 77.1%; p=0.48). For young adult patients who received augmented postinduction therapy that included two interim maintenance and DI phases, the 5-year EFS was 70.7% (SE 7.3%).

Five-year OS for patients on the augmented-intensity and standard-intensity arms was 83.2% (SE 6.8%) and 75.6% (SE 7.7%) respectively (p=0.14).

Patients 16–17 years and patients 18–21 years had identical 5-year EFS of 71.4%. Sex, race, mediastinal mass, platelet count, hemoglobin, and immunophenotype had no prognostic impact on survival outcome. Within the precursor B immunophenotype, young adults with a presenting WBC count $<50 \times 10^9$/L has a better EFS compared to those with a WBC count $>50 \times 10^9$/L (75.4% versus 43.9%; p=0.0004).

Toxicity

There were six induction deaths and seven deaths in remission. Deaths after induction failure, relapse or second malignant neoplasms were more frequent in the young adult patient group compared with young patients (80.3% versus 60% for patients 1–9 years and 68.5% for patients 10–15 years of age).

Conclusions

It was concluded that, as with children, young adults who had a RER to remission induction treatment benefit from early intensive postinduction therapy but do not benefit from a second interim maintenance and delayed intensification phase. Additionally, these results did not support a role for the routine use of allogeneic bone marrow transplantation in first remission for young adults with ALL.

PART 3

Supportive care
in pediatric oncology

CHAPTER 24

Colony-stimulating factors

Ananth Shankar

University College London Hospitals NHS Foundation Trust, London, UK

Commentary by Victoria Grandage

Myelosuppression is a common adverse consequence of the administration of many standard-dose chemotherapy regimens for both young and elderly patients with cancer. Although children tolerate the more intensive myelosuppressive regimens better than adult patients, infection remains a significant cause of morbidity and mortality [1].

Since the introduction of growth factors several decades ago, there have been numerous clinical trials investigating the potential benefits of adjunctive therapy with colony-stimulating factors (CSFs), the objective being amelioration or prevention of profound neutropenia and its potentially life-threatening infections. This in turn should lead to a decrease in antibiotic usage and duration of hospitalization. There was also an expectation that improved protocol compliance, reduced chemotherapy dose adjustments, and increased dosing intensity would afford an improvement in survival rates. The majority of these studies are in the adult setting. Granulocyte colony-stimulating factors (G-CSFs) have led to improved delivery of full-dose chemotherapy at a planned schedule, although this has not been generally shown to lead to a better response or improved overall survival [2]. However, in node-positive breast carcinoma and aggressive lymphoma, dose-dense regimens supported by G-CSF did improve disease-free and/or overall survival when compared to standard regimens [3, 4].

Many of the studies in children reported in this and the last edition show that although routine use of G-CSF decreases the incidence of febrile neutropenia and duration of hospitalization and may decrease delays in subsequent chemotherapy, this does not translate into reduced infectious morbidity and mortality or improve overall survival [5,6,7,8]. This is exemplified by the prospective randomized trial AML-BFM 98 (Study 2) which investigated the impact of G-CSF on hematopoietic recovery and infectious complications (primary endpoints) and on outcome (secondary endpoint) in children (aged 0–18 years) with *de novo* acute myeloid leukemia (AML). Patients with more than 5% blasts in day 15 bone marrow or with FAB M3 were not included. Between 1998 and 2003, 161 children with AML were randomized to receive G-CSF after inductions 1 and 2, whereas 156 patients were assigned to the control group. The duration of neutropenia after inductions 1 and 2 was significantly shorter in the G-CSF group (23 versus 18 days and 16 versus 11 days; $p=0.02$ and 0.001, respectively). G-CSF did not decrease the incidence of febrile neutropenia (72 and 36 patients versus 78 and 37 patients, respectively), microbiologically documented infections (27 and 25 patients versus 36 and 19 patients, respectively) or infection-associated mortality (5 versus 2 patients). Both groups had similar 5-year event-free survival (EFS; $59\%\pm4\%$ versus $58\%\pm4\%$).

Evidence-Based Pediatric Oncology, Third Edition. Edited by Ross Pinkerton, Ananth Shankar and Katherine K. Matthay.
© 2013 John Wiley & Sons, Ltd. Published 2013 by John Wiley & Sons, Ltd.

A particular concern regarding the use of G-CSF in AML is the possibility of inadvertent stimulation of the leukemia clone. A subgroup analysis of the above study suggested an increased incidence of relapse in the standard-risk (SR) group after G-CSF treatment (p=0.054). Concerned by this trend towards a higher incidence of relapse, the team intensively analyzed the AML-BFM 98 dataset and performed additional molecular analyses on leukemic blasts. They identified G-CSF receptor (G-CSFR) isoform IV overexpression as a significant and fundamental risk factor for AML relapse in children after G-CSF administration. Given this evidence and the lack of effect on the risk of infectious complications or outcome in children undergoing therapy for AML, one cannot advocate the routine use of G-CSF in this patient group.

In other patient groups there have been suggestions of a potentially increased risk of AML/myelodysplastic syndrome (MDS) with G-CSF administration in epidemiological studies. This was not observed in individual randomized trials. A recent analysis by Lyman *et al.* reported an increase in relative and absolute risk of AML/MDS of 1.92% and 0.41% respectively, related to G-CSF. It is not possible from this meta-analysis to determine whether the risk of AML/MDS is secondary to G-CSF or related to the higher total doses of chemotherapy [9,10].

Although little evidence exists to suggest that prophylactic G-CSF improves infectious morbidity or survival rates, it is often used to reduce hospitalization and improve the quality of life in a child undergoing cancer chemotherapy. A number of American guidelines in adult patients, including the National Comprehensive Cancer Network guidelines, suggest that a risk of febrile neutropenia of 20% or more for a given regimen is an indication for primary prophylaxis with G-CSF. Other centers use a cut-off of 40%. Other indications may include pre-existing neutropenia due to disease, extensive prior chemotherapy, previous irradiation to the pelvis or other areas containing large amounts of bone marrow, a history of recurrent febrile neutropenia while receiving earlier chemotherapy of similar or lesser dose intensity and conditions potentially enhancing the risk of serious infection, e.g. poor performance status, decreased immune function, open wounds, etc.

There are no current consensus guidelines in children.

The pegylated formulation of G-CSF (PEG G-CSF) has the advantage of a prolonged serum half-life of 15–80 h versus 3.5 h for recombinant G-CSF, thus having the advantage of a reduced dosing frequency. PEG G-CSF is usually given once per chemotherapy cycle, at least 24 h after the last dose of chemotherapy and at least 14 days before the next dose is due. For this reason it is not suitable for weekly regimens. Two recent studies (Studies 5 and 6) have looked at the use of PEG filgrastim versus standard filgrastim in pediatric and young adult patients with sarcoma. Both trials were randomized and compared a single dose of PEG filgrastim 100 µg/kg to filgrastim 5 µg/kg daily. They both showed that these doses were comparable in reducing the duration of severe neutropenia and the number of episodes of febrile neutropenia. There was no increase in adverse side-effects with the PEG filgrastim. On drug costs alone, PEG filgrastim is the more expensive agent based on one injection of PEG G-CSF and 10 for the recombinant G-CSF. However, the advantages of a single injection with regard to tolerability and ease of administration also need to be taken into account.

The area where G-CSF is used routinely is in peripheral blood stem cell mobilization, particularly for autologous rescue but also in some older sibling donors. It is also used routinely post hematopoietic stem cell transplantation to stimulate stem cell proliferation and hasten neutrophil recovery. In patients heavily pretreated with myelosuppressive chemotherapy or irradiation, G-CSF may fail to mobilize stem cells from the bone marrow. Plerixafor is emerging as a reliable alternative option in such situations in adult patients. It is an inhibitor of the CXCR4 chemokine receptor which plays an important role in holding hematopoietic stem cells in the bone marrow. Drugs that block the CXCR4 receptor appear to be capable of "mobilizing" hematopoietic stem cells into the bloodstream. Plerixafor is currently used in combination with G-CSF for autologous mobilization in patients who have failed to harvest. Robust data in support of the high efficacy and safety of plerixafor are available in adults with lymphoma and myeloma. Very little evidence is available on the usefulness of this drug in children. Potter *et al.* have recently reported their experience with plerixafor usage on five occasions in pediatric patients, with a success rate of 60%. They found no significant side-effects in any patient [11]. Further trials are necessary in children before plerixafor can be used routinely. A UK phase I/II trial in children with solid tumors is currently recruiting.

There are no recent trials in the use of recombinant erythropoietin (EPO) in children. There have been several small studies looking at heterogeneous populations receiving chemotherapy which suggest that EPO is effective at reducing transfusion requirements and it may be used in this setting when patients are unable to receive blood products for religious reasons. Certain tumors, e.g. Wilms and neuroblastoma, may express EPO receptors and therefore EPO use may have a detrimental effect on tumor growth and progression. There are a number of reports of randomized controlled trials of EPO use in adults with cancer that resulted in significantly reduced tumor-free survival and/or overall survival for those given EPO [12]. It is not known currently at what hemoglobin or what EPO dose the risk of tumor progression becomes significant so this growth factor should not be used routinely but within the context of clinical trials.

Thrombopoietin (TPO) is the physiological regulator of platelet production. It works by binding to its receptor on megakaryocyte precursors which activate a large number of downstream antiapoptotic and maturation pathways. "First-generation" recombinant forms of TPO were developed over a decade ago and were found to increase the platelet count in patients undergoing nonmyeloablative chemotherapy. Thrombopoietin did not improve platelet counts in patients undergoing stem cell transplantation or acute leukemia induction, presumably because of a lack of megakaryocyte progenitors in the bone marrow. Further development ended when neutralizing antibodies formed against one of the recombinant proteins. Subsequently, two "second-generation" TPO mimetics have been developed and are entering clinical practice: romiplostim and eltrombopag. Both increased the platelet counts in healthy subjects and in over two-thirds of patients with idiopathic thrombocytopenic purpura (ITP), before and after a splenectomy; responses were maintained for at least 1 year. Romiplostim and eltrombopag are now approved for the second-line treatment of patients with ITP. Adverse events have been few but long-term assessment for reticulin formation, increased bone marrow blasts, and thromboembolism is ongoing. Studies are under way to assess the efficacy of these drugs in the treatment of other thrombocytopenic disorders associated with chemotherapy, myelodysplasia, and chronic hepatitis [13].

References

1 Hann I, Visoli.C, Paesmans M, Gaya H, Glauser M. A comparison of outcome from febrile neutropenia episodes in children compared with adults: results from four EORTC studies. International Antimicrobial Therapy Comparative Group (IATCG) of the European Organisation for Research and treatment of Cancer. *Br J Haematol* 1997;**99**(3):580–8.

2 Gisselbrecht C, Haioun C, Lepage E *et al*. Placebo-controlled phase III study of lenograstim (glycosylated recombinant human granulocytes colony stimulating factor) in aggressive non-Hodgkin's lymphoma: factors influencing chemotherapy administration. Groupe d'Etude des Lymphomes de l'Adulte. *Leuk Lymphoma* 1997;**25**:289–300.

3 Citron ML, Berry DA, Cirrincione C *et al*. Randomised trial of dose dense versus conventionally scheduled and sequential versus concurrent combination chemotherapy as postoperative adjuvant treatment of node positive primary breast cancer: first report of Intergroup trial C9741. Cancer and Leukaemia Group B Trial 9741. *J Clin Oncol* 2003;**21**: 1431–9.

4 Pfreundschuh M, Trümper L, Kloess M *et al*. Two weekly or 3 weekly CHOP chemotherapy with or without etoposide for the treatment of elderly patients with aggressive lymphomas: results of the NHL-B2 trial of the DSHNHL. *Blood* 2004;**104**: 634–41.

5 Heath J, Steinherz PG, Altman A *et al*. Human granulocyte colony stimulating factor in children with high risk acute lymphoblastic leukaemia. A Children's Cancer Group Study. *J Clin Oncol* 2003;**21**:1612–17.

6 Sung L, Sung L, Nathan PC, Lange B, Beyene J, Buchanan GR. Prophylactic granulocyte colony stimulating factor and granulocyte macrophage stimulating factor decrease febrile neutropenia after chemotherapy in children with cancer. A meta analysis of randomised controlled trials. *J Clin Oncol* 2004;**22**:3350–6.

7 Pui CH, Boyett JM, Hughes WT *et al*. Human granulocyte colony stimulating factor after induction chemotherapy in children with acute lymphoblastic leukaemia. *N Engl J Med* 1997;**336**:1781–7.

8 Ozkaynak MF, Krailo M, Chen Z, Feusner J. Randomised comparison of antibiotics with and without granulocyte colony stimulating factor in children with chemotherapy-induced febrile neutropenia: a report from the Children's Oncology Group. *Pediatr Blood Cancer* 2005;**45**:242–3.

9 Tigue CC, McKoy JM, Evens AM, Trifilio SM, Tallman MS, Bennett CL. Granulocyte colony stimulating factor administration to healthy individuals and persons with chronic neutropenia or cancer: an overview of safety considerations from the research on adverse drug events and reports project. *Bone Marrow Transplant* 2007;**40**:185–92.

10 Lyman GH, Dale DC, Wolff DA *et al*. Acute myeloid leukaemia or myelodysplastic syndrome in randomised controlled trials of cancer chemotherapy with granulocyte colony stimulating factor: a systematic review. *J Clin Oncol* 2007;**25**:3158–67.

11 Aabideen K, Anoop P, Ethell ME, Potter MN. The feasibility of plerixafor as a second-line stem cell mobilizing agent in children. *J Pediatr Hematol Oncol* 2011;**33**(1):65–7.

12 Rizzo JD, Somerfield MR, Hagerty KL *et al*. Use of epoetin and darbepoetin in patients with cancer: 2007 American Society of Clinical Oncology/American Society of Hematology clinical practice guideline update. *J Clin Oncol* 2008;**26**: 132–49.

13 Kuhler D. New thrombopoietic growth factors. *Clin Lymphoma Myeloma* 2009;**9**(Suppl 3):S347–56.

Summary of previous studies

Granulocyte colony-stimulating factor

Use of growth factors such as granulocyte colony-stimulating factor (G-CSF), granulocyte macrophage colony-stimulating factor (GM-CSF) and erythropoietin has become common after chemotherapy for childhood malignancies.

In the randomized cross-over study in high-risk acute lymphoblastic leukemia (ALL) conducted by the Children's Cancer Study Group [1], previously untreated children with high-risk ALL (presenting white blood cell count [WBC] $\geq 50 \times 10^9$/L, hemoglobin ≥ 10 g/dL, T-cell phenotype with massive lymphadenopathy [>3 cm], splenomegaly extending below the umbilicus or a large mediastinal mass) were randomized to receive or not G-CSF (during either remission induction [RI] phase or consolidation block [CD]).

Granulocyte colony-stimulating factor was commenced 24 h after completion of intravenous chemotherapy and continued until the absolute neutrophil count (ANC) >2.5×10⁹/L for 2 consecutive days and subsequent chemotherapy commenced 48 h after stopping G-CSF. The dose of G-CSF was 5 μgm/kg subcutaneously and was administered daily. Outcome endpoints were time taken to ANC recovery >0.5×10⁹/L for 2 consecutive days, time taken for platelet recovery to $\geq 50 \times 10^9$/L, number of days of febrile neutropenia, number and type of documented infections, incidence of positive blood cultures, time taken to complete scheduled treatment blocks and event-free survival (EFS) and overall survival (OS).

Of the 287 eligible patients, 143 were randomized to receive G-CSF during RI phase while 144 received G-CSF during the first CD block. ANC recovery was significantly shorter for those who received G-CSF compared with the control groups (16.3 days versus 19.2 days; p=0.0003) with no evidence of carry-over effect in the cross-over analysis (p=0.99). Mean platelet recovery time was not significantly different between the G-CSF and control groups of patients (14.8 versus 14.5 days; p=0.70). There were no differences in episodes of neutropenic fever (p=0.41), number of serious infections (p=0.66), positive blood cultures (p=0.66), number of days of antibiotic usage (p=0.30) or the time taken to complete the RI phase of therapy or the CD block between the G-CSF and the control group of patients. The 6-year EFS rates were not statistically different among the four treatment groups of patients. It was concluded that children with high-risk ALL did not benefit from the prophylactic use of G-CSF.

Using G-CSF to improve chemotherapy dose intensity (CDI) and thereby improve DFS was the main objective of the report by Michel et al. [2]. Children with high-risk ALL (slow early responders [SER], high-risk cytogenetics) who were enrolled in the FRALLE 93 trial were included in this report. All eligible patients were randomized to receive G-CSF or not during the consolidation phase of therapy. CDI was calculated as the interval from day 1 of the first consolidation cycle to hematological recovery after the fifth consolidation block. G-CSF (5 μg/kg) was commenced 24 h after chemotherapy and continued until ANC >1×10⁹/L. The next scheduled chemotherapy course commenced 24 h after discontinuation of G-CSF and only if ANC >1×10⁹/L. Outcome endpoints were CDI, number of days of febrile neutropenia, number of days of IV antibiotic treatment, number of days of hospitalization, number of days of bone marrow aplasia, number of transfusions and DFS. Of the 67 randomized patients (G-CSF 34, no G-CSF 33), 55 were SER and the remaining 12 had high-risk cytogenetics. The intervals after course 1, 3, and 5 were significantly shorter in the G-CSF group. The duration of neutropenia, number of days of hospitalization and days of intravenous antibiotics were all reduced in the G-CSF group. The risk of septicemia per patient per course was 4% in the G-CSF arm compared to 11% in the no G-CSF arm (p=0.075). Although ANC recovery was more rapid in the G-CSF group, the duration of thrombocytopenia was significantly longer in the G-CSF group and this translated to greater number of platelet transfusions for patients randomized to receive G-CSF. There was no difference in the 3-year DFS rates between the two groups (G-CSF 47%±9% versus 55%±10% no G-CSF). The report concluded that prophylactic G-CSF during the consolidation phase of treatment was associated with improved and higher CDI although this did not translate to an improved DFS.

A meta-analysis of 16 randomized trials in childhood cancer is featured in the Sung et al. [3] report. Criteria for inclusion for meta-analysis were: study population consisted of children or data were extractable for < 18 years in studies that include children and adults, G-CSF given prophylactically before development of neutropenia/febrile neutropenia and identical chemotherapy preceded G-CSF and placebo administration or no chemotherapy. Outcome endpoints were occurrence of febrile neutropenia, duration of neutropenia, duration of parenteral antibiotic treatment, length of chemotherapy delay, amphotericin B usage and cost-effectiveness of G-CSF treatment.

While G-CSF significantly reduced the rate of febrile neutropenia episodes with a rate ratio of 0.8 (95% confidence interval [CI] 0.67–0.95; p=0.01), shortened the duration of neutropenia by 4 days, reduced duration of hospitalization by 2 days, lessened the use of amphotericin B usage and decreased the rate of documented infections, its prophylactic use did not result in lowered infection-related mortality (p=0.97). When tumor types were evaluated for efficacy of G-CSF, no differences were noted. When costs were calculated, three studies reported that the use of prophylactic G-CSF was associated with higher costs while three other studies documented the reverse. Quality of life was not reported in any of the 16 studies. The authors concluded that while the use of prophylactic G-CSF in children with cancer was associated with a reduction in the rate of febrile neutropenia (20%), documented infections (22%) and duration of hospitalization, this did not translate into a reduction in infection-related mortality.

The report by Pui et al. [4] is similar to the earlier studies as the primary objective of this study was to determine the efficacy of prophylactic G-CSF in preventing febrile neutropenia and consequent hospitalization among children with childhood ALL. Previously untreated eligible children and adolescents who were enrolled on the St Jude Total Therapy Trial XIIIA were included in this report. Patients were randomized to receive G-CSF or a placebo a day after completing remission induction therapy and G-CSF (10 μg/kg/day) was administered for 15 days or till postnadir ANC was $\geq 1 \times 10^9$/L for 2 consecutive days. Neutropenia was defined as ANC <0.5×10^9/L. The main outcome endpoints were rate of hospitalization, overall survival, and cost of supportive care.

The patients in the G-CSF treatment arm had a more rapid recovery from neutropenia than the placebo group (p=0.007). More importantly, the use of G-CSF did not hamper platelet recovery. While the hospitalization rates were similar in both treatment groups, the median hospital stay was significantly shorter in the group assigned to receive G-CSF (6 versus 10 days; p=0.011). Again, although the G-CSF group experienced fewer documented infections, the difference in the incidence of severe infections was not significantly different. The use of parenteral antibiotics and transfusions was similar in both groups. Even though the time to start the consolidation block was shorter in the G-CSF group, the 3-year EFS rates were similar in both groups of patients. Of note was the fact that there was no increase in the incidence of AML in the group randomized to receive G-CSF (5.1%, 95% CI 0.1–10 in the G-CSF arm versus 3.9%, 95% CI 0–8.4% in the placebo group; p=0.36). The median estimated cost of all supportive care was not significantly different between the two groups. The authors concluded that although prophylactic G-CSF was of some benefit for children with ALL as its use was associated with a faster neutrophil recovery and fewer documented infections, it did not reduce the rate of hospitalization or the cost of supportive care.

Continuing on the same theme of ameliorating chemotherapy-induced myelosuppression, Dibenedetto et al. [5] conducted a prospective randomized trial on the use of prophylactic G-CSF in children with intermediate-risk (IR) ALL. IR patients who achieved a complete remission (CR) after remission induction therapy were randomized to receive or not prophylactic G-CSF (10 μg/kg/day subcutaneously) 24h after completing the phase II block and G-CSF was continued until the ANC was >0.2×10^9/L. The primary endpoint was the efficacy of G-CSF in shortening the duration of the phase II block of therapy. Secondary endpoints were duration and severity of neutropenia, incidence of fever, duration of hospitalization, antibiotic usage, and the number of platelet and red cell transfusions.

Thirty-two patients were randomized to receive G-CSF (n = 14) or not (n = 18). While the anticipated duration of the phase II block was 29 days, only one patient in the G-CSF group and two in the control group completed the phase II block within this scheduled time. Median length of phase II was 37 days (range 29–65 days) in the G-CSF group compared to 36 days (29–55 days) in the control arm (p = NS). The number of febrile episodes, the duration of hospitalization, and the blood support requirements were also similar amongst the two groups of patients. The authors concluded that prophylactic G-CSF was unnecessary in children with ALL when the predicted period of neutropenia is small and the risk of infection low.

In an effort to improve EFS by reducing the duration of myelosuppression, Laver et al. [6] conducted a randomized study to assess the impact of prophylactic recombinant methionyl human G-CSF (r-metHuG-CSF) on the period of neutropenia, number of days of hospitalization, and delays in subsequent administration of chemotherapy in a cohort of patients with T-cell ALL (T-ALL) or advanced-stage lymphoblastic lymphoma (ASLL). The study population included all previously untreated children and adolescents < 22 years of age with either T-ALL or advanced-stage (III or IV) T-cell NHL. Patients were randomized to receive or not recombinant methionyl human G-CSF (10 µg/kg/day subcutaneously; r-metHuG-CSF) during the remission induction (RI) phase and two cycles of continuing therapy and this was commenced 24 h after completion of chemotherapy and continued until the ANC was >1 × 10^9/L. Fifty-six patients with T-ALL and 33 with ASLL were enrolled onto the study from April 1994 to December 1995.

Their results showed no significant difference in number of days of ANC less than 500/µL, hospitalizations, or delays in therapy in the induction phase. However, in the continuation therapy phase, the number of days of ANC less than 500/µL was significantly shorter (p = 0.017) on the G-CSF arm without significantly affecting the number of days of hospitalizations or delays in therapy. The authors concluded that r-metHuG-CSF did not significantly affect the period of neutropenia, hospitalization, or delays in therapy in the induction phase, whereas in the two cycles of continuation therapy, it significantly shortened the period of neutropenia.

A randomized, cross-over study on the prophylactic use of recombinant G-CSF following intensive chemotherapy to reduce chemotherapy-related myelosuppression and toxicity was the main aim of the Clarke et al. study [7]. All previously untreated children with ALL and T-NHL were eligible for inclusion on the study. Seventeen children with ALL or T-NHL and treated on standard protocols were randomized to receive G-CSF following either the first or second intensification blocks of chemotherapy. G-CSF was administered as a single daily subcutaneous injection of 5 µg/kg from day 9 following the start of intensification therapy, and continued until the neutrophil count exceeded 0.5 × 10^9/L for 3 days. Study endpoints were days of neutropenia (neutrophils < 1 × 10^9/L) and severity of neutropenia (neutrophils < 0.5 × 10^9/L), days in hospital, days of fever, and days on antibiotics.

The use of G-CSF resulted in a significant reduction in the number of days of neutropenia (95% CI 3.8–8 days; p = 0.0001), severity of neutropenia (95% CI 1.8–7.4 days; p = 0.002) and hospitalization days (95% CI 0.9–6.3 days; p = 0.01). Overall, a longer period of neutropenia was observed after the second intensification block (p = 0.0003; 95% CI 2.2–6.4 days), but this difference was not seen in children who received G-CSF and were significantly more likely to commence continuing therapy on schedule (p = 0.05). There was, however, no difference in the number of days of antibiotic treatment or in the number of days of fever. It was concluded that G-CSF reduced hematological toxicity of intensification chemotherapy in ALL/T-NHL and may allow improved compliance with chemotherapy scheduling.

Another prospective randomized cross-over study that evaluated the role of prophylactic G-CSF given after a 5-day intensification block in children with ALL was the Little study [8]. The main objectives were to determine if the prophylactic administration of G-CSF could reduce the rate of readmission to hospital for management of febrile neutropenia (FBN). Forty-six previously untreated children with ALL or T-NHL < 17 years of age treated on MRC ALL 97, UK ALL XI or UK CCSG 9504 NHL protocols were randomized to receive G-CSF following either the first or the second block of intensive chemotherapy in a cross-over study. For patients randomized to receive G-CSF (5 µg/kg/day subcutaneously), this commenced 24 h after completion of the last dose of chemotherapy and continued for a total of 10 days or until the ANC was $>10 \times 10^9$/L, whichever occurred sooner. Additionally, G-CSF was given electively at a similar dose intravenously to all patients admitted to hospital with FBN (or continued if the patient was previously randomized to G-CSF prophylaxis) and was continued until discharge or until the ANC was $>10 \times 10^9$/L, whichever occurred sooner. Outcome endpoints were hospital readmission rate for the management of FBN within 28 days of commencing the first or second intensification blocks, duration of hospital stay, duration of antibiotic and antifungal usage, blood product support, time to ANC recovery, and tolerability of G-CSF.

Readmission rate with FBN was significantly lower in the group that received prophylactic G-CSF (34/46; 74%) compared to 42/46 (91%) in the control arm (p=0.0386). Although resolution of fever was faster in the G-CSF group, this was not statistically significant. Similarly, there were no significant differences in the duration of hospitalization between the two groups (6 days in each group). The speed of ANC recovery and transfusion requirements were also similar in both G-CSF and control arms. While G-CSF was well tolerated, no significant differences were noted with regard to use of antibiotics, antifungals or antivirals between the two groups of patients. There was no demonstrable cost benefit derived from the prophylactic administration of G-CSF.

This study showed that the prophylactic administration of G-CSF following intensification chemotherapy for childhood ALL and T-NHL resulted in a significant reduction in the rate of readmission to hospital for the management of FBN.

The report by Delorme et al. [9] was an update of the second study reported in this chapter. The aim of this report was to provide an economic evaluation of the prophylactic use of G-CSF in the same cohort of patients. The following cost factors were measured: hospital stay, units of blood product used by category (red cell, platelets, etc.) number of days and prescribed doses for G-CSF, antibiotics, antifungals, and chemotherapy. Hospitalization unit cost was calculated as *per diem* cost for a pediatric hospital including overhead costs, salaries, and medical tests. Costing according to the resource category indicated that for the G-CSF group, hospitalization cost was significantly reduced ($21,883 versus $25,780) while costs of platelet transfusions were significantly higher ($2876 versus $1958).

The mean costs per course in the two randomized groups were not significantly different: $5848.80 versus $6181 and $7388.10 versus $6475.70 for R3 and COPADM, respectively. Finally, the mean total costs per child were not statistically different: $32,309 in the G-CSF group versus $31,569 in the non-G-CSF group. It was concluded that the use of prophylactic G-CSF did not increase the overall costs of treatment in children with ALL.

Another study that evaluated the economic costs and benefits of G-CSF was carried out by González-Vicent et al. [10] who conducted a prospective randomized trial in children following autologous peripheral blood stem cell transplantation (PBSCT) for both solid tumor and hematological malignancies. The conditioning regimen for solid tumor patients consisted of oral busulphan and IV melphalan while for ALL and AML patients it comprised total body irradiation plus IV cyclophosphamide and oral busulphan and IV cyclophosphamide respectively. Patients were randomly assigned to receive G-CSF ($10 \mu g$/kg/day) or not following stem cell reinfusion. Outcome endpoints include engraftment kinetics, supportive care, and treatment costs.

Of the 117 patients randomized, 51 were assigned to receive G-CSF and 66 patients formed the control group. ANC engraftment was quicker in the G-CSF group irrespective of the number of CD34+ cells infused, and the median time to achieve ANC $>0.5 \times 10^9$/L was 10 days in the G-CSF group compared to 11 days in the control arm (p<0.009). Although platelet engraftment was delayed in patients who were assigned to receive G-CSF, early and long-term platelet engraftment was similar in patients who received $<5 \times 10^6$/kg CD34+ cells with or without G-CSF. The control arm received significantly fewer platelet transfusions than patients in the G-CSF group. Although total costs were similar in both sets of patients, there was a trend towards higher costs in the G-CSF group. The report concluded that prophylactic G-CSF was of limited benefit in children receiving autologous peripheral blood stem cell transplantation for either hematological or solid tumor malignancies.

While the previous study investigated the cost-benefit analysis of prophylactic G-CSF in children undergoing PBSCT, the study by Kawano et al. [11] examined the clinical effectiveness of G-CSF in improving engraftment after PBSCT. In this prospective trial with a study population that mainly comprised children with ALL or neuroblastoma, a total of 74 children who underwent high-dose chemotherapy followed by autologous PBSCT were randomized at diagnosis to receive G-CSF (300 μg/m²/day IV) or not. G-CSF commenced a day after PBSCT and continued until ANC was >3× 10⁹/L. The cytoreductive therapy before transplant was the MCVAC regimen, consisting of ranimustine (MCNU, 450 mg/m²), ARAC (16 g/m²), etoposide (1600 mg/m²), and cyclophosphamide (100 mg/kg), which was used for patients with ALL. Patients with solid tumors received a combination of melphalan (180 mg/m²), etoposide (1600 mg/m²), and carboplatin (1600 mg/m²). Outcome endpoint was the speed of ANC engraftment.

The median time for ANC engraftment ($>0.5 \times 10^9$/L) was 11 days (8–20 days) in the G-CSF group and 12 days (9–49 days) in the control group (p=0.04 log-rank test). While in children with ALL, the time to ANC engraftment was identical in both the G-CSF and control groups, in the solid tumor patients ANC engraftment was significantly earlier in the G-CSF group (11 days versus 12 days; p=0.045). The median time for platelet engraftment ($>20 \times 10^9$/L) in the G-CSF and control groups was 22 days and 16 days respectively (p=0.009 log-rank test). There were no differences in the number of febrile neutropenic episodes in either group of patients. The report concluded that although prophylactic G-CSF marginally improved the speed of neutrophil engraftment in patients with solid tumors, this benefit was offset by the delayed platelet recovery.

The BFM group [12] conducted a randomized open-label study on the efficacy of recombinant G-CSF (rG-CSF) in improving chemotherapy dose intensity (CDI) by ameliorating chemotherapy-induced myelosuppression in children with high-risk ALL. Patients were randomized (after completion of remission induction) to receive nine cycles of chemotherapy (CT) followed by rG-CSF or nine cycles of CT alone. Children randomized to rG-CSF received 5 μg/kg/day subcutaneously from day 7 of each cycle and continued till day 20. If ANC on day 20 was $<0.2 \times 10^9$/L, G-CSF was continued until this ANC value was reached or a maximum of 28 days, whichever occurred earlier. G-CSF was stopped if ANC breached 30×10^9/L prior to the expected nadir of the white cell count and restarted when ANC was $<10 \times 10^9$/L. Outcome endpoints were reduction in the incidence of FBN with rG-CSF, duration of neutropenia, duration of hospitalization, IV antibiotic usage, incidence of mucositis, and overall CDI.

Of the 87 patients enrolled on the study, only 34 patients were randomized. The average incidence of FBN/cycle was significantly reduced in the rG-CSF group (17% versus 40%; p=0.007) as was the median total duration of FBN over the entire treatment period (6.2 days/patient versus 20.3 days/patient in the no G-CSF group; p=0.02). Similarly, the average incidence of neutropenia/cycle and the number of days of neutropenia/patient were also significantly reduced in the rG-CSF group (48% versus 87%; p=0.002) and (17.4 days versus 61.6 days; p<0.01). The average incidences of treatment cycle delays were significantly lower in the rG-CSF arm (29% versus 51%; p=0.007) and the median reduction in total treatment time was 10 days/patient (9.7 days G-CSF arm versus 19.7 days control arm). While the total duration of fever was shorter in the rG-CSF group of patients (7.1 days versus 12.6 days; p=0.04), the average incidences of infectious episodes were similar in both groups of patients. Although the incidence of infectious episodes were similar in the two groups, the incidence of culture positive infections was significantly reduced in the rG-CSF group [8 % vs. 15%; p=0.04]. Accordingly, the antibiotic usage was lower in the rG-CSF group (p=0.02). The report concluded that prophylactic G-CSF significantly reduced the incidence of FBN and thereby improved CDI in patients with high-risk ALL.

The effectiveness of prophylactic G-CSF in children with T-NHL was explored by Patte et al. [13] in their study in which children with NHL were randomized to receive or not G-CSF after induction chemotherapy. Children treated on any of the three NHL protocols, i.e. T-cell (LMT 89), B-cell (LMB 89) or ALCL (HM 91), were eligible for study enrollment. G-CSF was administered subcutaneously at a dose of 5 μg/kg/day for a minimum of 6 days or a maximum of 15 days, depending on the ANC. If ANC was $>0.5 \times 10^9$/L for 2 consecutive days, it was stopped or if the total WBC was $>20 \times 10^9$/L. Neutropenia was defined as ANC $<0.5 \times 10^9$/L.

Outcome endpoints were incidence of FBN, incidence of severe infections, duration of neutropenia, hospitalization, antibiotic usage and fever, incidence of grade 3–4 mucositis and thrombocytopenia, overall and event-free survival.

Of the 148 patients who were randomized, 75 were assigned to receive G-CSF and 73 to the control arm. Although the incidence of neutropenia was not significantly different between the two groups of patients, the duration of neutropenia was significantly shorter in the G-CSF group. There were no differences between the two groups with regard to incidence of FBN (89% versus 93%) after COPAD (M) 1, nor were there differences in the duration of hospitalization or antibiotic usage. OS and EFS were similar in both groups of patients. The report concluded that prophylactic G-CSF did not reduce the incidence of FBN, increase CDI or decrease treatment-related morbidity in children with NHL.

A variation in the prophylactic use of G-CSF was the study by Ozkaynak et al. [14] in which children were randomized to receive or not G-CSF only after the commencement of antibiotics for febrile neutropenia. Eligible patients were randomized within 24 h of commencing antibiotic treatment and G-CSF was administered either subcutaneously or intravenously. The primary outcome endpoint was duration of FBN while the secondary endpoints included number of days of antibiotic therapy, proportion of patients who developed septic shock, required antifungal treatment or had documented infections after start of antibiotic treatment.

Of the 67 patients enrolled on the study, 32 were randomized to receive G-CSF along with IV antibiotics while 34 received antibiotic treatment alone.

The median time to resolution of FBN was 4 days in the G-CSF plus antibiotic (AB) treatment arm compared to 13 days in the antibiotic alone arm. This effect was attributed to reduction in the duration of neutropenia. The duration of hospitalization was also shorter in the G-CSF+AB group. However, when the two treatment groups were compared there wereno differences in the number of days of antibiotic treatment (G-CSF group median 5.9 days versus 7.2 days; p=0.19), the addition of antifungal treatment or in the number of patients who went into septic shock. *The report concluded that the addition of G-CSF resulted in a faster resolution of FBN and was of some clinical use as it reduced the duration of hospitalization.*

References

1 Heath JA, Steinherz PG, Altman A *et al.*, for the Children's Cancer Group. Human granulocyte colony-stimulating factor in children with high-risk acute lymphoblastic leukemia: a Children's Cancer Group study. *J Clin Oncol* 2003;**21**:1612–17.

2 Michel G, Landman-Parker J, Auclerc MF *et al.* Use of recombinant human granulocyte colony-stimulating factor to increase chemotherapy dose-intensity: a randomized trial

in very high-risk childhood acute lymphoblastic leukemia. *J Clin Oncol* 2000;**18**:1517–24.

3 Sung L, Nathan PC, Lange B, Beyene J, Buchanan GR. Prophylactic granulocyte colony-stimulating factor and granulocyte-macrophage colony-stimulating factor decrease febrile neutropenia after chemotherapy in children with cancer: a meta-analysis of randomized controlled trials. *J Clin Oncol* 2004;**22**:3350–6.

4 Pui CH, Boyett JM, Hughes WT *et al.* Human granulocyte colony-stimulating factor after induction chemotherapy in children with acute lymphoblastic leukemia. *N Engl J Med* 1997;**336**:1781–7.

5 Dibenedetto SP, Ragusa R, Ippolito AM *et al.* Assessment of the value of treatment with granulocyte colony-stimulating factor in children with acute lymphoblastic leukemia: a randomized clinical trial. *Eur J Haematol* 1995;**55**:93–6.

6 Laver J, Amylon M, Desai S *et al.* Randomized trial of r-metHu granulocyte colony-stimulating factor in an intensive treatment for T-cell leukemia and advanced-stage lymphoblastic lymphoma of childhood: a Pediatric Oncology Group pilot study. *Leukemia Lymphoma* 1997;**26**:589–93.

7 Clarke V, Dunstan FD, Webb DK. Granulocyte colony-stimulating factor ameliorates toxicity of intensification chemotherapy for acute lymphoblastic leukemia. *Med Pediatr Oncol* 1999;**32**:331–5.

8 Little MA, Morland B, Chisholm J *et al.* A randomized study of prophylactic G-CSF following MRC UKALL XI intensification regimen in childhood ALL and T-NHL. *Med Pediatr Oncol* 2002;**38**:98–103.

9 Delorme J, Badin S, Le Corroller AG *et al.* Economic evaluation of recombinant human granulocyte colony-stimulating factor in very high-risk childhood acute lymphoblastic leukemia. *J Pediatr Hematol Oncol* 2003;**25**:441–7.

10 González-Vicent M, Madero L, Sevilla J, Ramirez M, Díaz MA. A prospective randomized study of clinical and economic consequences of using G-CSF following autologous peripheral blood progenitor cell (PBPC) transplantation in children. *Bone Marrow Transplant* 2004;**34**:1077–81.

11 Kawano Y, Takaue Y, Mimaya J *et al.* Marginal benefit/disadvantage of granulocyte colony-stimulating factor therapy after autologous blood stem cell transplantation in children: results of a prospective randomized trial. The Japanese Cooperative Study Group of PBSCT. *Blood* 1998;**92**:4040–6.

12 Welte K, Reiter A, Mempel K *et al.* A randomized phase-III study of the efficacy of granulocyte colony stimulating factor in children with high-risk acute lymphoblastic leukemia. Berlin-Frankfurt-Münster Study Group. *Blood* 1996;**87**:3143–50.

13 Patte C, Laplanche A, Bertozzi AI *et al.* Granulocyte colony-stimulating factor in induction treatment of children with non-Hodgkin's lymphoma: a randomized study of the French Society of Pediatric Oncology. *J Clin Oncol* 2002;**20**:441–8.

14 Ozkaynak MF, Krailo M, Chen Z, Feusner J. Randomized comparison of antibiotics with and without granulocyte colony-stimulating factor in children with chemotherapy-induced febrile neutropenia: a report from the Children's Oncology Group. *Pediatr Blood Cancer* 2005;**45**:242–3.

Granulocyte macrophage colony-stimulating factor

While G-CSF is a lineage specific factor that regulates neutrophil production alone, granulocyte macrophage colony stimulating factor (GM-CSF) is a multilineage factor and activates neutrophils, eosinophils and monocyte/macrophages and is theoretically more effective than G-CSF. The study by van Pelt et al.[1] aimed to determine whether the prophylactic administration of GM-CSF in children undergoing intensive chemotherapy for solid tumor malignancies reduced the duration of neutropenia. Chemotherapy protocols were disease specific and consisted of multiagent combination regimens that were myelosuppressive but not myeloablative. Patients were randomized before each pair of chemotherapy courses to receive GM-CSF or not after the first or second course of chemotherapy and if the treatment protocol comprised alternating courses of combination chemotherapy regimens, patients were randomized to receive GM-CSF or not after the first or second of each pair of identical chemotherapy courses (i.e. after the first and third courses or second and fourth courses). GM-CSF (5 µg/kg/day subcutaneously) commenced 24 h after the last course of chemotherapy and continued for a total of 10 days. Outcome endpoints included mean duration of neutropenia, number of documented infections, duration of febrile neutropenic episodes, and number of red cell and platelet transfusions.

Although GM-CSF significantly reduced the mean duration of neutropenia (mean reduction 2.2±0.6 days; p=0.003), it did not reduce the duration of leukopenia. There were no differences between the two groups with respect to the number of days of fever or the incidence of episodes of high fever that required IV antibiotics. Blood product requirements were similar between the GM-CSF and control groups. The authors concluded that while prophylactic GM-CSF significantly reduced the duration of neutropenia, it did not have any impact on the number of days of fever or reduce the need for transfusion support.

The next randomized trial on GM-CSF in children was the Calderwood study [2] in which children with poor-risk ALL were randomized to receive GM-CSF or a placebo during the CNS phase of treatment and the aim was to determine whether concurrent administration of GM-CSF will reduce the incidence of treatment-related neutropenia and its attendant complications. The CNS treatment phase was over 4 weeks and patients randomized to the GM-CSF arm received it at a dose of 5 µg/kg/day subcutaneously on days 5–11 and 19–25. The placebo group received a placebo injection subcutaneously on the same schedule. Outcome endpoints included ANC, number of days chemotherapy could be given, time to complete the CNS phase, the time to commence the next phase of therapy, duration of fever, number of days of antibiotic treatment, duration of hospitalization, and the severity and type of infections.

Twenty patients each were randomized to the GM-CSF and placebo groups. The mean ANC was slightly higher in the GM-CSF treatment arm during the two 7-day treatment cycles [days 5-11 and days 19-25] but not at any other time. 7/16 (44%) children in the GM-CSF arm received 20 or more days of chemotherapy compared to 4/19 (21%) patients in the placebo arm. There was no significant difference between the two groups of patients in the number of days to complete the CNS phase of treatment or to begin the next phase of treatment. There were no differences in any of the other outcome endpoints such as number of days of fever, length of hospitalization, duration of antibiotic therapy or severity and type of infections. The authors concluded that GM-CSF was ineffective in preventing chemotherapy-induced myelosuppression and complications associated with neutropenia in children with poor-risk ALL.

The use of GM-CSF to reduce chemoradiotherapy-related hematological toxicity and supportive care requirements in children with sarcoma was explored by Wexler et al. [3]. Children and young adults with sarcomas (Ewing sarcoma, rhabdomyosarcoma, etc.) were randomized to receive GM-CSF, the cardioprotectant dexrazoxane (DEXN), both GM-CSF and DEXN, or neither. Accordingly, 38 subsequent patients were randomized to receive 18 cycles of chemotherapy alone (18 patients) or the identical chemotherapy plus GM-CSF commencing with cycle 3 (20 patients). The dose of GM-CSF was initially 15 µg/kg but subsequently reduced to 5 µg/kg/day subcutaneously and commenced after the final dose of chemotherapy in a given cycle and continued until day 19 or until ANC was ≥0.5×10⁹/L for 2 consecutive days. Outcome endpoint was duration of grade 4 neutropenia (ANC <0.5×10⁹/L).

Even though the use of GM-CSF resulted in a significantly shorter period of grade 3 and 4 neutropenia (7 and 7 days respectively for the GM-CSF group versus 11 and 9 days for the control group; $p < 0.0001$), use of GM-CSF was associated with significantly greater thrombocytopenia, longer platelet recovery time ($p < 0.0001$) and greater platelet transfusion requirements ($p < 0.0001$). There were no differences seen between the GM-CSF group and the control group in the duration of hospitalization, infectious complications, average duration of fever, antibiotic usage or interval between chemotherapy cycles. EFS and OS were also similar between the GM-CSF and control groups. Clearly, GM-CSF was of minimal benefit in patients undergoing chemoradiotherapy for sarcoma as it did not reduce the severity or duration of neutropenia but was associated with significantly worsened thrombocytopenia.

The Burdach et al. [4] study, like the previous study, also explored the effectiveness of GM-CSF in children and adolescents with solid tumors (soft-tissue sarcoma, Ewing sarcoma or neuroblastoma). At diagnosis, patients were categorized into two groups: group 1 patients received GM-CSF (250 μg/m^2/day as continuous intravenous infusion, 48 h after the last dose of chemotherapy) after the first and third cycles of chemotherapy while group 2 patients received GM-CSF after the second and fourth cycles. The study ceased with the commencement of local radiotherapy. GM-CSF was continued until the ANC was $>1.0 \times 10^9$/L for 5 consecutive days or for a maximum of 14 days.

Duration of severe neutropenia ($<0.5 \times 10^9$/L) with GM-CSF was 1.9 ± 0.4 days compared to 5.7 ± 0.5 days without GM-CSF ($p = 0.0001$) per treatment cycle. In addition, during the entire treatment period, the duration of neutropenia ($<1.0 \times 10^9$/L) for each patient who received GM-CSF was 18.5 ± 4.1 days versus 34 ± 3.9 days without GM-CSF. Although there were no differences in the packed cell transfusion requirements in the two groups of patients with or without GM-CSF, the number of days that the platelet count was $<20 \times 10^9$/L was higher in patients who received GM-CSF (2.1 ± 0.4 days versus 1.2 ± 0.3 days; $p = 0.047$). While there were fewer documented infectious episodes during GM-CSF treatment (8 versus 14), there were no differences in the number of infections or in the number of days of antibiotic treatment. The authors concluded that although GM-CSF reduced the severity and duration of neutropenia, its use compromised platelet recovery.

References

1 Van Pelt LJ, de Craen AJ, Langeveld NE, Weening RS. Granulocyte-macrophage colony-stimulating factor (GM-CSF) ameliorates chemotherapy-induced neutropenia in children with solid tumors. *Pediatr Hematol Oncol* 1997;**14**:539–45.
2 Calderwood S, Romeyer F, Blanchette V et al. Concurrent RhGM-CSF does not offset myelosuppression from intensive chemotherapy: randomized placebo-controlled study in childhood acute lymphoblastic leukemia. *Am J Hematol* 1994;**47**:27–32.
3 Wexler LH, Weaver-McClure L, Steinberg SM et al. Randomized trial of recombinant human granulocyte-macrophage colony stimulating factor in pediatric patients receiving intensive myelosuppressive chemotherapy. *J Clin Oncol* 1996;**14**:901–10.
4 Burdach SE, Müschenich M, Josephs W et al. Granulocyte-macrophage-colony stimulating factor for prevention of neutropenia and infections in children and adolescents with solid tumors. Results of a prospective randomized study. *Cancer* 1995;**76**:510–16.

Erythropoietin

In numerous trials in adult cancer patients, treatment with recombinant erythropoietin (EPO) has been shown to increase hemoglobin levels, reduce red blood cell transfusion requirements, and improve quality of life. Much less has been published of its use in the prevention or treatment of cancer-associated anemia (CAA) in children, in whom chemotherapy is usually more intensive and likely to result in greater myelosuppression. The first study cited by Wagner et al. [1] was a single-center randomized trial that evaluated the usefulness of prophylactic EPO in reducing transfusion requirements in children with high-risk neuroblastoma. Eligible patients were randomized to receive G-CSF alone or G-CSF with EPO after each of the six cycles of intensive chemotherapy. Chemotherapy drugs used included cyclophosphamide, doxorubicin, etoposide, and cisplatin. G-CSF commenced 24 h after completion of the first cycle and on day 6 of the first cycle, patients were randomized to receive or not EPO 200 units/kg/day subcutaneously and continued until 2 days before the start of cycle 2. In subsequent cycles, EPO commenced 24 h after completion of chemotherapy. The aim was to maintain hemoglobin levels of patients between 10 and 13 g/dL. Patients with iron deficiency also received ferrous sulfate supplements (2 mg/kg/day). The main outcome measure was the total number of packed red cell transfusions received by patients randomized to EPO.

The median total of packed red cell transfusions per patient was 106.6 mL/kg (66.6–202.9) for the G-CSF group compared to 161 mL/kg (92–243.6) for the G-CSF+EPO group (p=0.05). The G-CSF+EPO group received more packed red cell transfusions compared to the G-CSF group (258 versus 207). When analysis was restricted to transfusions given when the hemoglobin was <8 g/dL, the median number of transfusions was higher in the G-CSF+EPO group compared to the G-CSF alone group (10 versus 8; p=0.044). There were no significant differences in the duration of neutropenia, number of platelet transfusions, total duration of induction therapy or survival outcome between the two groups of randomized patients. The report concluded that addition of EPO to G-CSF provided no extra benefit to high-risk neuroblastoma patients undergoing intensive induction chemotherapy.

The next study, by Csaki et al. [2], evaluated the safety, feasibility, and effectiveness of recombinant human EPO (rhEPO) in the prevention and treatment of chemotherapy-induced anemia in children with solid tumors. This was a prospective single-center randomized trial and eligible patients with Ewing sarcoma, osteosarcoma, soft tissue sarcoma or neuroblastoma were randomized to either a control group with no rhEPO or a rhEPO treatment group. Patients randomized to the rhEPO group received rhEPO at a dose of 150 U/kg subcutaneously three times a week for a minimum of 12 weeks or three chemotherapy cycles. Inclusion criteria included a life expectancy of >3 months, WHO performance status <3 and hemoglobin (Hb) value of <12 g/dL before the first dose of rhEPO. The main outcome measures were Hb levels and hematocrit (Hct) values in patients randomized to rhEPO, the total number of packed red cell transfusions in patients randomized to rhEPO, and safety profile of rhEPO.

While the mean Hb rates were higher in the rhEPO group from the fourth week of treatment, they reached statistical significance after the eighth week of therapy (13.11±1.13 g/dL versus 11.06±1.35 g/dL; p<0.05). Similarly, the mean Hct increased progressively in the rhEPO group and was significantly higher than the control group at week 8 (39.3±4.2% versus 33.2±2.1%; p<0.05). The mean precycle and midcycle Hb levels were also higher in the rhEPO group compared to the control group. Although the red cell transfusion requirements over the entire study period were similar in both groups of patients, when stratified by month of therapy, transfusion requirements in the rhEPO group were significantly lower in the third month of treatment (0 versus 4) compared to the control group. rhEPO had no significant effect on either platelet counts or platelet recovery. Performance status was improved in the rhEPO group with weight loss lower in the rhEPO group (0.7, range −5 to +1.5 kg) versus 2.5 kg (range -5.8 to +0.0 kg) in the control group. No significant adverse effects were reported after rhEPO administration. The authors concluded that recombinant human EPO safely and effectively ameliorated anemia and improved the performance status of children with malignant solid tumors who received intensive chemotherapy.

The single-center randomized study by Büyükpamukçu et al. [3] was similar to the earlier studies of EPO (epoetin alfa) in children as its main aim was to determine the efficacy and safety of EPO in the prevention and treatment of chemotherapy-induced anemia in those undergoing intensive treatment. The main outcome endpoints were the total number of packed red cell transfusions and tolerability of EPO in patients randomized to receive EPO.

Children randomized to receive EPO had a significant increase in their Hb levels by the end of the study (p=0.027) while there was no change in the Hb levels of patients in the control group. Consequently, patients randomized to the EPO group had significantly lower transfusion requirements compared to the control group (1 versus 8; p=0.008). The report concluded that epoetin alfa was safe and significantly improved hemoglobin levels and reduced transfusion requirements in children with solid tumors receiving intensive chemotherapy.

Porter et al. [4] reported on a single-center study that assessed the value of prophylactic rhEPO on the transfusion requirements in children with sarcomas undergoing intensive chemotherapy. Children were randomized to receive rhEPO (n=10) or a placebo (normal saline, n=9) for a 16-week study period. The dose of rhEPO was 150 IU/kg three times/week administered subcutaneously and the aim was to maintain the

Hb level between 11.5 and 16.5 g/dL. All patients received ferrous sulfate (6 mg/kg/day) during the entire study period. At the end of the 16-week study period all patients, including those randomized to the placebo arm, were offered rhEPO for the remainder of their treatment period. The main outcome endpoint was the number of packed red cell transfusions (mL/kg) in both groups of patients during the 16-week study period.

The median dose of rhEPO during the study period was 198 IU/kg three times per week and most patients received rhEPO intravenously. Patients who were randomized to rhEPO received significantly fewer red cell transfusions (median units transfused 4.5 versus 13 and median amount transfused 23 mL/kg versus 80 mL/kg; p=0.02) and platelet transfusions compared to the placebo group. Unsurprisingly, the number of donor exposures was also significantly less in the rhEPO group. All patients in the placebo group who subsequent to the 16-week study period received rhEPO had fewer packed red cell transfusions, with a median decrease of 33% (9–68%). No documented adverse effect related to rhEPO was reported in the study. *The report concluded that prophylactic rhEPO was safe and significantly reduced red cell transfusions in children with sarcomas undergoing intensive chemotherapy.*

The final report [5], again a single-center study, evaluated the effectiveness of once-daily rhEPO in maintaining Hb levels and thereby reducing transfusion requirements and improving quality of life of children during ALL maintenance therapy. Sixty children were randomly assigned to receive either epoetin alfa (rHuEPO; n=30) or no rHuEPO (n=30) during the maintenance phase of treatment. Both groups were matched with regard to age, sex, baseline Hb levels, remission status, chemotherapy regimens, and risk category of leukemia. The dose of rHuEPO was 450 IU/kg given once weekly subcutaneously for 12 consecutive weeks.

Among the 30 patients randomized to rHuEPO, the mean increase in Hb level from baseline to final evaluation was 3.08 ± 1.48 g/100 mL (p<0.001). An increase in Hb ≥2 g/dL occurred in 70% of patients (n=21) who were on study for 30 days or more. A response was observed in 90% of children randomized to rHuEPO. Epoetin alfa treatment significantly improved quality of life, as seen by improved mean cancer analog scale scores for energy levels, and ability to perform daily activities. rHuEPO was well tolerated. The report concluded that epoetin alfa was safe and well tolerated and significantly improved hemoglobin levels, reduced transfusion requirements and improved the functional status and quality of life of children during ALL maintenance treatment.

References

1 Wagner LM, Billups CA, Furman WL, Rao BN, Santana VM. Combined use of erythropoietin and granulocyte colony-stimulating factor does not decrease blood transfusion requirements during induction therapy for high-risk neuroblastoma: a randomized controlled trial. *J Clin Oncol* 2004;**22**:1886–93.

2 Csáki C, Ferencz T, Schuler D, Borsi JD. Recombinant human erythropoietin in the prevention of chemotherapy-induced anaemia in children with malignant solid tumours. *Eur J Cancer* 1998;**34**:364–7.

3 Büyükpamukçu M, Varan A, Kutluk T, Akyüz C. Is epoetin alfa a treatment option for chemotherapy-related anemia in children? *Med Pediatr Oncol* 2002;**39**:455–8.

4 Porter JC, Leahey A, Polise K, Bunin G, Manno CS. Recombinant human erythropoietin reduces the need for erythrocyte and platelet transfusions in pediatric patients with sarcoma: a randomized, double-blind, placebo-controlled trial. *J Pediatr* 1996;**129**:656–60.

5 Abdelrazik N, Fouda M. Once weekly recombinant human erythropoietin treatment for cancer-induced anemia in children with acute lymphoblastic leukemia receiving maintenance chemotherapy: a randomized case-controlled study. *Hematology* 2007;**12**:533–41.

New studies*

Study 1

Ladenstein R, Valteau-Couanet D, Brock P *et al.* Randomized trial of prophylactic granulocyte colony-stimulating factor during rapid COJEC induction in pediatric patients with high-risk neuroblastoma: the European HR-NBL1/SIOPEN study. J Clin Oncol 2010;**28**:3516–24.

Objectives

To determine whether the prophylactic use of G-CSF during the rapid dosing schedule in children with high-risk neuroblastoma decreases the incidence of febrile neutropenia.

Study design

This was a pan-European multicenter prospective randomized trial conducted between May 2002 and December 2005. Written informed consent for the study was obtained for all patients. The details of this study are reported in Chapter 5, Study 6.

Results

The mean number of FBN episodes in the G-CSF group was 2.3±2 (median 2) over the entire cycle compared to 3.0±2 in the control arm. There was a significant overall median and mean reduction in febrile episodes by 1 and 0.6 respectively (p=0.002). With regard to the secondary endpoints, patients randomized to receive G-CSF had eight fewer hospital days, two fewer febrile days, and 7.5 fewer antibiotic days.

Protocol compliance was significantly improved in the G-CSF group by a shorter time to completion of the course (p=0.005).

There was no significant difference in the incidence of severe bacterial or fungal infections. There was also no difference in the number of patients admitted to the intensive care unit between the two

groups of patients (G-CSF group five versus six in the control group). All four deaths were seen in the group randomized to receive G-CSF.

There was no difference in response rates between the two groups and similarly, prophylactic G-CSF made no impact on the success of peripheral blood stem cell harvest.

Toxicity

Grade 4 hematological toxicity was less in the G-CSF group (neutropenia), 50% versus 70% in the control group (p<0.001). The overall transfusion rate/course were similar in both groups. Patients randomized to G-CSF had a lower incidence of mucositis, nausea/vomiting, constipation, and weight loss.

Conclusions

It was concluded that prophylactic G-CSF did not affect response rates. It significantly reduced the incidence of febrile neutropenic episodes and number of hospital days, and protocol compliance was improved.

Study 2

Lehrnbecher T, Zimmermann M, Reinhardt D, Dworzak M, Stary J, Creutzig U. Prophylactic human granulocyte colony-stimulating factor after induction therapy in pediatric acute myeloid leukemia. **Blood** 2007;109:936–43.

Objectives

To determine the impact of the use of prophylactic G-CSF on hemopoietic recovery, infectious complications, and clinical outcome in children with *de novo* acute myeloid leukemia (AML).

---

*Relevant new studies only found for granulocyte colony-stimulating factor.

Study design

This study was part of the AML-BFM 98 trial and was a prospective multicenter randomized trial conducted between July 1998 and June 2003. Randomization was centrally performed using a permuted block method.

All patients except those with >5% blasts in the bone marrow on day 15 and those with FAB M3 AML were eligible for the G-CSF randomization done on day 15. Briefly, the treatment plan consisted of an 8-day AIE induction (cytarabine 100 mg/m^2 continuous IV infusion on days 1 and 2 followed by a 30 min infusion every 12 h on days 3–8, idarubicin 12 mg/m^2 IV on days 3–5, and etoposide 150 mg/m^2 IV on days 6–8 with intrathecal cytarabine on days 0 and 8). A second induction (HAM: cytarabine 3 g/m^2 IV every 12 h for 3 days, mitoxantrone 10 mg/m^2 IV on days 4–5 and intrathecal cytarabine on day 6) was given to all patients except those with FAB M3 AML and children with Down syndrome. Children were randomized to receive, or not, prophylactic G-CSF (5 μg/kg subcutaneously or IV infusion) on day 15 after the start of AIE and HAM respectively and those children randomized to receive G-CSF continued to receive it until the ANC was >0.5×10^9/L for 3 consecutive days.

Statistics

It was estimated that 135 patients per group had to be randomized to receive, or not, prophylactic G-CSF to detect a decrease of infectious complications by 15% in the G-CSF treatment group (power 80%, α 5% two-sided test). All analyses were based on intention-to-treat principle.

Results

One hundred and sixty-one patients were randomized to receive G-CSF while 156 were assigned to the control group that did not receive G-CSF. Compliance with treatment allocation was 90%; 18 patients in the control group received G-CSF whereas 14 patients randomized for G-CSF did not receive it.

Efficacy

Duration of neutropenia after both AIE and HAM was significantly shorter in the G-CSF group compared to the control group (median 18 versus 23 days, p=0.02, and 11 versus 16 days, p=0.001 respectively). This difference was particularly pronounced in the high-risk patients (median 18 versus 24 days, p=0.03, and

11 versus 15 days, p=0.008). G-CSF did not have any effect on platelet recovery.

Infectious complications

There was no difference between the G-CSF and control groups during induction in the incidence of either life-threatening sepsis (1 versus 5; p=0.12) or infection-associated mortality (5 versus 2; p=0.45). There was no difference between the groups in either the incidence of febrile neutropenic episodes without a source identified or the use of antifungal agents. In addition, the number of febrile days was not reduced by the administration of G-CSF.

Survival outcome

The administration of G-CSF had no impact on complete remission (CR) rates; 154/161 (95.7%) in the G-CSF group and 149/156 (95.5%) in the control group achieved CR (p>0.999). G-CSF use did not have any effect on the 5-year cumulative incidence of relapses or the 5-year risk of death in continuous clinical remission. There were no differences in the EFS (risk ratio 1.13; 95% CI 0.79–1.6; p=0.50) or OS (risk ratio 1.30: 95% CI 0.86–1.98; p=0.22) between the two groups of patients.

Toxicity

The use of G-CSF did not have any significant impact on the incidence of oral or pharyngeal mucositis (26.6% and 6.9% with G-CSF versus 23.6% and 5.2% without G-CSF; p=0.59). Similarly, no differences were seen between the two groups in the incidence of diarrhea, vomiting, hepatic or cardiovascular abnormalities.

Conclusions

It was concluded that G-CSF was of limited benefit for children undergoing induction treatment for AML as it did not have any impact on the incidence of infectious complications or improve survival outcome.

Study 3

Inaba H, Cao X, Pounds S *et al*. Randomized trial of 2 dosages of prophylactic granulocyte-colony-stimulating factor after induction chemotherapy in pediatric acute myeloid leukemia. *Cancer* 2011;**117**:1313–20.

Objectives

The main aim of this study was to determine whether a higher dose of G-CSF after induction therapy in children with AML will reduce the duration of neutropenia and frequency of documented infections, and improve survival outcome.

Study design

Patients enrolled on the St Jude AML 97 trial and remaining on trial after the window therapy were eligible for enrollment to the G-CSF study that began in May 1999. Briefly, this was a prospective randomized study that ran from March 1997 to June 2002 and included children below 22 years with previously untreated AML except those with acute promyelocytic leukemia. The AML 97 treatment protocol has been described previously in Chapter 13, Study 2.

The G-CSF study design was a double-blind randomization of patients to receive either 5 µg/kg or 10 µg/kg daily intravenously after induction courses DAV1 and DAV2. G-CSF intravenous infusions began 24 h after the last day of each chemotherapy cycle and continued until the ANC was $>0.5 \times 10^9/L \times 2$ days. The next chemotherapy cycle started 24 h after discontinuation of G-CSF. G-CSF was not administered to patients who were scheduled to undergo stem cell transplantation after DAV2 or to patients who had a poor response to DAV1 and thus were taken off the AML 97 protocol.

The primary outcome measure was the duration of neutropenia and the secondary outcomes included the number of days of G-CSF treatment and hospitalization, the cumulative episodes of febrile neutropenia, episodes of grade 2–4 infections, antibiotic courses including IV antibiotic courses and antifungal courses, number of red cell and platelet transfusions, the cost of supportive care, and estimates of EFS and OS.

Statistics

The study design assumed that 36 patients would provide 90% power to detect a 5-day difference in the number of neutropenic days at an α level of 0.05. Patient characteristics between G-CSF treatment arms were compared using the exact chi-square test. Outcome variables were measured during the period beginning with the end of each DAV course and ending with the start of the subsequent chemotherapy course. The median number of days of G-CSF treatment in the two

arms was compared separately for each induction cycle by using the Wilcoxon rank-sum test. A repeated-measures, mixed-effects model based on normal distribution was used to analyze the effect of G-CSF dosage on the number of days of neutropenia and hospitalization as well as the cost of supportive care. Proportional means models were used to compare the cumulative number of febrile neutropenia episodes, episodes of grade 2–4 infection, antibiotic therapy courses, intravenous antibiotic therapy courses, antifungal therapy courses, and erythrocyte and platelet transfusions with G-CSF treatment as fixed covariate. EFS was defined as the time between G-CSF randomization and disease recurrence, death, secondary malignancy or last follow-up. Remission induction failure was treated as an event at time 0. The Kaplan–Meier method was used to estimate the probability of EFS and OS; standard errors were estimated by the Peto method.

Results

Of the 47 patients randomized to the G-CSF part of the AML 97 trial, one patient was excluded because of physician choice. Forty-six patients were analyzed after induction course DAV1 and 36 after DAV2. Patient characteristics did not differ significantly in the two randomized treatment arms.

There were no significant differences between the two G-CSF treatment arms in the duration of G-CSF treatment after DAV1 or DAV2. The number of neutropenic days also did not differ significantly in the two treatment arms.

There were no significant differences in the number of FBN episodes or episodes of grade 2–4 infections between patients in the two treatment groups. The duration of hospitalization also did not differ significantly between the two arms.

There were no significant differences between the two treatment arms in the number of antibiotic therapy courses, intravenous antibiotic therapy courses, or antifungal therapy courses.

The number of red cell and platelet transfusions did not differ significantly between the two G-CSF arms.

There were no significant differences in any of the six categories of supportive care costs.

The 6-year EFS and OS rates were 52.2%±10% and 65.2%±9.6% (p=0.43) and 39.1%±9.7% and 52.2%± 11.4% (p=0.45) respectively for patients who received 5 µg/kg and 10 µg/kg daily.

Conclusions

It was concluded that the higher dose of G-CSF (10 µg/kg) was not superior to the standard dose of 5 µg/kg in children with AML receiving intensive chemotherapy.

Study 4

Ehlers S, Herbst C, Zimmermann M *et al.* Granulocyte colony-stimulating factor (G-CSF) treatment of childhood acute myeloid leukemias that overexpress the differentiation-defective G-CSF receptor isoform IV is associated with a higher incidence of relapse. *J Clin Oncol* 2010;**28**:2591–7.

Objectives

To determine whether the use of prophylactic G-CSF reduces infectious complications and improves outcome in children and adolescents with AML.

Study design

This study was part of the AML-BFM 98 trial (Creutzig U, *et al.* J Clin Oncol 2006;**24**:4499-4506).

The AML-BFM 98 was a randomized controlled phase III study and all patients irrespective of risk stratification were randomly assigned for prophylactic G-CSF treatment. Patients in the G-CSF group commenced prophylactic G-CSF (5 µg/kg/day subcutaneously) on days 15 and 28 of the treatment schedule and this was continued until the ANC was >500/µL on 3 consecutive days. This review focuses on children and adolescents with standard-risk (SR) AML. This group includes the FAB M1/M2 with Auer rods, M4eo or favorable karyotyes such as t(8;21), t(15;7), and inv(16) and those patients who had <5% blasts in the bone marrow on day 15. However, children with FAB M3 subtype were excluded, as they were not given G-CSF in the AML-BFM 98 trial.

Leukemic blasts were separated and analyzed for cell surface G-CSF receptor (G-CSFR) expression by four-color cytometry. Quantification of G-CSFR RNA isoform I and IV expression was by real-time quantitative reverse transcriptase polymerase chain reaction using probes specific for G-CSFR isoform I and isoform IV. This was determined in 50 (of 154) SR patients. G-CSFR overexpression was defined as expression level > than the median level (0.04 copies/*ABL* copy) in all analyzed SR patients. G-CSFR isoform IV was detectable in all samples but at a lower threshold than that of isoform I.

Statistics

Event-free survival was calculated from the date of diagnosis to the date of last follow-up or first event (failure to achieve remission, relapse, second malignancy or death from any cause). The cumulative incidences of relapse was calculated by the method of Kalbfleisch and Prentice and were compared between groups using the Gray test.

Results

Of the 154 patients categorized as standard risk, 59 were randomized to receive G-CSF and 79 to the control group. Of the 50 patients who had G-CSFR isoform I and IV quantitatively determined, 30 patients were in the G-CSF group and 20 were in the control no G-CSF group.

Of the 30 patients in the G-CSF group who had G-CSFR isoform IV surface expression, 16 had overexpression of G-CSFR isoform IV and they had an increased 5-year cumulative incidence of relapse compared to the 14 patients with low isoform IV expression (50% ±13% versus 14±10%; log-rank p=0.04). In patients not receiving G-CSF (n=20), the level of isoform IV expression affected the cumulative relapse rate (0% ±0% in patients with high expression [n=11] versus 18% ±12% in patients with low expression [n=9]; p=0.19).

Multivariate analyses of the G-CSF subgroup, including G-CSFR isoform IV overexpression, sex, and favorable cytogenetics, showed that patients with G-CSFR isoform IV overexpression had poorer 5-year EFS (p=0.031) and higher relapses (p=0.049).

Analyses according to the Medical Research Council trial (favorable cytogenetics only) with respect to G-CSFR isoform IV expression displayed the same trend but was not statistically significant in the 5-year incidence of relapse due to small patient numbers.

G-CSFR isoform IV expression in patients who had relapsed was 100-fold higher than in their initial diagnostic samples.

Conclusions

It was concluded that children and adolescents with AML who overexpress G-CSFR isoform IV had a higher relapse rate when given prophylactic G-CSF after induction therapy.

Study 5

Spunt SL, Irving H, Frost J et al. Phase II, randomized, open-label study of pegfilgrastim-supported VDC/IE chemotherapy in paediatric sarcoma patients. *J Clin Oncol* 2010;**28**:1329–36.

Objectives

To compare the efficacy and safety of a single subcutaneous dose of pegylated G-CSF (pegfilgrastim) against standard G-CSF (filgrastim) in reducing the incidence of chemotherapy-induced neutropenia in children receiving treatment for sarcoma.

Study design

This was a multicenter randomized open-label trial conducted between 2000 and 2007 in the USA and Australia. Children were grouped in three age strata: 0–5, 6–11 and 12–21 years, and an age stratum was closed to accrual after two successive groups of six patients within the age stratum achieved ANC recovery.

Previously untreated children with biopsy-proven sarcoma were randomly assigned in a 6:1 ratio to receive a single pegfilgrastim (PEGFIL) dose of 100 μg/kg or a daily dose of 5 μg/kg/day of filgrastim (FIL). Children randomized to FIL received 5 μg/kg/day subcutaneously beginning 24 h after completion of chemotherapy and continued until either the postnadir ANC was $\geq 10 \times 10^9$/L or until 24 h before the start of the next chemotherapy cycle while those assigned to PEGFIL received 100 μg/kg subcutaneously at 24 h after completing chemotherapy. An ANC count $\geq 1 \times 10^9$/L and a platelet count $\geq 100 \times 10^9$/L were necessary to start each treatment cycle. A surface lasmon resonance Biacore 3000 (Biacore, Piscataway, NJ) affinity assay was used to quantify antibodies capable of binding to FIL and PEGFIL. Samples testing positive for binding antibodies were then tested for neutralizing antibodies using a cell-based neutralizing antibody test.

Statistics

The calculations for sample size were based on an assumption of normally distributed durations of neutropenia documented in other published studies. The minimum sample size for the study (12 PEGFIL and two FIL in each of the three age strata) was calculated to be 42. This sample size allowed a difference in the duration of grade 4 (ANC $<0.5 \times 10^9$/L) neutropenia

between the two treatment groups to be estimated with a distance from the estimate to the 95% confidence bounds of 1.3 days (the assumed standard deviation was 1.5 days) for cycles 1 and 3. The primary efficacy endpoint was the duration of grade 4 neutropenia during cycles 1 and 3 while safety was evaluated across all four chemotherapy cycles.

Results

Forty-four patients were enrolled on the study with 38 and six children being randomized to PEGFIL and FIL respectively. The median age, age distribution, race/ethnicity, weight, baseline ANC, and baseline platelet counts were similar in the two treatment groups. There were four patients between the ages of 28 days and 23 months enrolled in the study. Only 37 of the 38 patients randomized to receive PEGFIL received it, as one patient was withdrawn before it was administered due to concerns about the protocol required blood draws. Eighty-four percent (n=32) and 50% (n=3) of patients assigned to PEGFIL and FIL respectively completed all planned cycles of chemotherapy and study drug treatment.

After the first and third cycles of chemotherapy, the median duration of grade 4 neutropenia in the PEGFIL group was 5 and 7 days respectively compared to 6 and 7 days respectively for the FIL patient group. The median time to ANC recovery after the first cycle of chemotherapy was 14 days in both treatment groups. Over the course of the study, 25 (68%) patients in the PEGFIL group developed febrile neutropenia compared to five patients (83%) in the FIL group. In the PEGFIL group, the median duration of grade 4 neutropenia was inversely related to the age group in both cycles 1 and 3.

The maximum median PEGFIL concentration was achieved 24–48 h after PEGFIL administration and was sustained until ANC nadir was reached while with regard to FIL, even though the median serum concentrations declined rapidly after the first dose, after repeated administrations, the daily trough concentrations of FIL increased until ANC nadir was reached. Both PEGFIL and FIL serum concentrations declined rapidly after ANC recovery. Children assigned to FIL had elevated ANC beyond the normal range because of continued administration of FIL during the neutrophil recovery phase. Children in the age group 0–5 years had a higher exposure to PEGFIL than the other two cohorts because they had the longest duration of neutropenia.

Toxicity

Adverse events attributable to PEGFIL and FIL were reported in 22% and 33% of patients respectively, with bone pain being the most commonly reported (11% PEGFIL, 17% FIL). There were no significant differences in the overall safety profile between the treatment arms or across the age groups in the PEGFIL treatment arm. The presence of antibodies had no effect on the clinical outcome or the pharmacokinetics of PEGFIL.

Conclusions

It was concluded that a single dose of pegfilgrastim (100 μg/kg subcutaneously) administered once per chemotherapy cycle was comparable to daily injections of filgrastim in reducing chemotherapy-induced neutropenia and also had a similar safety profile.

Study 6

Fox E, Widemann BC, Hawkins DS *et al.* Randomized trial and pharmacokinetic study of pegfilgrastim versus filgrastim after dose-intensive chemotherapy in young adults and children with sarcomas. *Clin Cancer Res* 2009;**15**:7361–7.

Objectives

To compare the effectiveness, tolerance, and pharmacokinetics of a single dose of pegfilgrastim (PFG) to daily filgrastim (FG) in children and young adults with sarcomas treated with dose-intensive combination chemotherapy.

Study design

This was a two-center prospective randomized trial conducted between December 2000 and December 2005.

Patients aged < 26 years with Ewing sarcoma family of tumors, alveolar rhabdomyosarcomas, stage III or IV embryonal rhabdomyosarcoma, unresectable peripheral nerve sheath tumor or synovial sarcoma were eligible for study entry. All patients had to have had normal cardiac, renal and full blood counts (neutrophil $>1.5 \times 10^9$/L, hemoglobin >9 g/dL and platelets $>100 \times 10^9$/L) for study enrollment. Patients who had received

chemotherapy and/or radiotherapy or who had bone marrow infiltration were excluded from the study. Similarly, pregnant or breastfeeding patients were also excluded. Randomization was done centrally and was not stratified for age, diagnosis or baseline characteristics. Severe neutropenia was defined as ANC <500/mcl and ANC recovery as postnadir ANC >500/mcl.

Patients were randomized at study entry to receive a single dose of PFG (100 μg/kg subcutaneous [SC]) 24–36 h after completion of each chemotherapy cycle or FG (5 μg/kg/dose SC) daily starting 24 h after each cycle of chemotherapy and continuing till the ANC was $\geq 10^4$/mcl. Each patient had the same treatment (i.e. PFG or FG) assignment throughout the entire treatment. Chemotherapy treatment consisted of 14 cycles of six cycles of vincristine, doxorubicin, and cyclophosphamide (VDC) and eight cycles of ifosfamide and etoposide (IE). The duration of severe neutropenia during cycles 1–4 and cycle duration for all cycles were compared. Local treatment (surgery and/or radiotherapy) for the primary tumor commenced after cycle 5. Pharmacokinetics of PFG and FG and CD34 stem cell mobilization were studied on cycle 1. Toxicity was graded according to the National Cancer Institute Common Toxicity Criteria v.2. Any toxicity (hospitalization for FBN, number of red cell and platelet transfusions, mucositis, documented or suspected infections) that was possibly, probably or definitely related to the growth factors was reported for cycles 1–4.

Statistics

The sample size was estimated based on standard methods for a two-group t test of equivalence of mean and equal SDs and sample size. A Wilcoxon rank-sum test was used to test if the duration of neutropenia differed significantly (overall p < 0.05) between the arms when the durations from the two V_3DC cycles (vincristine [one dose per week for 3 weeks], cyclophosphamide, doxorubicin) and the two IE cycles were averaged and tested separately. Differences in toxicity, pharmacokinetic parameters, CD34 stem cell mobilization, and days of FBN were also compared by the same Wilcoxon rank-sum test. Differences in the duration of neutropenia between the V_3DC cycles and IE cycle were tested for statistical significance by a Wilcoxon signed-rank test separately for the two treatment arms. All p-values were two-tailed and presented with adjustment for multiple comparisons.

Results

Thirty-four patients were enrolled on the study. Two patients in the PFG arm did not complete the initial four cycles of chemotherapy and this was unrelated to any adverse events. For patients randomized to the FG arm, the mean number of daily doses of FG was 13 (7–27)/cycle for the two cycles of V_3DC and 10(6–24)/cycle for the two IE cycles.

Duration of neutropenia was significantly longer after the V_3DC (cycles 1 and 3) than after the IE cycle (cycles 2 and 4) for both PFG (p<0.001) and FG (p<0.001) treatment arms.

During the first four cycles, the number of days of severe neutropenia was not significantly different between the two treatment arms for either the V_3DC (PFG: median 5.5 [range 3–8] versus FG: median 6.0 [range 0–9]; p=0.76) or IE cycles (PFG: median 1.5 [range 0–4] versus FG: median 3.75 [range 0–6.5]; p=0.11). The median cycle duration for both VDC and IE cycles was 21 days for patients in both PFG and FG treatment arms. No patient required a dose reduction due to delayed recovery of blood counts.

The median (range) prenadir peak for patients in the PFG treatment arm was 20,100/mcl (2300–94,900/mcl) compared to 10,700/mcl (1400–39,400/mcl) (p=0.024) for patients in the FG treatment group while the postnadir peak for patients in the PFG arm was 8000/mcl (2400–28,200/mcl) compared to 20,400/mcl (2200–47,400/mcl) for the FG treatment group (p<0.001).

Twelve of 17 patients in the PFG group experienced 18 episodes (29% of cycles) of grade 3 FBN during the first four cycles of chemotherapy and required hospitalization compared with 15/17 patients and 32 episodes (47% of cycles) of FBN on the FG arm. Stem cell mobilization did not differ between the two treatment groups.

Both PFG and FG were well tolerated and adverse events (AE) due to growth factor administration during the first four cycles of chemotherapy were similar in both treatment groups. No dose modifications to growth factor therapy were needed as a result of AE on either treatment arm. One patient in the PFG arm developed acute leukemia 20 months after completion of chemotherapy.

The serum concentration of PFG peaked 2h after administration and then declined before a second peak after day 7 when ANC was at its nadir. Absorption (T_{max}) and apparent clearance (CL/F) were significantly different (p<0.001) in the PFG compared to the FG arm. Substantial interpatient variability was observed with both PFG and FG.

Conclusions

It was concluded that a single dose of pegfilgrastim was well tolerated and was as effective as filgrastim in reducing both the duration of severe neutropenia and the number of episodes of febrile neutropenia, including documented infections after dose-intensive chemotherapy with VDC and IE.

CHAPTER 25

Cardioprotection in pediatric oncology

Ananth Shankar

University College London Hospitals NHS Foundation Trust, London, UK

Commentary by Gill A. Levitt

Cardiac disease in childhood cancer survivors has been recognized as a major cause of premature deaths and morbidity. Anthracyclines and cardiac radiation are the main offenders and recognition has been documented since the 1970s [1,2]. Recent late mortality studies from the UK and French collaboration [3] and the American Childhood Cancer Survivor Study (CCSS) [4] have reported a 4.4-(95% confidence interval [CI] 1.3–15.3) to 3.1-(95% CI 1.6–5.8) fold increased risk of premature death associated with doses of anthracyclines in excess of 360 and 401 mg/m^2 respectively.

Further evidence has been reported in long-term morbidity studies, although there is a wide variation in incidence. Kremer *et al.* [5,6] conducted a systematic review of published studies between 1996 and 2000 and reported an incidence of acute heart failure between 0% and 16% and of subclinical cardiac dysfunction between 0% and 57%. This extreme variation is in part due to variable total anthracycline dose, follow-up interval, and differences in the definition of cardiac disease.

Prevention of anthracycline cardiotoxicity has been addressed by various groups and three systematic reviews have been conducted [7,8,9]. The obvious method of reducing cardiotoxicity is to reduce the number of patients who receive anthracyclines; at present approximately 60% are exposed. The addition of anthracyclines to many protocols in a nonrandomized way in the 1980s coincided with the marked improvement in survival. The jury is still out regarding the need to incorporate anthracyclines into certain treatment regimens and it is now difficult to perform randomized trials to answer the question [10]. The Childhood Acute Lymphoblastic Leukaemia Collaborative Group [11] performed a meta-analysis on acute lymphoblastic leukemia (ALL) trials started between 1972 and 1984 that randomized the use of anthracyclines and methods of reducing cardiotoxicity (use of dexrazoxane, type of anthracycline used, method of administration, bolus versus infusion). Anthracycline use was shown to be beneficial in preventing bone marrow relapse but did not change the event-free survival (EFS) and there was a nonsignificant increase in early deaths in the anthracycline group. The Cochrane review on treatment with anthracyclines versus without supported the ALL data but there were too few trials to come to any conclusion for solid tumors [10]. More detailed risk stratification may result in fewer patients receiving anthracyclines, as recently demonstrated in an International Society of Paediatric Oncology (SIOP) renal tumor randomized study in which there was no beneficial effect of the addition of anthracyclines in stage II–III intermediate-risk Wilms tumor [12].

Reduction of cardiotoxicity using different administration regimens has been effective in adult studies but has not been found to be effective in children [13], although the studies performed have been in patients receiving moderate doses of anthracyclines. However,

---

Evidence-Based Pediatric Oncology, Third Edition. Edited by Ross Pinkerton, Ananth Shankar and Katherine K. Matthay.
© 2013 John Wiley & Sons, Ltd. Published 2013 by John Wiley & Sons, Ltd.

there is anecdotal evidence in the treatment of hepato-blastoma that the change from bolus dosing to 48-h infusion reduced the need for cardiac transplantation in these high-risk patients (young age and high doses – 480 mg/m^2) [14].

The use of cardioprotective agents has been addressed in a number of systematic reviews. They all comment on the methodological limitations of randomized studies, namely the definition of cardiac outcomes varies, blinding of patients and outcome assessors, completeness of follow-up, and small sample number. The only agent reported to show benefit was dexrazoxane [7,8,9]. Dexrazoxane (ethylene diamine tetra-acetic acid) is a cyclic derivative of the chelating agent EDTA which readily penetrates cell membranes. It was initially developed as a chemotherapy drug because it interferes with topoisomerase II activity; it is notable that inhibition occurs at a different site to epipodophyllotoxin action. Subsequently, it was noted in mice to protect against anthracycline cardiotoxicity. Its action is thought to be due to the chelating proper-ties preventing the formation of harmful iron-mediated free radical generated oxygen free radicals which are released after anthracycline administration [15].

The assessment of dexrazoxane as a cardioprotective agent falls into two categories: first, whether it provides a useful cardioprotective effect and second, whether its use affects event-free survival by decreasing the effi-cacy of anthracyclines, reducing dose intensity of the treatment regimen or causing life-threatening toxicity. A large breast cancer study suggested there was a reduction in survival in those patients in the dexrazox-ane group but subsequent longer follow-up studies have not found a decrease in efficacy and no childhood cancer study has identified a problem [16,17,18].

The toxicity of dexrazoxane centers around its adverse effect on bone marrow. Increased myelosuppression has been reported in both adult and childhood studies [16, 19]. The more worrisome toxicity was reported in 1997 by Tebbi [20] in the results of a randomized trial of the use of dexrazoxane in pediatric Hodgkin disease (HD) patients, showing an increased number of patients developing acute myeloid leukemia (AML)/myelodys-plastic syndrome (MDS) 2.55%±1.0% within the dexrazoxane-treated group compared with 0.85%±0.6% (p=0.06) in the control group. The regimen also included etoposide and doxorubicin, both topoisomerase inhibi-tors although acting at different sites. It is conceivable that

there is a synergistic effect along with a dose–response effect. The chromosomal aberrations seen in the HD patients were also cited in the patients treated with a related oral compound, razoxane, used in the 1980s for treatment of psoriasis and colon cancer [21].

The big question is whether this finding translates to other tumor types or is particular to HD and/or the use of etoposide in treatment. The American ALL studies in which patients did not receive etoposide showed no evidence of an increase in AML/MDS [22,23] although the Salzer study [23] suggested an increase with longer follow-up of 10 years to 4.2%±2.2% in the dexrazoxane arm compared with 1.3%±0.9% (p=0.15) in the control group.

The European Medicine Agency discussed this issue in 2010 and made a decision in July 2011 that "Dexrazoxane is now contraindicated for use in chil-dren and adolescents up to age 18 years due to evidence of serious harm in this age-group". Use is restricted to adults with advanced or metastatic breast cancer who have previously received a minimum cumulative dose of 300 mg/m^2 doxorubicin or 540 mg/m^2 epirubicin. The dose ratio for dexrazoxane to be used in combina-tion with doxorubicin has been halved. Dexrazoxane is no longer indicated for use in patients with malignan-cies other than breast cancer [24].

The real question, which may never be answered in Europe, is whether the increased risk of second malignant neoplasm (SMN) outweighs the risk of life-threatening cardiotoxicity. For the low-to-moderate anthracycline dose regimes (>360 mg/m^2) this is probably true but where high-dose anthracyclines are required or the patient has a genetic susceptibility to anthracycline-related cardiotoxicity, this question needs to be answered.

References

1 Van Hoff DD, Layard MW, Basa P et al. Risk factors for doxorubicin-induced congestive heart failure. Ann Intern Med 1979;97:710–17.

2 Cohn KE, Stewart JR, FajardoLF, Hancock EW. Heart disease following radiation. Medicine (Baltimore) 1967;46:281–98.

3 Tukenova M, Guibout C, Oberlin O et al. Long-term overall and cardiovascular mortality following childhood cancer: the role of cancer treatment. J Clin Oncol 2010;28:1308–15.

4 Mulrooney DA, Yeazel MW, Kawashima T et al. Cardiac out-comes in a cohort of adult survivors of childhood and adoles-cent cancer: retrospective analysis report of the Childhood Cancer Survivor Study cohort. BMJ 2009;339:b4606.

5 Kremer LCM, van Dalen EC, Offringa M, Voute PA. Frequency and risk factors of anthracycline-induced heart failure in children: a systematic review. *Ann Oncol* 2002;**13**: 503–12.

6 Kremer LCM, van der Pal HJH, Offringa M, van Dalen EC, Voute PA. Frequency and risk factors of subclinical cardiotoxicity after anthracycline therapy in children: a systematic review. *Ann Oncol* 2002;**13**:819–29.

7 Smith LA, Cornelius VR, Plummer CJ *et al.* Cardiotoxicity of anthracycline agents for the treatment of cancer: systematic review and meta-analysis of randomised controlled trials. *BMC Cancer* 2010;**10**:337.

8 Bryant J, Picot J, Baxter L, Levitt G, Sullivan I, Clegg A. Clinical and cost effectiveness of cardioprotection against the toxic effects of anthracyclines given to children with cancer: a systematic review. *Br J Cancer* 2007;**96**:226–30.

9 Van Dalen E, Caron HN, Dickinson HO, Kremer LC. Cardioprotective interventions for cancer patients receiving anthracyclines. *Cochrane Database Syst Rev* 2011;**6**:CD003917.

10 Van Dalen EC, Raphael MF, Caron HN, Kremer LC. Treatment including anthracyclines versus treatment not including anthracyclines for childhood cancer. *Cochrane Database Syst Rev* 2011;**1**:CD006647.

11 Childhood Acute Lymphoblastic Leukaemia Collaborative Group (CALLCG). Beneficial and harmful effects of anthracyclines in the treatment of childhood acute lymphoblastic leukaemia: a systematic review and meta-analysis. *Br J Haematol* 2009;**145**:376–88.

12 Lipshultz SE, Giantris AL, Lipsitz SR *et al.* Doxorubicin administration by continuous infusion is not cardioprotective: the Dana-Farber 91-01 Acute Lymphoblastic Leukemia protocol. *J Clin Oncol* 2002;**20**:1677–82.

13 Pritchard-Jones K, Graf N, Bergeron C *et al.*, for the SIOP Renal Tumours Study Group. Doxorubicin can be safely omitted from the treatment of stage II/III intermediate risk histology Wilms tumour: results of the SIOP WT 2001 randomised trial. *Pediatr Blood Cancer* 2011 **157**:741 (abstract O137).

14 Levitt G, Anazodo A, Burch M, Bunch K. Cardiac or cardiopulmonary transplantation in childhood cancer survivors: an increasing need? *Eur J Cancer* 2009;**45**:3027–34.

15 Hershko C, Pinson A, Link G. Prevention of anthracycline cardiotoxicity by iron chelation. *Acta Haematol* 1996;**95**:87–92.

16 Swain SM, Whaley FS, Gerber MC *et al.* Cardioprotection with dexrazoxane for doxorubicin in woman with breast cancer. *J Clin Oncol* 1997;**15**:1318–32.

17 Schwartz CL, Constine LS, Villaluna D *et al.* A risk-adapted, response-based approach using ABVE-PC for children and adolescents with intermediate- and high-risk Hodgkin lymphoma: the results of P9425. *Blood* 2009;**3**(114):2051–9.

18 Wexler LH, Andrich MP, Venzon D *et al.* Randomized trial of the cardioprotective agent ICRF-187 in pediatric sarcoma patients treated with doxorubicin. *J Clin Oncol* 1996;**14**:362–72.

19 Lipshultz SE, Scully RE, Lipsitz SR *et al.* Assessment of dexrazoxane as a cardioprotectant in doxorubicin-treated children with high-risk acute lymphoblastic leukaemia: long-term follow-up of a prospective, randomized, multicentre trial. *Lancet Oncol* 2010;**11**:950–61.

20 Tebbi CK, London WB, Freidman D *et al.* Dexrazoxane-associated risk for acute myeloid leukemia/myelodysplastic syndrome and other secondary malignancies in pediatric Hodgkin's disease. *J Clin Oncol* 2007;**25**:493–500.

21 Gilbert JM, Hellmann K, Evans M *et al.* Randomized trial of oral adjuvant razoxane (ICRF 159) in resectable colorectal cancer: five-year follow-up. *Br J Surg* 1986;**73**:446–50.

22 Vrooman LM, Donna D, Neuberg SD, Stevenson KE. The low incidence of secondary acute myelogenous leukemia in children and adolescents treated with dexrazoxane for acute lymphoblastic leukemia: a report from the Dana-Farber Cancer Institute ALL Consortium. *Eur J Cancer* 2011;**47**:1373–9.

23 Salzer WL, Devidas M, Carroll WL *et al.* Long-term results of the Pediatric Oncology Group studies for childhood acute lymphoblastic leukemia 1984–2001: a report from the Children's Oncology Group. *Leukemia* 2010;**24**:355–70.

24 Drug Safety Update, July 2011, issue 12: A3.

Summary of previous studies

Dexrazoxane is a cardioprotectant that significantly reduces the incidence of adverse cardiac events in adults treated with doxorubicin-containing regimens. Clinical evidence for the efficacy of dexrazoxane as a cardioprotectant in children, especially from randomized clinical trials, is limited. The Lipshultz *et al.* [1] report was a multicenter randomized controlled trial conducted by the Dana-Farber Cancer Institute (DFCI) in children and adolescents with previously untreated high-risk ALL. The primary objective of the study was to determine whether dexrazoxane reduced anthracycline-associated cardiac damage. Patients were randomized to receive doxorubicin (DOX) alone or dexrazoxane (DXN; 300 mg/m^2) immediately followed by DOX. All patients received two doses of DOX (30 mg/m^2) during remission induction followed by eight further doses (30 mg/m^2) during the treatment course. No DOX was given after 9 months of treatment. The main outcome measure determined the frequency of elevated cardiac troponin T levels between the two groups of patients. Cardiac troponin T was considered elevated if the value was >0.01 ng/mL and extremely elevated if the value was 0.025 ng/mL. Serum samples for cardiac troponin T levels were collected at standardized times (at diagnosis before DOX, daily after DOX during remission induction, 7 days after DOX during remission induction, and at the end of therapy).

Elevations of troponin T occurred in 35% of the patients (55 of 158). Compared to patients treated with doxorubicin alone, fewer patients in the DOX plus DXN group had elevations in the troponin T levels (21% versus 50%; p<0.001) and extremely elevated troponin T levels (10% versus 32%; p<0.001). Ten percent of patients had elevated cardiac troponin T levels prior to commencement of DOX treatment and even after exclusion of children with pretreatment elevated troponin T levels, DXN had a significant cardioprotective effect. Echocardiogram data showed no significant differences between the two groups of patients with respect to mean left ventricular dimension, fractional shortening or contractility before,

during or after DOX treatment. The 2.5-year EFS was 83% in both groups of patients. The report concluded that dexrazoxane prevented or reduced cardiac injury, as reflected by elevations in troponin T that was associated with the use of doxorubicin for childhood ALL without compromising the antileukemic efficacy of doxorubicin.

This report has been updated recently – see Study 1 in the New Studies section of this chapter.

The report by Wexler *et al.* [2] was a multicenter randomized study in children and young adults with sarcoma undergoing intensive anthracycline-containing chemotherapy. Eligible patients underwent a computer-generated 1:1 factorial randomization to receive dexrazoxane (DXN), granulocyte colony-stimulating factor (G-CSF), both or neither. The chemotherapy drugs included vincristine, doxorubicin (DOX), cyclophosphamide, ifosfamide, and etoposide. Radiotherapy used for local tumor control commenced at week 12 after five courses of chemotherapy. The dose of DXN was 20 times the dose of DOX that was given intravenously 15 min before DOX administration. Multi-gated acquisition (MUGA) scans using technetium 99m pertechnetate-labeled red blood cells were used to determine doxorubicin cardiotoxicity. These were performed at baseline and at 6–12 weeks after 210, 310, 360, and 410 mg/m^2 cumulative doses of doxorubicin. Dose-limiting cardiotoxicity was defined as a reduction in the left ventricular ejection fraction (LVEF) to <45% or a decrease in the LVEF by <20 percentage points from the baseline or clinical evidence of congestive cardiac failure. The main outcome measure was to determine short-term cardiotoxicity by measuring the change in the resting LVEF.

Of the 39 eligible children included in the report, two were randomized to receive DXN with chemotherapy (DXN group) and 19 to chemotherapy alone (control group). The mean decrease in LVEF/100 mg/m^2 of doxorubicin was 2.7% points in the control group compared to 1% point in the DXN group (p=0.02). Of the 15 patients who received a cumulative dose of 410 mg/m^2 (control group 5%, DXN group 10%),

LVEF in the control group was 44%±2.8% compared to 53.9%±2.2% in the DXN group (p=0.03). The control group developed dose-limiting cardiotoxicity much earlier than the DXN group (p<0.01). The number of patients who developed cardiotoxicity after 210, 310 and 410 mg/m^2 was 5, 7, and 10 compared to 0, 2 and 4 in the DXN group. LVEF returned to normal in three out of four patients at the time of the first follow-up MUGA scan compared to none of seven in the control group who had a follow-up MUGA scan (p=0.02). While more patients in the DXN group had grade 3 or higher thrombocytopenia after cycle 1 (11/23) versus 3/18 in the control group (p<0.05) after cycle 6 (9/14) versus 1/9 in the control group (p<0.001) and also significantly lower nadir platelet counts after cycles 4 and 6 of chemotherapy, no significant nadirs in the absolute neutrophil count (ANC) were seen. The 2-year EFS rates were 39% and 43% for the control and DXN groups respectively and were not statistically significant. The report concluded that dexrazoxane was cardioprotective in children and young adults with sarcomas undergoing intensive anthracycline-containing chemotherapy and did not adversely affect chemotherapy response or chemotherapy tolerability.

Acute doxorubicin-induced cardiotoxicity can be prevented in adults by continuous infusion of the drug, but mechanisms of cardiotoxicity are different in children. Lipshultz et al. [3] in their report compared cardiac outcomes in children with high-risk ALL receiving bolus or continuous infusion of doxorubicin to determine which of the two modes of infusion offered better cardioprotection. Eligible patients were randomized to receive either a continuous 48-h infusion (CI) or a bolus 1-h infusion (BI) of 30 mg/m^2 doxorubicin. Irrespective of their clinical status, all patients underwent echocardiography (ECHO) at predetermined intervals and this included measurements of left ventricular dimensions, thickness, and fractional shortening. Patients who were still receiving doxorubicin before their last follow-up ECHO or had their dose of doxorubicin reduced due to cardiac-related problems were excluded from analysis.

Of the 121 evaluable patients, 64 were randomized to receive CI of doxorubicin and 57 received BI of doxorubicin. Baseline ECHO results were similar in both groups of patients. The median time for postdoxorubicin ECHO from diagnosis was 1.5 years and this was similar in both treatment groups. In both the CI and BI groups, median left ventricular (LV) wall thickness decreased by 0.3 SD, which was significantly below normal. LV peak systolic wall stress was also significantly elevated in both groups of patients. Five-year EFS rate were 89%±3.9% and 87.4%±4.5% for the bolus and continuous infusion group of patients respectively (p=0.5). It was concluded that continuous infusion of doxorubicin over 48h for children with ALL did not offer any cardioprotective advantage over a short bolus infusion. Both regimens were associated with significant progressive subclinical cardiotoxicity.

References

1 Lipshultz SE, Rifai N, Dalton VM et al. The effect of dexrazoxane on myocardial injury in doxorubicin-treated children with acute lymphoblastic leukemia. N Engl J Med 2004;**351**:145–53.

2 Wexler LH, Andrich MP, Venzon D et al. Randomized trial of the cardioprotective agent ICRF-187 in pediatric sarcoma patients treated with doxorubicin. J Clin Oncol 1996;**14**:362–72.

3 Lipshultz SE, Giantris AL, Lipsitz SR et al. Doxorubicin administration by continuous infusion is not cardioprotective: the Dana-Farber 91-01 Acute Lymphoblastic Leukemia protocol. J Clin Oncol 2002;**20**:1677–82.

New studies

Adverse effects of cardio-protectant (dexrazoxane)

Study 1

Lipshultz SE, Scully RE, Lipsitz SR *et al*. Assessment of dexrazoxane as a cardioprotectant in doxorubicin-treated children with high-risk acute lymphoblastic leukaemia: long-term follow-up of a prospective, randomized, multicentre trial. *Lancet Oncol* 2010;**11**: 950–61.

Objectives

This report follows up on the Lipshultz *et al*. (2004) study covered in the Summary of Previous Studies section above. It detailed the long-term follow-up results of high-risk ALL patients who were randomized to receive doxorubicin with or without the cardioprotectant dexrazoxane.

Study design

One hundred children were assigned to doxorubicin alone (66 analyzed) and 105 to doxorubicin plus dexrazoxane (68 analyzed).

Results

Five years after completion of doxorubicin chemotherapy, the mean left ventricular fractional shortening and endsystolic dimension Z-scores were significantly worse than normal for children who received doxorubicin alone (left ventricular fractional shortening -0.82; 95% CI −1.31 to −0.33; endsystolic dimension 0.57, range 0.21–0.93) but not those who also received dexrazoxane (left ventricular fractional shortening −0.41, -0.88 to 0.06; endsystolic dimension 0.15, −0.20 to 0.51). The protective effect of dexrazoxane relative to doxorubicin alone on the left ventricular wall thickness (difference between the two groups 0.47, range 0.46–0.48) and thickness to dimension ratio (0.66, range 0.64–0.68) were the only statistically significant characteristics at 5 years. Subgroup analysis revealed that at 5 years, dexrazoxane cardioprotection with regard to LV fractional shortening (girls 1.17, 95% CI 0.24–2.11, boys −0.10, 95% CI −0.87 to 0.68; p=0.04) and LV thickness to dimension ratio was seen in girls but not boys (girls 1.15, 95% CI 0.44–1.85 versus boys 0.19, 95% CI −0.42 to 0.81; p=0.046).

With a median follow-up for recurrence and death of 8.7 years (range 1.3–12.1 years), EFS was 77% (95% CI 67–84) for children in the doxorubicin alone group and 76% (95% CI 67–84) for children who received doxorubicin with dexrazoxane (p=0.99).

Conclusions

It was concluded that dexrazoxane provided long-term cardioprotection without compromising oncological efficacy in children with high-risk ALL treated with doxorubicin. Furthermore, this long-term cardioprotective effect was greater in girls than in boys.

Study 2

Vrooman LM, Neuberg DS, Stevenson KE *et al*. The low incidence of secondary acute myelogenous leukaemia in children and adolescents treated with dexrazoxane for acute lymphoblastic leukaemia: a report from the Dana-Farber Cancer Institute ALL Consortium. *Eur J Cancer* 2011;**47**:1373–9.

Objectives

The purpose of the study was to determine whether the use of dexrazoxane as a cardioprotectant in children with high-risk ALL increased the risk of second malignant neoplasms including AML and MDS. Although the report included three consecutive multicenter trials, this review focuses on the first DFCI trial protocol 95-10 (1996–2000).

Study design

In the DFCI ALL Consortium Trial (1996–2000), newly diagnosed high-risk ALL patients were randomly assigned to receive doxorubicin (30 mg/m^2, cumulative dose 300 mg/m^2) preceded by dexrazoxane (300 mg/m^2, 10 doses) or the same dose of doxorubicin without dexrazoxane during induction and intensification phases. Risk stratification was according to the National Cancer Institute (NCI) age and white blood cell count (WBC) criteria. Patients were considered to have high-risk ALL if their presenting WBC count was $>50 \times 10^9$/L, age ≥ 10 years, with central nervous system (CNS) involvement at diagnosis, mediastinal involvement and/or T-cell disease or Philadelphia-positive ALL.

Briefly, the treatment was divided into four phases.
1 Remission induction (4 weeks) that consisted of vincristine, doxorubicin, oral prednisone, methotrexate, and intramuscular (IM) L-asparaginase.
2 CNS intensification phase that consisted of intrathecal (IT) chemotherapy, 18 Gy cranial irradiation, doxorubicin, vincristine, and 6-mercaptopurine.
3 Thirty-week intensification phase including L-asparaginase, vincristine, steroid pulses, 6-mercaptopurine and doxorubicin.
4 A continuation phase consisting of vincristine, steroids, 6-mercaptopurine, and methotrexate.
The total cumulative dose of doxorubicin was 300 mg/m². Dexrazoxane was administered by rapid infusion immediately prior to each dose of doxorubicin during the induction and intensification phases.

Reporting of second malignancies
A second malignancy (SMN) was defined as any malignancy occurring after the primary diagnosis of ALL and was intended to include skin cancers, meningioma, AML/MDS or any other malignancy. SMNs following relapse were not included in this analysis because of the possibility of incomplete ascertainment of SMN following relapse and the potential impact of relapse therapy on the development of SMN.

Statistics
The rate of SMNs along with the standard error of that rate was estimated using the method of cumulative incidence as implemented in the *cmprsk* package in R. Patients who were last known to be alive without relapse and without SMN were censored in the cumulative incidence analysis.

Results
One hundred and five high-risk patients in protocol 95-01 were randomly assigned to receive dexrazoxane with doxorubicin. Four patients were excluded from final analysis (three did not achieve a complete response [CR] and one died during remission induction).

The number of SMNs observed was 0 in the 95-01 trial (median follow-up 9.6 years; range 1.3–13.6 years). In fact, in the two succeeding trials, 00-01 and 05-01 (in which all high-risk and very high-risk ALL patients were electively given, not randomized to, dexrazoxane), only one patient developed a SMN. With a median follow-up of 3.8 years (range 0.2–13.6 years, all three trials included), the overall 5-year estimated cumulative incidence of SMNs for all 533 patients was 0.24 (95% CI 0.02–1.29%).

Conclusions
It was concluded that the use of dexrazoxane as a cardioprotectant was safe and the occurrence of secondary AML was a rare event.

Study 3

Tebbi CK, London WB, Friedman D *et al*. Dexrazoxane-associated risk for acute myeloid leukemia/myelodysplastic syndrome and other secondary malignancies in pediatric Hodgkin's disease. *J Clin Oncol* 2007;25: 493–500.

Objectives
The main purpose of the study was to evaluate the safety, incidence, and risk of AML/MDS when dexrazoxane (DXN) was used as cardioprotectant during treatment in children and adolescents with Hodgkin lymphoma (HL).

Study design
Patients younger than 21 years with HL enrolled on the Pediatric Oncology Group (POG) 9426 and POG 9425 trials were included in the study. Patients received two doxorubicin, bleomycin, vincristine, etoposide (ABVE) (POG 9426) or three doxorubicin, bleomycin, vincristine, etoposide-prednisolone, cyclophosphamide (ABVE-PC) cycles (POG 9425) before response evaluation at 8–9 weeks after start of treatment. Early responders proceeded to receive 25.5 Gy (POG 9426) involved-field radiotherapy (IF RT) or 21 Gy regional-field treatment (POG 9425). Two additional doses of chemotherapy were given to slow responders before radiation. G-CSF at 5 µg/kg/day

was used to maintain dose intensity. Patients were randomly assigned to receive or not receive intravenous DXN (300 mg/m^2) on any day that doxorubicin or bleomycin was administered.

Statistics

All analyses were performed for the baseline comparability of the randomly assigned treatment groups. Cumulative incidence (CI) rates were calculated considering competing relapses and deaths. The time to an event was calculated from date of enrollment until first occurrence of relapse, progressive disease, SMN, death or until last contact. SMN was calculated from enrollment date until date of SMN or last contact if no SMN was reported. Treatment comparisons of cumulative incidence rates were made using a modified χ^2 test, with p-values of <0.05 considered statistically significant. Standardized incidence ratios (SIRs) of observed to expected malignancies were calculated using race, age, and sex-specific incidence rates of the Surveillance and End Results (SEER) Program of the National Cancer Institute (Bethesda, MD). For secondary analysis of SMN as a first event, patients were considered at risk of SMN from enrollment date until first occurrence of a relapse, progressive disease, SMN, death or until last contact if no event occurred. For a given diagnosis (AML, MDS, papillary carcinoma thyroid or osteosarcoma), the incidence of SMN was standardized by comparison to the incidence of those diagnoses in the general population. Otherwise, the SIRs were calculated by standardizing in comparison to the incidence of any malignant diagnosis. Treatment comparisons of SIRs were made using a log-linear model (Poisson regression model with a log-link function) and p-values of <0.05 were considered statistically significant. Excess absolute risk (expressed per 1000 person-years) was calculated as an additional indicator of the impact of cancer diagnosis and therapy on the cohort compared with the general population.

Results

POG 9426 (October 1996–September 2000) enrolled 262 eligible patients while POG 9425 (March 1997–February 2001) enrolled 216 eligible patients. Analyses of baseline comparability found no differences between the DXN-positive and DXN-negative groups in terms of sex (p=0.9253), race (p=0.1652), diagnos-

tic stage (p=0.9233), age (p=0.2710) or follow-up time (p=0.3299). There were statistically significant differences in the proportion of early responders or EFS rates between the DXN groups.

Secondary AML/MDS

Five patients developed AML and three developed MDS on the POG 9426 and 9425 trials at a median time of 26 months (range 12–48 months). This was higher when compared to the general population (SIR 406.89; 95% CI 175.67–801.73). Additionally, the incidence of AML/MDS was higher among those who received DXN (SIR 613.6; 95% CI 225.2–1335.6) compared to those who did not receive DXN (SIR 202.37; 95% CI 24.5–731.0; p=0.0990). Eight of the patients who developed SMN were in the DXN group; five were slow responders while the remaining three were rapid responders.

All SMNs

In addition to the eight patients who developed AML/MDS, two patients developed solid tumors: osteosarcoma outside the radiation field at 34.5 months after diagnosis and papillary thyroid carcinoma within the radiation field at 38.9 months after diagnosis. Overall, there were eight SMNs (six AML/MDS and two solid tumors) in the DXN group compared to two in the non-DXN group (one AML and one MDS). At a median follow-up of 58 months, the 4-year CI of any SMN was 3.43% ± 1.2% with DXN versus 0.85% ± 0.6% without DXN (p=0.60). Among the DXN patients, the SIR for any SMN was 41.86× that of the general population and statistically significantly higher than the SIR of 10.08 in the non-DXN group after age, sex, and race standardization (95% CI 18.07–82.48 and 1.22–36.44 respectively; p=0.0231). Overall, the excess absolute risk was 4.79 excess malignancies per 1000 person-years of patient follow-up (3.83 excess absolute risk for AML/MDS, 0.46 excess absolute risk for papillary carcinoma, and 0.47 excess absolute risk for osteosarcoma per 1000 person-years of patient follow-up).

Analysis of SMN as first event

The 4-year CI of AML/MDS as a first event was 2.10% ± 0.9% with DXN versus 0.42% ± 0.4% with DXN (n=239; p=0.1052). A secondary analysis of the eight patients who developed SMN as a first event (excluding the two patients who developed SMN after relapse) showed that the 4-year CI of SMN was 2.98% ± 1.1% with DXN versus 0.42% ± 0.4% without DXN (p=0.0355). As slow responders received more chemotherapy, resulting in higher cumulative doses of doxorubicin, etoposide, bleomycin and cyclophosphamide, an analysis of risk number of chemotherapy cycles was also performed. Neither the number of chemotherapy cycles nor the increased cyclophosphamide exposure appeared to increase the risk of SMN.

Conclusions

It was concluded that the use of dexrazoxane as a cardioprotectant when combined with the Hodgkin chemotherapy used in the POG 9426 and 9425 trials probably increased the incidence of SMN, especially AML/MDS.

Efficacy of anthracyclines in pediatric oncology

Study 4

Childhood Acute Lymphoblastic Leukaemia Collaborative Group (CALLCG). Beneficial and harmful effects of anthracyclines in the treatment of childhood acute lymphoblastic leukaemia: a systematic review and meta-analysis. *Br J Haematol* 2009;145:376–88.

Objectives

This systematic review assessed the efficacy and cardiotoxicity of anthracyclines (ANCYN) in the treatment of childhood ALL.

Objectives and study design

Individual patient data from randomized trials that commenced before 2000 that involved unconfounded treatment comparisons of anthracycline therapy were evaluated. Trials were included if at least 50% of patients were up to 21 years of age. The variables considered were addition or not of ANCYN to standard therapy, type of ANCYN, mode of ANCYN administration, and the presence or not of a cardioprotectant. Trials were identified after detailed search of databases including EMBASE and MEDLINE. Additional hand searching was undertaken of major cancer and medical journals, review articles, meeting abstracts, and reference lists of published trials.

Checked data on each patient aged ≤21 years included sex, presenting WBC count, immunophenotype, treatment allocation, site of first relapse, dates of birth, diagnosis, randomization of treatment, first remission, relapse, death or last contact, and the date and type of any second malignancy. All data were checked for internal consistency, balance between the treatment groups by initial features, randomization dates and length of follow-up and consistency with publications on the trials.

Primary outcome measures included were EFS and overall survival (from date of randomization). Secondary outcome measures were no remission (defined as deaths without achievement of remission), bone marrow (BM) relapse including combined relapses, non-BM relapses, death in remission, relapse-free interval (time to any relapse). When relapses were analyzed, those patients who died prior to achieving a remission were excluded while deaths in remission were censored. Data were obtained only for first relapse and thus analyses of a particular type of relapse were censored at relapse of any other type.

Statistics

All analyses were from time of randomization to event within the trial with observed minus expected (O-E) number of events and its variance obtained by the log-rank method. These O-E values were then added over all trials to produce a total (T) with variance (V) equal to the sum of separate variances. These were used to calculate an overall odds ratio (OR) or ratio of event rates, and its 95% confidence interval equal to exponent (T/V ± 1.96/$\sqrt{V}$). All p-values were two-sided and considered significant when <0.05.

Results

Data were not available for two trials (SWOG 690/691 and the ALGB 6801 trials).

Addition of an anthracycline

Six trials were reviewed. Cumulative doses in all six trials were all <100 mg/m^2 daunorubicin, 80 mg/m^2 doxorubicin or 60 mg/m^2 plus 35 mg/m^2 doxorubicin. In three of the trials reviewed, all patients received cranial irradiation. Patients who received anthracyclines had a lower incidence of BM relapses (OR 0.77; 95% CI 0.60–1.00; p=0.05) and a nonsignificant reduction in non-BM relapses (OR 0.88; 95% CI 0.63–1.25;

p=0.5), resulting in an improved relapse-free interval (OR 0.81; 95% CI 0.66–1.00; p=0.05). However, there was a nonsignificant increase in induction failures (p=0.3) and deaths in remission (31 versus 21; OR 1.45; 95% CI 0.84–2.48; p=0.2) in these patients. Five-year EFS was 56.7% in the anthracycline group versus 52.8% without anthracycline with a long-term difference of 3.7% (95% CI -3.2 to 10.6).

Type of anthracycline

Although four trials were reviewed, one was excluded as it was for patients with relapsed disease. While the FRALLE 93 trial randomized children between two doses of daunorubicin (DNR) or two doses of idarubicin (IDA) in remission induction, a third dose of the randomized anthracycline was given for patients not in marrow remission on day 21. All patients received doxorubicin (DOX) in intensification. Cumulative doses in these trials were $60 mg/m^2$ of DNR plus $35 mg/m^2$ of DOX or $80 mg/m^2$ of DOX (DFCI 73001); 80 (or 120) mg/m^2 DNR plus $75 mg/m^2$ of DOX or 16 (or 24) mg/m^2 of IDA plus $75 mg/m^2$ of DOX (FRALLE 93), and $240 mg/m^2$ of DOX or $120 mg/m^2$ DOX plus $180 mg/m^2$ of epirubicin. No significant differences in outcome measures were found.

Methods of administration

Three trials that included 437 patients compared slow infusion (24 or 48 h) with a short 1-h infusion or bolus injection. Median follow-up was 8 years for all trials reviewed. Cumulative doses were $600 mg/m^2$ of DNR, $330 mg/m^2$ of DOX and 60 or $120 mg/m^2$ of DOX plus $144 mg/m^2$ of DNR respectively. No significant differences in outcome were found nor any different effect in any subgroup. The DFCI ALL 91-001 trial reported that both regimens were associated with progressive subclinical cardiotoxicity. Although the MSK-NY-II reported that four children who received bolus anthracycline injection had clinically significant reduction in their cardiac function, this was not statistically significant (p=0.10).

Cardioprotectant use

Two trials that included 568 children comparing anthracycline with the addition of cardioprotectant to the same anthracycline treatment were reviewed. Median follow-up was 6 years. DOX was the anthracycline used in both trials and the cumulative doses were $300 mg/m^2$ and $360 mg/m^2$. There were no significant differences seen for any of the outcome endpoints. The 5-year EFS rates were 77% with and 77.5% without cardioprotectant (95% CI -7.7 to 6.8%).

Conclusions

It was concluded that the limited data from all the reviewed trials did not demonstrate differences in clinically evident cardiotoxicity with the variables studied. While anthracyclines were effective in preventing bone marrow relapses, this did not translate into improved EFS. Also, the evidence on the type of anthracycline, method of administration, or the use of cardioprotectant was insufficient to exclude important differences.

Study 5

Van Dalen EC, Raphaël MF, Caron HN, Kremer LC. Treatment including anthracyclines versus treatment not including anthracyclines for childhood cancer. *Cochrane Database Syst Rev* 2011;1:CD006647.

Objectives

The primary objective of the report was to compare the survival in children with any type of malignancy who received anthracyclines (ANCYN) as part of their treatment with the survival in children who did not receive ANCYN during their treatment. Secondary objectives included evaluation of tumor responses and cardiotoxicity profile in patients of both treatment groups.

Study design

Only randomized controlled trials (RCTs) comparing treatment of childhood cancer with and without ANCYNS were included in the review. While most of the trials reviewed were conducted in children, some included both children and adults but in these trials, children constituted the majority of the trial participants. The maximum age of participants did not exceed 30 years. In the reviewed trials, interventions other than ANCYNs (radiotherapy and/or surgery) were the same in both treatment groups. Although the timing of different aspects of treatment differed between the study groups, the cumulative effect of therapy other than ANCYNs did not differ by >25%

between the study groups. Additionally, prior treatment (where this was applicable) was comparable in both treatment groups.

Electronic searches of MEDLINE/PubMed (from 1966 to March 2010), EMBASE/Ovid (from 1980 to March 2010) and the Cochrane Central Register of Controlled Trials (CENTRAL) (Cochrane Library 2010, Issue 2) was performed to extract relevant RCTs. Information about trials not registered in CENTRAL, MEDLINE or EMBASE either published or unpublished was located by searching the reference lists of relevant articles and review articles. Also included were SIOP and ASCO conference proceedings from 2002 to 2009. Additionally, ongoing trials in the ISRCTN register and the National Institutes of Health register were also screened. Data collection was not restricted by language. Details of reasons for exclusion of any study were clearly stated. Final inclusion of studies was determined by agreement by the two independent reviewers. Data on the following were extracted from all the included trials: study design, number of trial participants including those excluded, randomized and evaluated, age and sex of participants, type of tumor, disease stage, primary or recurrent disease, prior treatment, type of anthracycline, cumulative dose of anthracycline, ANCYN peak dose defined as maximal dose received in 1 week, infusion duration of ANCYN, other treatment including radiotherapy, other chemotherapy agents, surgery, outcome measures, and duration of follow-up.

Statistics

Analysis was based on intention-to-treat principle. If this was not possible, this was stated and analysed "as treated." A random effects model for the estimation of treatment effects was used throughout the review. All results were presented with the corresponding 95% confidence interval. Data were analyzed separately for different types of tumor and, where possible, for different stages and histology. When a particular study outcome was not assessed in >50% of the patients due to an attrition bias, the results were not reported in the outcome measure.

Results

Not all articles allowed data extraction for all the outcome endpoints.

Overall survival

Acute lymphoblastic leukemia

Data on this outcome measure could be extracted from only three trials, that included 912 patients. They showed no significant difference between treatment not including and including ANCYNs (hazard ratio [HR]1.22; 95% CI 0.95–1.57; p=0.13). No heterogeneity was observed.

Wilms tumor

Data on overall survival (OS) could only be extracted from one trial (n = 316 patients). Data were presented for patients with stage II and III disease with favorable histology, stage II and III disease with unfavorable histology, and stage IV disease. Combining all patients, analysis showed a significant difference in favor of treatment that included ANCYN (HR 1.85; 95% CI 1.09–3.15; p=0.02). While for patients with stage II and III disease with favorable histology and stage IV disease, the analyses showed no significant difference between the two treatment groups, for patients with stage II and III disease with unfavorable histology, a significant difference in favor of treatment that included ANCYN was seen (HR 3.1; 95% CI 1.03–9.28; p=0.04). In contrast to the early results, long-term follow-up data showed no significant difference between treatment groups for patients with stage II and III disease with favorable histology or unfavorable histology and for stage IV patients (HR 1.27; 95% CI 0.77–2.11; p=0.34). It was not possible to perform an intention-to-treat analysis for stage IV patients due to variance with the original published data.

Rhabdomyosarcoma and undifferentiated sarcoma

Data could be extracted only from one trial (n=413) with data for stage III and IV patients presented separately. The combination of both treatment groups showed no significant difference between the groups (HR 1.04; 95% CI O.83–1.29; p=0.76). The same was true when each clinical group was analyzed separately. No heterogeneity was detected.

Ewing sarcoma

Overall survival was evaluable only in one trial. Not all patients were evaluable from this trial and not all data for analysis for OS were provided. Nevertheless, there was evidence of a significant survival advantage for patients who received ANCYN compared to those who did not (p=0.02).

Non-Hodgkin lymphoma
Overall survival could not be evaluated since data could not be reliably extracted for analysis.

Hepatoblastoma
Overall survival was evaluated in one trial (n=255). OS was not different between the two treatment groups (HR 1.14; 95% CI 0.41–3.16; p=0.80).

Event-free survival
Acute lymphoblastic leukemia
Data on EFS were extracted from two trials. Outcome analysis showed no significant difference in EFS rates between the two treatment groups (+ANCYN versus – ANCYN; p=0.77).

Wilms tumor
Combining the data of all patients (i.e. stage II–III favorable and unfavorable histology and stage IV disease), outcome analysis showed significantly improved EFS in patients who received treatment that included ANCYNs (HR 2.21; 95% CI 1.44–3.4; –=0.0003). While the long-term outcome data showed a significant difference in EFS in favor of the use of ANCYNs (HR 1.72; 95% CI 1.09–2.72; p=0.02) for patients with stage II or III with favorable or unfavorable histology (HR 1.80; 95% CI 1.04–3.12; p=0.04), no significant difference in EFS was observed for patients with stage IV disease between the two treatment groups.

Rhabomyosarcoma and undifferentiated sarcoma
The EFS could not be evaluated, as data were not reliably extracted.

Ewing sarcoma
The EFS was evaluated in one trial. While only a proportion of patients were eligible for inclusion in the review, there was evidence of a significantly improved EFS for children treated with ANCYNs as compared to those who did not receive ANCYNs (p=0.01).

Non-Hodgkin lymphoma
Data on EFS were evaluable in only one trial (n=284). Analysis did not show any significant difference in EFS between the two treatment groups.

Hepatoblastoma
The EFS was evaluated in only one trial (n=255). No difference in EFS was seen between the two treatment groups (HR 0.81; 95% CI 0.42–1.55; p=0.52).

Tumor response
Acute lymphoblastic leukemia
Data were evaluated from two studies. The meta-analysis did not show any significant difference in response rates between the ANCYN and non-ANCYN group of patients (relative risk [RR] 1.02; 95% CI 0.99–1.06; p=0.22).

Wilms tumor
No information on tumor response was available.

Rhabdomyosarcoma and undifferentiated sarcoma
Data on tumor response were evaluable in only one trial. This did not show any significant difference between the two treatment groups (p=0.95).

Ewing sarcoma and non-Hodgkin lymphoma
No information was available on tumor response.

Hepatoblastoma
This was evaluable in only one trial (n=255). The analysis showed no significant difference between treatment not including and including ANCYNs (RR 1.02; 95% CI 0.96–1.08; p=0.61).

Cardiotoxicity
Cardiac death
Data on cardiac deaths were only available from two trials (n=410) of patients with Wilms tumor or Ewing sarcoma. The meta-analysis did not show any significant difference between treatment not including and including ANCYNs (RR 0.41; 95% CI 1.04–3.89; p=0.44).

Congestive cardiac failure (CCF)

Information on CCF was available only from one trial (n = 413) of patients with rhabdomyosarcoma or undifferentiated sarcoma. Again, analysis did not show any significant difference in CCF rates between the two treatment groups (RR 0.33; 95% CI 0.01–8.02; p = 0.49).

Asymptomatic cardiac dysfunction

Data on asymptomatic cardiac dysfunction were available in only one trial (n = 255). However, due to the high risk of attrition bias (reported in only 49% of the patients), the results of this study were not evaluated.

Conclusions

The authors concluded that while RCTs in ALL did not show any evidence that a treatment program including anthracyclines improved either OS or EFS, evidence of absence does not necessarily suggest there is evidence of no effect. In the case of Wilms tumor, rhabdomyosarcoma/undifferentiated sarcoma, Ewing sarcoma, NHL and hepatoblastoma, as only one RCT was available and evaluable, no definite conclusions could be drawn about the antitumor efficacy of anthracyclines in these tumors. No definitive conclusions on the efficacy of anthracyclines could be drawn about other childhood malignancies, as no RCTs were available for analysis.

CHAPTER 26

Infections in pediatric and adolescent oncology

Ananth Shankar and Sara Stoneham

University College London Hospitals NHS Foundation Trust, London, UK

Commentary by Julia E. Clark

Introduction

Fever is often a marker of infection and in the context of chemotherapy-induced neutropenia, creates great concern, as bacterial infections can be rapidly progressive and have in the past had a significant mortality and morbidity. With the recognition that early antibiotic intervention is vital, the previous high mortality has significantly improved but deaths still occur.

An understanding of the variety of pathogens involved in rapid overwhelming sepsis is vital for informing antibiotic choices. In the 1960s and 1970s gram-negative bacteria initially dominated, with *Pseudomonas*, *Klebsiella* spp. and *E.coli* all having potential for rapid progression and death. With the increasing use of indwelling central venous catheters and thus breaches in skin integument, gram-positive isolates were increasingly recognized. Although coagulase-negative staphylococci are now the most frequently encountered and are the least pathogenic, other gram-positive bacteria such as *Staph.aureus*, group A streptococci and *Strep.pneumoniae* can produce severe overwhelming infection. Drug-resistant gram-positive bacteria are increasingly problematic, although their incidence varies widely across continents, with methicillin-resistant *Staph. aureus* (MRSA) a much more significant pathogen in the US and some parts of Europe than in the UK.

With the historical predominance of gram-negative infections, antibiotic cover initially concentrated on combinations of aminoglycosides with β-lactams, cephalosporins and more recently carbapenems. Many different combinations of these have traditionally been used within individual centers, with each center deciding on local antibiotic choices, guided by local availability, microbiologist and personal physician preferences, experience, cost and local known bacterial prevalence and antibiotic resistance rates.

As gram-positive infection rates increased, empiric febrile neutropenia therapies incorporated cover for both gram-negative and significant gram-positive pathogens. It was still recognized, however, that gram-negative bacteria were associated with greater mortality.

Each center developed its own protocols for treatment regimens and for definitions of febrile neutropenia. Little good evidence informed policies and interventions. This individualization of supportive care by center contrasts starkly with the collaborative approach to chemotherapy and treatment of children with cancer across developed countries.

Having identified this as an issue, trials of antibiotic treatment of children have appeared over the last few years, providing a first evidence base to compare and rationalize treatment. No single antibiotic regimen has been shown to be superior in adult trials and no antibiotic combination will fit all, as local antibiotic availability, pathogens, and resistance patterns must also be considered. The aim should be to deliver the most

---

Evidence-Based Pediatric Oncology, Third Edition. Edited by Ross Pinkerton, Ananth Shankar and Katherine K. Matthay.
© 2013 John Wiley & Sons, Ltd. Published 2013 by John Wiley & Sons, Ltd.

effective, safe, convenient and cost-effective regimen for the local center. Antibiotic regimens need to provide pseudomonal and other gram-negative cover but include some gram-positive activity also.

Previous reliance on aminoglycosides as part of ensuring antipseudomonal cover has limited the development of monotherapy. This is attractive, and in adults as effective, as multidrug combinations. An adult meta-analysis found that β-lactam monotherapy is as effective with fewer side-effects than combined β-lactam and aminoglycoside treatment. Study 7 and Study 13 explore this in children, confirming equivalence of monotherapy with either piptazobactam or carbapenem alone, with a combination of piptazobactam and an aminoglycoside. Neither study documented significant side-effects in either arm.

Monotherapy providing both antipseudomonal activity and gram-positive cover is therefore the logical pathway to follow. But which agent? With many available and more added steadily over the years, no one antibiotic has been found to be superior. The randomized controlled trials (RCTs) identified here provide evidence for equivalence between piptazobactam and cefozopran (Study 6), piptazobactam and imipenem (Study 8), piptazobactam and cefoperazone (Study 9), piptazobactam and cefepime (Study 15). Study 12 demonstrated a slightly better but nonsignificant clinical response to meropenem compared with ceftazidime. Interestingly, this reflects concerns articulated around the activity of ceftazidime on gram-positive bacteria, within the Infectious Diseases Society of America (IDSA) guidelines. Although all the studies examined here are RCTs, numbers remain individually small with each trial generally conducted within an individual center.

Risk stratification

Most children with febrile neutropenia respond quickly to rapid and empiric antibiotics without a problem. It is clear, however, that the risk for dissemination of infection or complications varies with underlying disease, current illness presentation, chemotherapy regimen, degree and duration of neutrophil suppression and presence or absence of central venous catheter (CVC). Recognizing that many children may receive prolonged aggressive intravenous therapy when at low risk of severe bacterial infection,

developing ways to identify children at "high and low" risk of infection has been attempted. Risk assessment/ risk clarification or risk prediction rules are increasingly used to tailor modified antibiotic treatment for low-risk patients. As described in Study 11, many different rules are used in clinical practice, all incorporating variables within the child, episode, laboratory tests and presence or absence of CVC. No clear combination of variables predicts low or high risk, though all appear safe in terms of serious outcomes.

Studies 10 and 14 explore using oral instead of intravenous (IV) regimes in low-risk patients. Both studies are relatively small with, as expected, very low rates of active infection and are therefore difficult to draw definite conclusions from. Study 10 compares oral therapy right from the start of the febrile neutropenia episode with intravenous antibiotics, noting no difference in outcome. Study 14 gives both groups an initial one day of intravenous therapy and then compares an oral regime which has antipseudomonal cover with an IV regime which does not. In this study, children with definite bacteremia were excluded from continuing with the oral regimen. On the limited data that these studies provide, it does appear that in very highly selective groups at very low risk of gram-negative and gram-positive infections, combinations of oral antibiotics which include both gram-positive and gram-negative cover are safe. Larger numbers are needed to demonstrate this effectively. Care needs to be taken that the oral and IV groups compared have comparable antibiotic efficacy.

Fungal infection

Fungal infections rarely are identified in early febrile neutropenia, but are frequently a cause of prolonged fever with neutropenia. *Candida* is associated with hematogenous spread, often from colonization of mucosal surfaces. Molds take hold more often after a prolonged neutropenia of greater than 2 weeks. Fungal infections are rightly feared, as established proven fungal infection can be extremely difficult to treat, with a high morbidity and mortality. The antifungal drugs available for treatment are more limited than antibiotics, with long durations of treatment required. Unfortunately, specific data on antifungal prophylaxis or treatment of children have been limited, mainly derived from pediatric subgroup analyses from predominantly adult trials.

That three pediatric trials are described (Studies 1, 2 and 5) with a fourth, a Cochrane review (Study 4) is a great step forward.

Antifungal prophylaxis

Prevention is better than cure and, historically, fluconazole prophylaxis has been used in high-risk patients perceived to be at risk of invasive fungal infections. As *Candida* is a widespread colonizer of human mucosa, invasive candidal infections are well recognized in children undergoing chemotherapy. Adult trials and meta-analyses have established that fluconazole does decrease the incidence of invasive *Candida* infections in high-risk adult patients with cancer. However, fluconazole is not effective for molds and therefore would not be expected to decrease the frequency of mold infections. Thus, fluconazole would not be expected to be useful in children with prolonged neutropenia when *Aspergillus* infections are more likely. From this argument arose the concept for Study 3. This study, despite being in a high-risk population with good numbers of patients in each arm, had relatively few episodes of invasive fungal infection (55) and showed no difference in the rate of invasive fungal infection between fluconazole and voriconazole. As with many antifungal studies, relatively few children were included; only 24 received fluconazole and 27 voriconazole. It is increasingly apparent that voriconazole (and indeed other azole) efficacy is related to maintaining adequate drug levels. One possible explanation for the unexpected failure of voriconazole to decrease invasive fungal infections compared with fluconazole may be that this study did not encompass therapeutic drug monitoring and thus could not ensure adequate drug levels.

Study 5 compared fluconazole to oral nystatin. Although showing no difference in invasive candidal infection in either group, this was a very small study with 50 patients in both arms and is too small to conclude equivalence.

In practice, the concern around mold infections as well as *Candida* infections has meant that, historically, most children at very high risk of fungal infection, when offered antifungal prophylaxis, received itraconazole. Study 2 randomized 44 children with itraconazole against 43 given placebo after autologous stem cell transplant. In this small single-center study, no episode of invasive fungal infection (IFI) occurred in the short time frame observed (30 days), making it difficult to interpret the potential benefit. The absence of IFI is reassuring, suggesting that the fungal risk in this group of children was sufficiently low to make prophylaxis less attractive. Reassuringly, there was no difference in side-effects between itraconazole and placebo.

These three studies, although providing some welcome additional information on the efficacy of prophylaxis in children with high-risk cancer, are individually too small or flawed to give a good evidence-based answer. Prophylaxis policies are not informed by strong pediatric evidence and pediatric recommendations are derived from adult studies. Voriconazole and posaconazole are variously suggested for those at highest risk, with itraconazole next. There is concern that tolerability of itraconazole is poor and absorption, and thus consistent levels, are difficult to achieve. However, no studies on children have looked at either voriconazole or posaconazole levels in prophylaxis. None of the studies (Study 2, 3 or 5) help to move this discussion onwards as relatively small numbers of children are included, with very low fungal infection rates and without examining effective drug levels in the population studies.

Empirical antifungal therapy

Suspicion is raised when a child has persistent neutropenia and a fever despite more than 4 days of empirical antibiotic therapy. At this stage, empirical antifungal therapy can be started and often is in high-risk patients. Study 1 deserves note as one of the first pediatric, multicenter, antifungal RCTs. This study compared caspofungin with liposomal amphotericin in 82 children with comparable outcomes. National and international guidelines agree that both liposomal amphotericin and caspofungin be recommended as empirical therapy. This study adds at least some pediatric data to these recommendations.

The data from Study 1 were included in Study 4, a first meta-analysis of antifungal use in pediatric patients. Seven studies were identified but despite this, numbers of children remained low and confusingly covered both empirical and proven fungal infection. A huge limitation in gaining appropriate and relevant data in children appears to be that although numerous studies are available comparing different combinations of first-line antifungals, pediatric subgroup analysis is rarely provided. There are, therefore, many limitations to this meta-analysis. Within these, however, similar results to adult studies are obtained. No difference in outcome as measured by mortality was seen between liposomal amphotericin and conventional amphotericin or caspofungin. Lipid preparations have a reduced nephrotoxic effect.

Thus, this Cochrane review (Study 4) found no differences in mortality and morbidity between different antifungal treatments in children with neutropenia and prolonged fever (as a proxy for suspected fungal infection) or with *Candida* or invasive candidiasis. On the basis of this, liposomal amphotericin or caspofungin are equivalent and either can be considered. Interestingly, the role of voriconazole in empirical treatment of suspected fungal infection has very limited evidence in children. This must be borne in mind when examining well-recognized guidelines, as all of these suggest voriconazole as a recommended first-line treatment followed by liposomal amphotericin for invasive pulmonary aspergillosis.

Central venous catheter infections

Central venous catheter infections are increasingly recognized as being important in terms of morbidity and occasionally mortality and are avoidable with exemplary infection control and central venous line care. Many centers now monitor catheter-related bloodstream infections (CRBSI) and catheter-associated infections (CAI) rates in both short- and long-term CVCs. There is a good literature on reported CVC infection rates within pediatric hematology oncology patients, with quoted rates varying from around one to over seven per 100,000 line-days. Many centers incorporate multiple infection control practices as "bundling" to reduce CVC rates. These local strategies for insertion, management, and removal of catheters optimize infection control. Techniques include sterile insertion technique, use of 2% chlorhexidine as wipes and dressings, aseptic no-touch technique for accessing devices, daily site inspection, and chlorhexidine-impregnated catheter dressings.

Within very vulnerable populations with indwelling catheters and immunosuppression and, therefore, multiple risk factors such as chemotherapy, neutropenia and bone marrow transplant, other strategies to decrease infection rates have been explored. These have variously included antiseptic-impregnated, silver-impregnated, and antibiotic-impregnated catheters, antibiotic locks, and urokinase locks. Antibiotic locks have been the most frequently studied and it is pleasing that the Cochrane review (Study 20) in 2010 could identify five pediatric trials. That the baseline risk of 1.7 bloodstream infections per 100,000 catheter-days was low is also reassuring and when rates of catheter infections are low, it appears that the extra additional benefit confirmed by an antibiotic lock is of only limited benefit.

Study 19 compares minocycline and edetic acid (M-EDTA) with heparin in a small group of children with portacaths. Although at first sight this study is encouraging, the baseline heparin group infection rate of 6.3 per 1000 compared to the M-EDTA rate of 1.09 per 1000 is far too high as a comparative group. Portacath CRBSIs are documented as being less frequent than even tunneled CVCs and this high background rate would be expected to improve with most interventions. There is therefore no evidence on the basis of this study that M-EDTA would be of additional benefit when rates were lower. Study 20 concluded the same about urokinase and decreasing dressing changes.

With the increasing, widespread acceptance that uniform procedures and education around catheter care insertion and management can dramatically decrease CRBSIs, the ability to conduct RCTs on these interventions in a specific pediatric cancer population diminishes rapidly. There are, therefore, no RCTs exploring these interventions in children with cancer. It is increasingly important that centers looking after children with catheters on chemotherapy monitor their local CVC infection rates and local bacterial isolate and resistant patterns of bacteria. In the future, RCTs of further inventions such as comparison of different strengths of antibiotic locks, other antibiotics or antiseptics such as tauraline locks need to be introduced only in the context of optimal line care packages being in place. This will allow comparison between trials and give a true indication of the additional benefit of any intervention.

Antibiotic and antifungal regimes are dependent as far as possible on a good evidence base for best and safest antimicrobial but may require adjustment depending on local epidemiology. To this end, centers where children with immunocompromise are managed should have a good antimicrobial stewardship program and specialist infectious disease knowledge.

New studies

Fungal infections

Study 1

Maertens JA, Madero L, Reilly AF *et al.*, for the Caspofungin Pediatric Study Group. A randomized, double blind, multicenter study of caspofungin versus liposomal amphotericin B for empiric antifungal therapy in pediatric patients with persistent fever and neutropenia. *Pediatr Infect Dis J* 2010;**29**:415–20.

Objectives

The main aim of this study was to compare the safety, tolerability, and efficacy of caspofungin with liposomal amphotericin in the empirical treatment of suspected invasive fungal infections in neutropenic children with persistent fever.

Study design

This was a prospective randomized double-blind study conducted in 117 centers in the USA and Europe between June 2004 and September 2007. Children between 2 and 17 years of age were enrolled on the study if they had received chemotherapy for cancer or had undergone hematopoietic stem cell transplantation (HSCT) and also had received parenteral antibiotics for at least 96h and were persistently neutropenic (absolute neutrophil counts [ANC] < 500/mm³) and febrile (temperature > 38.0 °C).

Patients with inadequately managed bacterial infections or documented invasive fungal infections at the time of enrollment were excluded. Other exclusion criteria were serum bilirubin > 3 times upper normal limit, aspartate aminotransferase (AST)/alanine aminotransferase (ALT) > 5 times upper normal limit and patients on cyclosporine or rifampicin.

Randomization was stratified according to risk category and blinding was maintained by means of a double-blind, double-dummy procedure. Patients who had undergone allogeneic bone marrow or peripheral stem cell transplantation or were on treatment for relapsed acute leukemia were categorized as high-risk patients. Randomization was performed by a computer-generated schedule on a 2:1 ratio and patients were assigned to receive IV caspofungin (70 mg/m² loading dose and then 50 mg/m²/day with a maximum of 70 mg/day) plus placebo (corresponding to ambisome) or ambisome (3 mg/kg/day) or plus placebo (corresponding to caspofungin). The dosage of caspofungin and ambisome could be increased in children who had persistent fever exceeding 5 days and with deteriorating clinical condition on the discretion of the treating physician – ambisome to 5 mg/kg/day and caspofungin to 70 mg/m² (maximum 70 mg/day).

Antifungal treatment was continued for an additional 72h after resolution of neutropenia for a maximum of 28 days in children without documented invasive fungal infection but for children who had invasive fungal infection, it was recommended that treatment be continued for at least 14 days or at least for an additional 7 days after resolution of neutropenia.

Treatment was considered successful if all the following criteria were met: successful treatment of fungal infection, absence of breakthrough fungal infection during treatment or within 7 days of completing treatment, survival for 7 days after completing treatment, no premature discontinuation of therapy because of drug-related toxicity or lack of efficacy, and resolution of fever during neutropenia.

Statistics

The main safety evaluation was the proportion of patients with one or more (clinical and/or laboratory) drug-related adverse events during the study therapy plus 14 days post treatment. The proportion of patients and its respective 95% Clopper Pearson exact confidence interval (Proc–StatXact 5, Cytel Software Corporation, Cambridge, MA) were calculated for both treatment groups. The main efficacy analysis was conducted in a modified intention-to-treat population comprising patients with persistent febrile neutropenia who received at least one dose of the study antifungal agent. The main efficacy evaluation was the proportion of patients who had an overall favorable response defined as meeting all the five response criteria. Observed proportions and their respective 95% Clopper Pearson exact confidence intervals (CIs) were calculated for the overall response and for each of the five individual components. Observed proportions were within each treatment group according to risk strata and the estimated proportions of patients with a favorable response was calculated using the Cochran Mantel Haenzel weights adjusted to risk strata and the their respective 95% CIs.

Results

Of the 83 patients randomized (caspofungin 57 patients and ambisome 26 patients), only 82 received the study therapy (one patient in the caspofungin group was not treated). Baseline demographics were balanced between the two groups and most patients in the study were categorized as low risk. Previous antifungal prophylaxis as well as the type of antifungal prophylaxis was also similar between the two treatment groups of patients. The median duration of therapy was 11.6 days (range 3–36) and 11.4 days (range 1–55) in the caspofungin and ambisome groups respectively. The study drug dosage was increased in three patients in the caspofungin group (1.8%) versus two patients in the ambisome group (7.7%).

The overall drug-related clinical adverse events were similar in both randomized groups. Although three patients died during treatment, none of the deaths was drug related and all deaths occurred 7 days after end of therapy. However, the drug-related laboratory adverse events were lower in the caspofungin group (3.6%) compared to the ambisome group (11.5%). None of the drug-related laboratory adverse events led to discontinuation of treatment in either group. The most common laboratory adverse event was hypokalemia in both treatment groups of children.

Although patients randomized to caspofungin had a better overall favorable response (46.4%) compared to ambisome (32%), the 95% CIs overlapped as the study was not powered to detect a statistically significant difference between the two treatment groups. Although in the low-risk group, the overall favorable response was similar (caspofungin 41.5% versus 44.4% ambisome), patients randomized to caspofungin had a better overall response in the high-risk group of patients compared to those in the ambisome group (9/15; 60% versus none; 0%). In both treatment groups, higher efficacy responses were seen in acute

myeloid leukemia (AML) patients than in acute lymphoblastic leukemia (ALL) patients, solid tumors or other hematological malignancies.

Although there were no differences between the two treatment groups with respect to three efficacy components (successful treatment of baseline fungal infections, absence of breakthrough infections and survival for at least 7 days after completion of treatment), response rates for successful completion of therapy and resolution of fever during treatment were slightly higher in the caspofungin group. Premature discontinuation of therapy occurred in 3.6% of patients in the caspofungin group compared to 12% in the ambisome group.

Conclusions

It was concluded that ambisome and caspofungin were comparable in tolerability, safety, and efficacy as empirical antifungal therapy in children with persistent febrile neutropenia.

Study 2

Kim YJ, Sung KW, Hwang HS *et al.* Efficacy of itraconazole prophylaxis for autologous stem cell transplantation in children with high-risk solid tumors: a prospective double blind randomized study. *Yonsei Med J* 2011;**52**:293–300.

Objectives

The primary aim of the study was to evaluate in a randomized manner the efficacy of itraconazole prophylaxis in preventing IFI in children undergoing autologous HSCT (AHSCT) after high-dose chemotherapy (HDCT).

Study design

This single-center randomized study was conducted between April 2006 and March 2008 and included 55 children with high-risk solid tumors who underwent AHSCT as part of their treatment. All patients were randomized in a double-blind manner to receive either itraconazole prophylaxis (2.5 mg/kg/dose twice daily×2 days followed by 2.5 mg/kg/dose daily) or a placebo. Both itraconazole and placebo were commenced when the ANC fell $< 0.5 \times 10^9$/L after HDCT.

All antibiotics including itraconazole were discontinued after 3 consecutive days when the patient was afebrile (<37.5°C) with no evidence of documented infection and an ANC >0.5×10⁹/L. Tests for serum *Aspergillus* antigen was performed in a few patients.

Patients were assessed for development of IFI for a period of 30 days after AHSCT and all adverse events were recorded until 30 days after AHSCT or at the time of discharge. Costs between the two groups were compared in terms of duration of hospitalization and cost of total treatment during the transplantation period including the cost of antimicrobial agents.

Statistics

While the chi-square test was performed to compare the frequency of factors that were thought to have increased the risk of fungal infections, the student's *t* test was performed to compare the total duration of fever, antibiotic usage, duration of hospitalization, and treatment costs. Differences in the frequencies of various toxicities between the two groups were analyzed using the chi-square test.

Results

Although 87 transplant episodes were included in this report (43 in the prophylactic group and 44 in the placebo group), two patients were excluded because of early death and, hence, only 85 transplant episodes were analyzed. Patient characteristics between the two groups were similar and the clinical parameters for developing an invasive fungal infection were comparable between the two groups of patients.

While no case of probable, possible or proven case of fungal infection occurred in either group of patients, duration of fever >38°C was significantly shorter in the group who received itraconazole prophylaxis (4.7 ± 2.4 days versus 6.5 ± 3.5 days; p=0.007). Additionally, the number of patients who had fever >7 days as well as the number of patients who required second-line antibiotics were lower in the itraconazole prophylaxis group. Multivariate analysis revealed that prophylactic use of itraconazole was associated with shorter duration of fever.

There were no differences in the development of serious adverse events between the two groups of patients even though the itraconazole prophylaxis group received itraconazole for a longer duration (13.9 ± 2.8 days versus 8.9 ± 3.8 days; p < 0.001).

Although the duration of hospital stay was shorter in the prophylaxis group, this was not statistically significant. Similarly, there were no significant differences in the total cost of treatment during hospitalization or in the total cost of antimicrobial agents.

Conclusions

It was concluded that even though itraconazole prophylaxis led to shorter duration of fever as well as reduced need for antibiotic usage, the results were not sufficiently robust to recommend the routine use of itraconazole as antifungal prophylaxis in children undergoing stem cell transplantation for solid tumors.

Study 3

Wingard JR, Carter SL, Walsh TJ *et al.*, for the Blood and Marrow Transplant Clinical Trials Network. Randomized, double blind trial of fluconazole versus voriconazole for prevention of invasive fungal infection after allogeneic hematopoietic cell transplantation. *Blood* 2010;**116**:5111–18.

Objectives

The main aim of this randomized study was to compare fluconazole versus voriconazole in preventing invasive fungal infections after allogeneic bone marrow transplantation. The study included adults and children and while results in the report are all inclusive, personal communication from the author (RW) has provided some additional information in those <18 years of age.

Study design

This randomized multicenter trial of fluconazole versus voriconazole was conducted between November 2003 and September 2006 in 35 centers participating in the Blood and Marrow Transplant Clinical Trials network. Patients ≥2 years of age who met the trial eligibility criteria were randomly assigned to voriconazole or fluconazole before transplantation. Exclusion criteria included prior invasive yeast infection within 8 weeks of study entry, mold infection within 4 months of study entry, uncontrolled bacterial or viral infection at the time of study entry or were receiving treatment known to have adverse interaction with voriconazole and fluconazole.

The study drugs were masked by overencapsulation and doses were fluconazole 400 mg/once daily and voriconazole 200 mg twice daily. Where possible, both medications were administered orally within an hour of a meal and where oral administration was difficult, intravenous formulations were used. Children <12 years of age received lower doses. Study drugs were continued from days 0 to 100 post transplantation. However, for patients who were receiving prednisolone 1 mg/kg/day (or an equivalent steroid dose), or those who received a T-cell-depleted graft and required graft-versus-host disease prophylaxis or had a CD4 count <200/μL on days 90–100, antifungal prophylaxis continued to day 180 post transplantation. Early study withdrawal was mandated if unequivocal IFI was documented, development of grade 3 or 4 toxicity attributable to study drugs or relapse of disease. All patients who were withdrawn from the study prematurely received open-label fluconazole prophylaxis.

A short course of empirical antifungal therapy (maximum 14 days) with either an amphotericin B formulation or caspofungin during clinical evaluation to confirm or exclude IFI was permitted. However, during this empirical antifungal treatment, the randomized study drug was continued.

Proven IFI was defined as histopathological or cytopathological demonstration of fungal molds or yeast in deep tissue with clinical and radiological consistent with an infection. Presumptive IFI was defined as presence of at least one clinical criterion for lower respiratory tract infection for possible IFI and bronchoscopic examination that excluded another etiology.

The primary endpoint was failure-free survival (FFS) at day 180 post transplantation while the secondary endpoints were incidence of IFIs, time to IFI, 6-month and 1-year relapse-free survival (RFS) and overall survival (OS), frequency, time to and duration of empirical antifungal therapy, frequency of severe adverse events and incidence of acute and chronic graft-versus-host disease.

Statistics

Randomization was performed in a 1:1 ratio using permuted random blocks for the voriconazole and fluconazole arms and stratified by treatment center and donor type (sibling versus unrelated donor). Primary analysis was performed on an intention-to-treat principle with a two-sided hypothesis. FFS, OS, and RFS were estimated using the Kaplan–Meier life table method. The Gray test was used to compare the two

treatment arms. The Cox proportional hazards models were used to assess risk factors for FFS and IFI. Patients who did not experience an event were censored at last follow-up visit. A significance level of 0.10 was used in a stepwise model selection.

Results

Six hundred patients were randomized (voriconazole n=305 and fluconazole n=295). Baseline factors (i.e. patient, disease, and transplant characteristics) were balanced in the treatment arms. Only 8% were under the age of 18 (similar in both groups). While the OS for the whole cohort was 80.6% at 6 months and 69% at 12 months, age <18 years in both treatment arms was associated with better OS. There were no differences in the OS at 180 days (p=0.67) or at 12 months (p=0.59) between the two groups.

Fifty-five patients developed IFI (proven 14, probable 24 and presumptive 17) by day 180 post transplantation. The cumulative incidence rates of IFIs at day 180 and 1 year post transplantation were 11.2% and 7.3% (p=0.12) and 13.7% and 12.7% (p=0.59) for the fluconazole and voriconazole treatment arms respectively. There were no differences in the rate of proven and probable IFIs at 100, 180, and 365 days between the two treatment arms. Similarly, FFS rates were comparable for the two treatment arms (p=0.49). Age <18 years was associated with better fungal-free survival in both treatment groups.

There were no significant drug toxicities reported. Photopsia was the most common adverse effect reported (18 in the fluconazole arm and 21 in the voriconazole arm).

Conclusions

It was concluded that both fluconazole and voriconazole were similarly efficacious when administered prophylactically to prevent invasive fungal infections in allogeneic hematopoietic transplant recipients.

Study 4

Blyth C, Hale K, Palasanthiran P, O'Brien T, Bennett M. Antifungal therapy in infants and children with proven, probable or suspected invasive fungal infections. *Cochrane Database Syst Rev* 2010;**2**:CD006343.

Objectives

To review systematically and summarize the effects of different antifungal therapies in children with proven, probable or suspected invasive fungal infections.

Study design

The authors considered all randomized and quasi-randomized trials. Neonates and children older than 16 were excluded from the analysis.

Proven or probable invasive fungal infection was defined as clinical illness consistent with infection plus either radiological, histopathological or microbiological evidence of invasive fungal disease. Suspected invasive fungal infection was defined pragmatically as an individual clinician's choice to prescribe a systemic antifungal agent based on the clinical suspicion of invasive fungal infection in the absence of a confirmed diagnosis.

Trials including any of the following agents were considered: conventional amphotericin B deoxycholate; lipid preparations of amphotericin B; amphotericin B colloidal dispersion (ABCD); amphotericin B lipid complex (ABLC); 5-fluorocytosine; azoles; echinocandins or monoclonal antibodies. The authors considered any dose designed to have a therapeutic effect and accepted trials that compared different systemic antifungal agents or combination of agents, no treatment or inactive placebo. Trials considering antifungal prophylaxis were excluded.

The outcome measures considered were classified into primary and secondary outcomes. Primary outcomes included all-cause mortality, invasive fungal infection-related mortality, and complete resolution of invasive fungal infection. Secondary outcomes included a range of adverse reactions and toxicities commonly associated with antifungal agents, partial response or progression, with quality-of-life considerations and cost included in the criteria.

The authors searched electronic databases as follows: Cochrane Central Register of Controlled Trials, MEDLINE, EMBASE, and CINAHL. Other sources were considered including letters, abstracts, and unpublished trials. To extend their search, they contacted experts in the field and leading authors in an attempt to minimize publication bias.

All analyses from a synthesized database were performed using the RevMan 5.0 software.

Results

Trials were selected for inclusion by two review authors. Of a total of 3305 potentially relevant trials, only 30 were deemed eligible for full-text review. Of these, only seven were either performed in children or had sufficient pediatric subgroup analysis to satisfy the inclusion criteria.

The seven trials analyzed were as follows. Four RCTs enrolling 395 children comparing a liquid preparation of amphotericin B with conventional amphotericin in patients with prolonged neutropenic sepsis. A single study compared caspofungin with liposomal amphotericin B in suspected fungal infection. Micafungin was compared with liposomal amphotericin B in children with invasive candidiasis. The final trial enrolled 43 children to compare enteral fluconazole with enteral itraconazole in children with proven invasive fungal infection.

There was no significant difference found in all-cause mortality or mortality related to fungal infection across all groups. Complete resolution of documented fungal infections was recorded in only two patients. Most episodes were documented by fever resolution.

The probability of a fever resolution with a lipid preparation compared with conventional amphotericin B was of borderline significance relative risk (RR) of fever resolution with a lipid preparation was 1.23; 95% CI 1.00–1.52; p=0.05).

No progression of fungal disease was reported. Three trials reported breakthrough fungal infection. Pooled analyses demonstrated that no significant differences in breakthrough infection rates were observed between use of lipid or conventional amphotericin. (RR 0.67; 95% CI 0.24–1.84; p=0.43). Although patients randomized to caspofungin did not demonstrate breakthrough infection when compared with the 4% who received liposomal amphotericin, this did not fall within significance (RR 0.15; 95% CI 0.01–3.61; p=0.24).

Comparison of conventional and liposomal amphotericin preparations demonstrated that similar numbers of patients discontinued therapy for reasons of toxicity or lack of efficacy. The only significant differences in secondary outcome measures in children with fever and neutropenia were reduced (a) nephrotoxicity and (b) chills with lipid preparations of amphotericin B when compared with conventional amphotericin B; and (c) increased chills with ABCD compared with conventional amphotericin B. No significant differences were found in any of the other analyses. No study addressed quality of life or cost.

Conclusions

Few significant differences were observed in pediatric antifungals trials in children with prolonged fever and neutropenia and candidemia and candidiasis. No differences in mortality or efficacy were observed. However, there were noted to be numerous deficiencies in the pediatric literature. Pediatric data are insufficient to address the role of triazole drugs particularly in children with prolonged fever and neutropenia and candidemia or invasive candidiasis. The authors concluded that further RCT antifungal trials enrolling children are required.

Study 5

Groll A, Just-Nuebling G, Kurz M *et al.* Fluconazole versus nystatin in the prevention of Candida infections in children and adolescents undergoing remission induction or consolidation chemotherapy for cancer. *J Antimicrob Chemother* 1997;40:855–62.

Objectives

To assess the efficacy and safety of oral fluconazole against oral nystatin in preventing *Candida* infections in children undergoing remission induction or consolidation therapy for cancer.

Study design

Fifty patients between the ages of 6 months and 16 years were enrolled to an open prospective, randomized single-center pilot study in which patients were randomized to receive either fluconazole 3 mg/kg/day once daily or oral nystatin 50,000 iu/kg/day q6h. Chemoprophylaxis commenced at the start of a cycle. It was continued until resolution of neutropenia for that episode or throughout each cycle. Endpoints for assessment were incidence of superficial fungal infections, initiation of empirical antifungal infection for suspected systemic fungal infection, confirmed systemic fungal infections and orointestinal colonization at baseline, during and after end of prophylaxis.

Off-study criteria included prophylaxis failure, initiation of antifungal therapy, or grade 3–4 drug

toxicities. No patient had a documented fungal infection at enrollment or had been on any antifungal treatment within the week prior to enrollment.

Mycological evaluation was obtained at baseline and then weekly and at the end of prophylaxis. Assessment was made via stool samples and oropharyngeal swabs.

Statistics

Statistical evaluation was performed by chi-squared analysis or Fisher exact test. Continuous variables were compared by the Mann-Whitney U test.

Results

The most common underlying disease conditions were hematological malignancies (30/50). The nystatin group had a higher percentage of patients with hematological malignancies (19 versus 11; $p < 0.05$) along with a lower mean age (5 versus 7.4 years; $p < 0.05$) and more frequent steroid administration (14 versus 9; $p =$ not significant). The fluconazole group received more frequent broad-spectrum antibiotic therapy (11 versus 6) and more often exhibited ANC < 500/mL (14 versus 10).

The mean duration of prophylaxis was 31 days with fluconazole and 30 days with nystatin. Twenty-one out of 25 in the fluconazole and 20/25 in the nystatin group had a successful outcome from chemoprophylaxis. Mild and transient oropharyngeal candidiasis was observed in two and three of the patients in the fluconazole and nystatin groups respectively. One patient randomized to fluconazole and two to nystatin required empirical treatment with amphotericin B. One patient assigned to fluconazole developed tissue-proven *Candida* colitis. Noncolonized patients at the start remained yeast free with no differences between the two arms. Patients colonized at the start remained colonized but at the end of the study those on nystatin harbored more yeasts ($p = 0.05$). *Candida albicans* was isolated in 95% of involved cases. No *Candida* species resistant to nystatin or fluconazole were identified in any patient. No significant differences in toxicity were seen.

Conclusions

Fluconazole was as safe and effective as nystatin in controlling yeast colonization and in preventing superficial and invasive *Candida* infections and the empirical use of amphotericin B in children and adolescents undergoing intensive chemotherapy for cancer.

Bacterial infections

Study 6

Ichikawa M, Suzuki D, Ohshima J *et al.* Piperacillin/tazobactam versus cefozopran for the empirical treatment of pediatric cancer patients with febrile neutropenia. *Pediatr Blood Cancer* 2011;**57**:1159–62.

Objectives

The study aimed to evaluate the efficacy and safety of piperacillin/tazobactam (PIP/TAZ) and cefozopran (CZOP) monotherapy in pediatric cancer patients with febrile neutropenia (FBN).

Study design

This was a single-center prospective randomized open comparative study conducted between January 2009 and June 2010.

Children and adolescents younger than 19 years of age were enrolled on the study if they had received chemotherapy for hematological or solid tumor malignancies. An episode of fever was defined as a temperature of ≥37.5 °C taken on two separate occasions 1 h apart or a single axillary temperature >38°C. Neutropenia was defined as an ANC <500/mm³. Exclusion criteria for study enrollment were:

- patients older than 19 years of age
- recent antimicrobial treatment within the last 14 days before start of treatment
- oral fluconazole or intravenous micafungin therapy for documented invasive fungal infections at the time of enrollment
- fever due to blood product transfusions due to administration of granulocyte colony-stimulating factor (G-CSF)
- known allergic conditions
- renal/hepatic impairment
- protocol violations.

Some patients were randomized more than once if they had a separate FBN episode that was treated at 2 weeks earlier.

After clinical evaluation and routine investigations together with chest x-ray and cultures of blood, urine, and stool, including wound and cerebrospinal fluid (CSF) if appropriate, patients were assigned to receive IV PIP/TAZ (125 mg/kg q8h or CZOP 25 mg/kg q6h). Antibiotic treatment was continued until patients had remained afebrile for 5 days and signs of infection had resolved. Antibiotics were modified according to culture sensitivities or if there was worsening of the child's clinical status. Success of treatment was defined as resolution of fever and symptoms within 120 h of start of antibiotic treatment with no recurrence after stopping treatment.

Outcome endpoints included duration of fever and neutropenia, the need for modification of antibiotic treatment, and deaths.

Statistics

The Mann-Whitney U test was used to compare independent continuous variables. While the Pearson chi-square test was used to compare categorical data, the Fisher exact test was used to compare small numbers. A p-value <0.05 (two-tailed) was considered statistically significant.

Results

A total of 119 febrile episodes were documented in 49 patients in this study. There were no significant differences in the clinical characteristics between the two randomized groups of patients.

While blood cultures were positive in 24 (20.2%) of the episodes, there were no differences in the blood culture positivity rates amongst the two randomized groups of patients. The percentage of susceptible bacteria isolated from blood was not significantly different between the groups (10/14 in the PIP/TAZ group versus 4/10 in the CZOP group) and there were no difference in the success rates between the PIP/TAZ and CZOP treatment arms. During the study period, no modifications were made to the initial randomized antibiotic regimens because of adverse side-effects in either group. The duration of fever or antibiotic therapy was similar in both groups of patients.

Conclusions

It was concluded that piperacillin plus tazobactam and cefozopran were both similarly effective and equally safe in the initial empirical treatment of febrile neutropenia in children with cancer.

Study 7

Zengin E, Sarper N, Kılıç SC. Piperacillin/tazobactam monotherapy versus piperacillin/tazobactam plus amikacin as initial empirical therapy for febrile neutropenia in children with acute leukemia. *Pediatr Hematol Oncol* 2011;28:311–20.

Objectives

To compare the efficacy and safety of piperacillin/tazobactam (PIPTAZ) versus PIPTAZ plus amikacin in the treatment of febrile neutropenia in children with acute leukemia.

Study design

This was a single-center prospective randomized trial conducted between March 2007 and March 2008. Children and adolescents with acute leukemia (AL) who developed febrile neutropenia (FBN) were randomized to receive either PIPTAZ (360 mg/kg/day) versus the same dose of PIPTAZ plus amikacin (15 mg/kg/day as a single dose). If patients still had a fever 96 h after commencement of empirical antibiotic treatment, teicoplanin (10 mg/kg/dose) was added in the absence of any positive cultures and if fever persisted beyond 120 h or if there was clinical suspicion or radiological evidence of an invasive fungal infection, amphotericin B (conventional or liposomal) was added. All antimicrobials were discontinued after 7 afebrile days if the patient had shown clinical improvement or a documented infection was deemed eradicated.

Catheter-related bacteremia was defined as isolation of the same pathogen from the central venous catheter and peripheral blood while catheter infection was defined as isolation of the pathogen from blood drawn from the catheter. Clinically documented infection was considered when there was a focus of infection on clinical examination but without microbiological confirmation. Proven IFI was defined when there was a positive culture and/or histology whereas probable IFI was based on clinical and radiological findings. Possible infection was considered when there was no clinical or microbiological evidence of infection in a febrile episode.

Success of an intervention was defined as resolution of fever and other signs of infection and/or eradication of the micro-organism and maintenance of response for at least 7 days after discontinuation of treatment.

Success without modification was eradication of the pathogen with initial empirical therapy while modification was defined as addition of teicoplanin and or other antimicrobials including antifungals and/or antiviral agents to the empirical therapy. Protocol failure was defined as withdrawal of the empirical therapy and introduction of new agents due to failure to control the infection and treatment failure was defined as persistence of fever or infection or infection-related death despite modification or substitution of empirical treatment with new antimicrobials.

Statistics

Comparisons between the two groups were analysed by the chi-square, Fisher exact and Mann-Whitney tests. Statistical significance was determined at $p < 0.05$.

Results

All gram-positive isolates were sensitive to teicoplanin whereas one gram-negative isolate from the urine was resistant to PIPTAZ. Among the gram-negative isolates, there was no isolate that was sensitive only to amikacin. Although not statistically significant, the number of catheter isolates was higher in the PIPTAZ arm.

In the PIPTAZ and PIPTAZ plus amikacin arms, there were 20 (25) febrile episodes and 17 (22) episodes respectively. Treatment success was similar in both arms. Additionally, the number of clinical and microbiologically documented infections, addition of glycopeptides, and the duration of neutropenia/hospitalization were not different with or without central venous catheters between the two groups.

There were 18 febrile episodes (10 PIPTAZ and 8 PIPTAZ plus amikacin) after high-dose cytosine arabinoside chemotherapy. Success rates were similar with both treatment arms ($p > 0.05$).

Treatment success without modification was 44.4%. There were no significant differences between the two treatment arms with regard to median duration of FBN, defervescence of fever, duration of antibiotic treatment, modification of empirical therapy or treatment success ($p > 0.05$).

Toxicity

No serious adverse events were observed in either treatment arm. One patient in the PIPTAZ plus amikacin arm experienced nephrotoxicity that subsided after discontinuation of amikacin. This patient did not receive amphotericin B.

Conclusions

It was concluded that empirical therapy with piperacillin/tazobactam alone was effective in the treatment of febrile neutropenic episodes in children with acute leukemia and the addition of amikacin did not improve treatment success.

Study 8

Vural S, Erdem E, Gulec SG, Yildirmak Y, Kebudi R. Imipenem-cilastatin versus piperacillin-tazobactam as monotherapy in febrile neutropenia. *Pediatr Int* 2010;**52**:262–7.

Objectives

The primary am of the study was to compare the safety and efficacy of imipenem-cilastatin (IC) with piperacillin-tazobactam (PT) in the empirical therapy for febrile neutropenia in children with cancer.

Study design

This was a single-center prospective randomized study that was conducted between January 2005 and January 2006. The study population included children with acute leukemia, lymphoma, and solid tumors and all were treated as inpatients during their febrile neutropenic episodes. Prophylactic antibiotics were not given routinely to any of the patients either before or during the study except that patients with either leukemia or lymphoma received trimethoprim-sulfamethoxazole for *Pneumocystis carinii* prophylaxis. Febrile episodes were categorized as microbiologically documented infections, clinically documented infections or fever of unknown origin.

Febrile neutropenia was defined as fever (axillary temperature of 38.5°C once or axillary temperature >38°C twice 4h apart or a single oral temperature >38.3°C or an oral temperature >38.0°C lasting for an hour or more) occurring in a patient who had an ANC $<0.5 \times 10^9$/L.

Children with febrile neutropenia were randomized to receive empirical antibiotic therapy with either PT (360 mg/kg/day) or IC (60 mg/kg/day) regimens.

If temperature persisted beyond 72 h after start of empirical therapy, amikacin (15 mg/kg/day) was added and if no response was seen after 96 h of antibiotic treatment, teicoplanin (10 mg/kg) was added to the tthree-drug antibiotic combination. When a micro-organism was isolated, antibiotic treatment was changed according to culture results. Amphotericin was added empirically if fever persisted >7 days.

Antibiotics were continued until the patient became afebrile and achieved an ANC $<0.5 \times 10^9$/L. Antibiotics were also discontinued in children if they were afebrile for 7 days or more even if they remained neutropenic. G-CSF was not routinely used during FBN episodes.

Treatment was considered successful if the fever and clinical signs of infection resolved and if a micro-organism was isolated, it was eradicated from the blood or the site(s) of isolation. On the other hand, treatment was deemed a failure if the signs and symptoms resolved only after the addition of another antibiotic and/or antifungal agent or if the primary infection recurred within a week after discontinuing empirical therapy or if the isolated micro-organism was primarily resistant to the empirical antibiotic therapy or if a death occurred during the FBN episode.

Statistics

Statistical differences between the two study groups were evaluated using the chi-square test; a p-value <0.05 was considered statistically significant. All patients enrolled on the study were randomized and analysis was according to the principle of intention to treat.

Results

During the study period, 99 FBN episodes were recorded in 63 study patients (27.3% in children with acute leukemia, 30.3% in patients with non-Hodgkin lymphoma and 42% in children with solid tumors). The period of neutropenia varied between 2 and 38 days (median 5 days). Demography (age, sex) and clinical characteristics (classification of infections, duration of neutropenia and ANC count) of patients were similar in both randomized groups.

While the overall success and failure rates were 67% and 33% respectively, this was 62% and 38% respectively in the IC group versus 71% and 29% respectively in the PT group of patients (p>0.05). Although the success of empirical treatment was not affected by sex, primary disease or initial neutrophil count, it was strongly correlated to remission of primary disease (p < 0.0002) and duration of neutropenia (p < 0.02).

Microbiologically and clinically documented infections were observed in 19% and 49% respectively of patients in the IC antibiotic group compared to 12% and 53% respectively in the PT group (p > 0.05).

Toxicity

No major adverse effects were observed in either group and treatment was not discontinued in any patient due to adverse side-effects.

Conclusions

It was concluded that monotherapy with either piperacillin/tazobactam or imipenem-cilastatin combination was equally effective in the treatment of febrile neutropenia in children.

Study 9

Karaman S, Vural S, Yildirmak Y, Emecen M, Erdem E, Kebudi R. Comparison of piperacillin tazobactam and cefoperazone sulbactam monotherapy in treatment of febrile neutropenia. *Pediatr Blood Cancer* 2012;**58**:579–83.

Objectives

The main aim of this study was to compare the efficacy of cefoperazone-sulbactam (CS) with piperacillin-tazobactam (PIPTAZ) for initial treatment of febrile neutropenia in children undergoing treatment for childhood cancer.

Study design

This was a single-center randomized prospective study that was conducted between January 2008 and January 2009. The study population included patients aged between 1 and 18 years who were undergoing treatment for acute leukemia or solid tumors. Exclusion criteria were hypotension and multiorgan failure or patients who had received IV antibiotics during the preceding 48 h. Prophylactic antibiotics were not administered routinely for any patient group except for those who had acute lymphoblastic leukemia, who received trimethoprim-sulfamethoxazole for prevention of *Pneumocystis carinii* infection. Patients

were evaluated at the third, fourth, and seventh day as well as at the end of therapy for clinical efficacy and adverse effects.

Fever was defined as either a single oral temperature ≥38.3°C or sustained temperature over 1 h of ≥38.0°C.

Neutropenia was defined as an ANC ≤0.5×10⁹/L or 1×10⁹/L that was expected to drop to ≤0.5×10⁹/L within 24–48 h.

Duration of neutropenia was defined as from onset of fever to resolution of neutropenia.

Resolution of clinical signs and fever without primary treatment modification was defined as success while addition of another antibiotic and/or antifungal agent or the death of a patient due to infection was defined as a failure of empirical therapy.

Patients were randomized to either PIPTAZ (360 mg/kg/day) or CS (100 mg/kg/day) when they developed FBN. Treatment was given on an inpatient basis and if fever persisted >72 h after start of empirical antibiotic therapy, amikacin (15 mg/kg/day) was added with the addition of teicoplanin (10 mg/kg/day) at 96 h if patients were still febrile. Antibiotic treatment was changed to carbapenem in children whose clinical status deteriorated and amphotericin B was added to the antibiotic cocktail in those who had persistent fever beyond 7 days. Children with high-risk acute lymphoblastic leukemia, non-Hodgkin lymphoma and neuroblastoma received G-CSF as primary prophylaxis.

While antibiotics were discontinued if the ANC was >0.5×10⁹/L for 2 consecutive days if fever resolved it was also stopped after 7 days even if the patient remained neutropenic provided the clinical status was improving with resolution of fever.

Statistics

Statistical differences between the two study groups were assessed by chi-square test for categorical variables and by the student *t* test for continuous variables. Two-tailed p-values were used; p-value <0.05 was considered significant. All analysis of results was based on the principle of intention to treat.

Results

Fifty-five patients were enrolled on this study and there were no protocol violations reported. There was no difference between the two groups in terms of age, sex, remission status, type of malignancy, ANC count, duration of neutropenia or presence of grade

3–4 mucositis. In 24% of all documented febrile neutropenic episodes, a micro-organism was isolated, of which 54% were gram-negative bacteria, 28% gram-positive bacteria, and 8% fungal. All isolated gram-negative bacteria were sensitive to PIPTAZ and CS. Modification of empirical treatment was necessary in 41% of all FBN episodes.

Empirical therapy with CS was used in 50 FBN episodes while PIPTAZ was used in 52 FBN episodes. While the overall success rate was 59%, success rate in the CS group was 56% (95% CI 0.41–0.70) compared to 62% (95% CI 0.47–0.75) in the PIPTAZ group (p=0.57). Modification of empirical treatment was not significantly different between the two treatment groups (p>0.05). There were no deaths due to FBN in either group of patients. No patient was readmitted with recurrent fever in the 10-day follow-up period after discontinuation of either CS or PIPTAZ treatment.

Conclusions

It was concluded that both piperacillin-tazobactam and cefoperazone-sulbactam monotherapy were equally safe and efficacious in the initial treatment of febrile neutropenia in children with cancer.

Study 10

Gupta A, Swaroop C, Argarwala S, Pandy R, Bkashi S. Randomised controlled trial comparing oral amoxicilin-clavulanate and ofloxacin with intravenous ceftriaxone and amikacin as outpatient therapy in paediatric low risk febrile neutropaenia. *J Paediatr Haematol Oncol* 2009;**31**:635–41.

Objectives

To compare efficacy and safety of intravenous and oral outpatient treatments for pediatric patients with low-risk febrile neutropenia.

Study design

Single institutional prospective, open-label RCT in pediatric low-risk febrile neutropenia conducted between January 2006 and December 2007 at the Dr B R A Institute Rotary Cancer Hospital. Inclusion criteria were patients aged 2–15 years; ANC <500/µL; one

episode of fever >38.3 °C or above or two episodes of fever above 38°C within last 24h; normotensive; no clinical evidence of lower respiratory tract infection and no x-ray findings compatible with infection; presence of reliable caretakers living less than 1h away from hospital with telephone contact.

Exclusion criteria were clinically unwell child requiring hospitalization; previous history of invasive fungal infection; prophylactic use of growth factors; stem cell transplantation and other intensively myelosuppressive regimens. Informed consent was taken. Randomization was achieved using a computer spreadsheet program. Patients were randomized to either receive outpatient ofloxacin 7.5 mg/m^2 12 hourly and amoxicillin-clavulanate 12.5 mg/m^2 8 hourly versus outpatient intravenous ceftriaxone 75 mg/kg and amikacin 15 mg/kg once daily. Compliance was monitored via daily telephone contact. A daily treatment log was maintained by parents and checked at each clinical review. Antibiotics were continued until the patient had been afebrile for >48h and had an ANC >550/µL. Patients with positive blood cultures received at least 10 days of appropriate antibiotic therapy.

Admission back to hospital was considered if: the patient had fever >3 days with a positive blood culture, life-threatening complications related to treatment, worsening clinical status or non-resolution of fever.

Results

One hundred and twenty-three episodes in 88 patients were randomized; 119 were evaluable. Of these, 1/3 patients were leukemia patients in maintenance and the rest were solid tumors. Successful outcomes were recorded in 55/61 (90.16%) and 54/58 (93.1%) in the oral and IV arms respectively with no significant difference between the two arms.

Success was achieved without modification in 50/61 (81.96%) episodes in the oral arm and 52/58 (89.65%) in the intravenous arm. There were three hospitalizations, all in the oral arm, but no patient required intensive care and none died.

There were six in the oral arm and four in the IV arm. Failures were associated with perianal infection, bacteremia, febrile neutropenia onset before day 9 of chemotherapy, and vincristine, actinomycin D and cyclophosphamide (VAC) chemotherapy regimen. All gram-positive isolates were successes but both of the gram-negative isolates were failures. Diarrhea in the IV arm and VAC chemotherapy in the oral arm were predictors of failure in subgroup analysis.

Conclusions

There is no significant difference in outcome between oral amoxicillin-clavulanate plus ofloxacin and intravenous ceftriaxone and amikacin for low-risk febrile neutropenia in pediatric patients.

Study 11

Phillips B, Wade R, Stewart LA, Sutton AJ. Systematic review and meta-analysis of the discriminatory performance of risk prediction rules in febrile neutropaenic episodes in children and young people. *Eur J Cancer* 2010;**46**:2950–64.

Objectives

The main aim was to identify and critically appraise and synthesize the evidence on the discriminatory ability and predictive accuracy of existing clinical decision rules (CDRs) in febrile neutropenia episodes in children and young people undergoing treatment for malignant disease.

Study design

The review was conducted in accordance with "systematic reviews": CRD's (Center for Reviews and Dissemination) guidance for undertaking reviews in healthcare and registered on the Health Technology Assessment (HTA) registry of systematic reviews: CRD 32009100453. Studies that aimed to derive or validate a CDR in children and young people (0–18 years) presenting with FBN (both prospective and retrospective) were included. However, those using a case–control approach were excluded. The following databases from inception to February 2009 were examined: MEDLINE, MEDLINE In-Process and other nonindexed citations, EMBASE, CINAHL, Cochrane Database of Systematic Reviews, HTA Database, Cochrane Central Register of Controlled Trials (CENTRAL), Conference Proceedings Citation Index – Science (CPSI-S) and Literatura Latinoamericana y del Caribe en Ciencias de la Salud (LILACS). Two reviewers independently screened the title and abstract of studies for inclusion and then the full text of

retrieved articles. Data were extracted by one reviewer and checked by the other.

Statistics

For tests that produced three level results (low, medium and high risk) an approach based on previous meta-analysis of three-level CDR results was used. The random effects meta-analysis was undertaken using the WinBUGS 1.4.3 to estimate the proportions of individuals classified as low, medium and high risk in the bacteremic and nonbacteremic groups. Heterogeneity between study results was explored through consideration of study populations, study design, predictor variables assessed and outcomes chosen, although the small number of studies in each category limited this approach. Sensitivity analysis was undertaken by comparing results when the original (derivation) dataset was included and excluded. In areas where a quantitative synthesis was difficult, a narrative approach was used.

Results

Twenty studies (eight prospective, 11 retrospective and retrospective analysis of prospectively collected data) that described 16 different CDRs were included in the review. Age range of patients varied between 1 month and 23 years, a wide range of malignancies was included, and 7840 episodes of FBN were described and outcomes were summarized in five clusters: death, critical care requirement, serious medical complication, significant bacterial infection, and bacteremia. The 20 studies varied in quality; 13 definitions of FBN were used with 12 definitions of fever and four of neutropenia. However, most of the variations were at the lower risk part of the spectrum.

Clinical decision rules performance was examined by analysis of the tabulated CDR performance data and graphically with plots of sensitivity and specificity. A meta-analysis of studies that used identical CDR was undertaken for two cases; the "Rackhoff" rule (that of absolute monocyte count and temperature) to examine bacteremia and the "Santolaya" rule for serious infectious complications.

The Rackhoff rule discriminates between three groups of individuals at low, moderate, and high risk of bacteremia. A sensitivity analysis using this rule showed poor discriminative ability. Assuming a 22% overall prevalence of bacteremia (the average proportion of included studies in the review), the predictive values were low risk 6% (95% CI 1–34%), medium risk 18% (95% CI 3–37%) and high risk 49% (95% CI 6–84%).

Application of the Santolaya rule appeared to show moderate ability to discriminate between low- and high-risk groups when considering the outcome of bacterial infections. Using the average invasive bacterial infection (IBI) rate of 47%, the probability of IBI in the low-risk group was 13% (95% CI 9–13%) and 72% (95% CI 68–75%) in the high-risk group.

Assessing potential sources of heterogeneity, it appeared that derivation studies generally had better accuracy compared to validation studies. All analyses were confounded by correlation of location, population, outcome, and rule. Examination of detailed content of all rules showed that they usually addressed four main domains: patient-related factors, treatment including presence of a central venous catheter and type of chemotherapy, episode-specific clinical features, and episode-specific laboratory tests, and these were all various markers of bone marrow function. No study compared different approaches.

Conclusions

It was concluded that no CDR was more effective or reliable than any other and practical application of many of these CDRs within an inpatient environment was likely to be safe but without further research, uncertainty will remain as to the efficiency of the CDR in use.

Study 12

Fleischhack G, Hartmann C, Simon A *et al.* Meropenem versus ceftazidime as empirical monotherapy in febrile neutropaenia of paediatric patients with cancer. Br *J Antimicrob Chemother* 2001;**47**:841–53.

Objectives

To assess the efficacy and safety of meropenem versus ceftazidime as empirical monotherapy for febrile neutropenia in paediatric cancer patients.

Study design

Prospective, open, randomized, two-center comparative trial with two parallel study arms. Patients were included if they had received conventional or high-dose chemotherapy for primary, refractory or relapsed solid tumor or for a hematological malignancy. All consecutive patients with a fever >38.5°C >4h or over 39°C, ANC <0.5×10⁹/L (or if expected to fall <0.5×10⁹/L within 48h of admission) and presumed infection. Patients excluded were those receiving any antibacterial therapy 48h prior to admission other than prophylaxis.

To minimize potential differences between the two arms, three stratification variables were used: treatment center, chemotherapy intensity, and age of patient. Patients were then randomly allocated to initial monotherapy of either meropenem (60 mg/kg/day in three divided doses) or ceftazidime (100 mg/kg/day also in three divided doses).

Nonresponse within 48h in the ceftazidime arm led to the addition of teicoplanin. In the meropenem arm, teicoplanin was only added if documented gram-positive infection was found. If nonresolution of febrile neutropenia persisted at 96h, all patients were commenced on meropenem and teicoplanin and an antifungal agent. Modification of antimicrobial therapy for documented resistant organism was permitted and documented. Duration of therapy was at the clinician's discretion. However, all culture-proven infections were treated for a minimum of 7 days. Patients all received a minimum of 72h of IV antibiotics and continued for a minimum of 24h after resolution of fever.

Febrile episodes were classified into fever of unknown origin, microbiologically documented infection and clinically documented infection according to site or cause.

Response criteria were classified under two headings. For fever of unknown origin (FUO), response was defined when fever resolved and if no further antimicrobial therapy was required within the subsequent 7 days. For clinical or microbiologically documented infections, complete resolution of fever with resolution of clinical signs and eradication of microbiological etiology and no further antibiotic therapy within 7 days required.

Patients were primarily analyzed on an intention-to-treat basis. After excluding those who failed treatment, a second analysis was performed.

Results

Three hundred and forty-five out of 375 episodes in 169 patients were documented and evaluable. There were no significant differences documented between the characteristics of the episodes between the two arms, nor classification of the febrile episodes. In both arms about half were classified as FUO; 90/172 in the meropenem arm and 93/170 in the ceftazidime arm were microbiologically or clinically documented infections.

In the intention-to-treat analysis the overall success rates were comparable (both 99.4%). Two patients failed, of whom one died within 12 h of commencement of treatment with ceftazidime for polymicrobial septic shock. In the other patient, cessation of fever was not achieved until 25 days after corticosteroid intervention. This patient was considered to either have a drug fever or an autoimmune process confounding the febrile neutropenia.

Of significance, 96/172 in the meropenem arm (55.8%) and 68/170 (40%) in the ceftazidime arm responded to initial monotherapy (p=0.003). For patients classified as FUO, a significantly higher proportion responded to monotherapy in both groups when compared to documented clinical or microbiological infectious subgroups (meropenem 63/82 versus 33/90; p=0.000, and for the ceftazidime arm 0/77 versus 28/93; p=0.004). There were no significant differences between the two arms for types, sites and sources of documented infections. The initial response rate was not significantly different depending on underlying disease diagnosis.

One hundred and fifty-nine and 160 episodes were evaluable.

Similar success rates were noted with initial monotherapy and response to escalation of therapy. In patients with bacteremia, *in vitro* susceptibility to meropenem and ceftazidime was seen in 100% and 98.5% of all gram-negative organisms tested. However, the clinical responses *in vivo*, of 56% (meropenem arm) and 47.1% (ceftazidime arm), were significantly lower. Of 58 gram-positive isolates tested *in vitro*, 21 were resistant to oxacillin (thus conferring implied resistance to ceftazidime or meropenem) but although the clinical response in the ceftazidime arm was lower than the meropenem arm, it did not reach significance.

The duration of fever, antimicrobial therapy, and hospitalization was significantly longer in the ceftazidime arm. Comparison of the two treatment arms depending on initial ANC ($>$ or $<0.1\times10^9$/L) revealed significant differences in the meropenem arm only (p=0.038, 0.021, and 0.026). Long-term neutropenia, i.e. >10 days ANC $<0.5\times10^9$/L, was associated in

both arms with a longer duration of all parameters (p=0.0001). There was no significant difference in relapse rate or time to relapse between the two arms, with relapse patients generally having an ANC of $<0.1\times10^9$/L. There was also no observed difference in the rate of adverse events between the two arms.

Conclusions

Meropenem was more successful in the group classified as FUO. In bacteremic episodes caused by coagulase-negative *Staphylococcus*, the response to either meropenem or ceftazidime was poor and modification of treatment was required for successful resolution. However, empirical monotherapy with either meropenem or ceftazidime provides a safe, well-tolerated option for children with cancer and early febrile neutropenia episodes.

Study 13

Yildrim I, Aytac S, Ceyhan M *et al.* Piperacillin/tazobactam plus amikacin versus carbapenem monotherapy as empirical treatment of febrile neutropaenia in childhood haematological malignancies. *Paediatr Haematol Oncol* 2008;**25**:291–9.

Objectives

To compare the efficacy of piperacillin/tazobactam (PTA) and amikacin against carbapenem (C) monotherapy for the empirical treatment of febrile neutropenia in children diagnosed with ALL or AML.

Results

A randomized, prospective noninferiority single-center trial. Patients were considered eligible if they had a diagnosis of ALL or AML between the ages of 2 and 16 years of age and presented with febrile neutropenia. Only one episode per patient was evaluated, the first episode if patients had more than one. Patients were randomized to receive either 80 mg/kg piperaciilin and 10 mg/kg tazobactum 6 hourly with amikacin 7.5 mg/kg 12 hourly (PTA) or either meropenem or imipenem at 20 mg/kg 8 hourly. If patient remained febrile at 72 h, a glyopepetide was added and amikacin was added to the carbopenem group as well. If persistently unwell at day 5, antifungal cover with amphotericin B was added. Treatment was modified according to cultures. The minimum length of treatment was 7 days and antibiotics were stopped after 4 days without a fever.

Ninety-nine febrile episodes were randomized to receive either PTA or C. Response to treatment was evaluable in 87 episodes (46 PTA and 41 C). There was no statistically significant difference found for age, sex, ANC, hematological diagnosis, remission or relapse status, presence or absence of a central venous catheter, numbers in receipt of a colony-stimulating factor or numbers with a microbiologically confirmed diagnosis between the two groups; 21.8% of all patients had positive cultures. The most common positive isolate was *Staphylococcus epidermidis*, which was positive in 9/19. All isolates except one *Klebsiella pneumoniae* (resistant to carbapenem) were sensitive to both PTA and C *in vitro*. None of the outcomes measured showed difference approaching statistical significance. Addition of a glycopepetide was required in 52.1% in the PTA group and 51.2% in the C group. Equivalent numbers in both groups went on to receive antifungal therapy (17.3% and 14.5%). Duration of neutropenia between groups was similar.

Conclusions

Piperacillin/tazobactam is as effective as carbapenem monotherapy for the empirical treatment of febrile neutropenia in hematological malignancies. This supports evidence already present in the literature demonstrating equivalence in solid tumors.

Study 14

Paganini H, Gomez S, Ruvinsky S *et al.* Outpatient, sequential, parenteral-oral antibiotic therapy for lower risk febrile neutropaenia (LRFN) in children with malignant disease. *Cancer* 2003;**97**(7):1775–80.

Objectives

To determine the efficacy of parenteral-oral outpatient therapy in the management of children with LRFN who were undergoing treatment for malignant diseases.

Study design

A single-center prospective randomized controlled trial was conducted between August 2000 and April 2002. After patients were assessed for eligibility,

they were randomized to receive either ceftriaxone 100 mg/m²/day single dose plus amikacin 15 mg/kg/day single dose on day 1 followed by oral ciprofloxacin 20 mg/kg/day in two divided doses or ceftriaxone plus amikacin on day 1 followed by daily IV ceftriaxone. All patients were ambulatory. Cessation of antibiotic therapy was allowed once the patient's neutrophil count >100/mm³ and they were afebrile for 24 h.

Results

Five hundred and fifty-seven episodes in 420 patients were seen in the institution during the study timeframe but only 177 episodes in 135 patients met the inclusion criteria. Of those patients included, the median age was 7.5 years (range 1.6–15.8 years) and there were no significant differences in gender, presence of indwelling central venous catheter, use of hematopoietic growth factors or underlying disease. The excluded patient group comprised predominantly patients with ALL or AML with a predicted neutropenia episode lasting longer than 7 days; 60% of those excluded presented with an overt clinical site of infection.

In the study group, the origin of the febrile episode could be identified in over two-thirds of all patients, with the majority being localized and mild. Viruses were the micro-organisms most commonly identified. The clinical course and outcome were recorded with both regimens being tolerable and equally efficacious; 5% of children in group A and 7% in group B required hospitalization due to failure of ambulatory care. There were no deaths or intensive therapy unit admissions and tolerance of both regimens was similar.

Conclusions

Using previously well-described risk stratification criteria for febrile neutropenic episodes allows identification of a cohort of patients that can successfully be managed in an ambulatory setting. Differences of note in this study were the exclusion of all patients with documented bacteremia and the fact that this cohort comprised predominantly patients with ALL rather than solid tumors. A significant proportion of patients included had the offending organism identified. In this cohort of risk-stratified patients. both regimens used were equally efficacious.

Study 15

Corapcioglu F, Sarpa N, Zengin E. Monotherapy with piperacillin/tazobactam versus cefepime as empirical therapy for febrile nuetropaenia in paediatric cancer patients. *Paediatr Haematol Oncol* 2006;**23**:177–86.

Objectives

To compare efficacy, safety, and cost of piperacillin/tazobactam (pip/tazo)with cefepime monotherapy in children with febrile neutropenia.

Study design

Single-center, prospective randomized trial in which patients were consecutively randomized to receive either pip/tazo (80 mg/kg, 10 mg/kg) q6h or cefepime 50 mg/kg q8h. Treatment stopped once fever had subsided and ANC >500/mm- and eradication of microbiological and clinical infection. After 96 h of unremitting fever, teicoplanin was added. Empirical amphotericin B addition was not allowed before the fifth day of empirical antibiotic therapy.

Statistics

Analyses were performed using the chi-squared test or Fisher exact test and Mann-Whitney U tests were used for comparison. Univariate-multivariate analysis was used for evaluation of variables determining treatment response and cost.

Results

Fifty episodes in 27 patients were evaluable. The treatment groups were comparable with regard to underlying disease (overall 60% of the study group had a diagnosis of leukemia); whether in remission or not; presence of central venous catheter; use of hematopoietic stem cell growth factors; and absolute neutrophil count. Of note, 68% of the study group had an expected neutropenia duration >10 days.

There were nine bacterial isolates (six gram positive, all sensitive to glycopeptides, and three gram negative sensitive to both pip/taz and cefepime). Although there was no infection-related mortality, overall 35 different therapeutic modifications were made in 24 episodes. No significant difference could be demonstrated between treatment success and modification rate between groups; empirical changes were more frequent in the cefepime group. No severe

adverse events were recorded and all minor toxicities were reversible.

The median costs of each episode including antimicrobial drug, hospitalization, supportive therapy, and daily therapy costs were not significantly different between the two groups. In multivariate analysis, the duration of neutropenia was the most important factor for determining duration of fever and hospitalization.

Conclusions

Although this was a small study group, the authors concluded that piperacillin/tazobactam empirical monotherapy in pediatric febrile neutropenia is as effective as cefepime monotherapy and incurs similar costs.

Study 16

Kutluk T, Kurne O, Akyuz C *et al.* Cefepime versus meropenem as empirical therapy for neutropaenic fever in children with lymphoma and solid tumours. *Paediatr Blood Cancer* 2004;**42**:284–6.

Objectives

To evaluate the efficacy of monotherapy with cefepime with meropenem in febrile neutropenia episodes in children with lymphoma or solid tumors.

Study design

Single-centre, prospective randomized trial comparing cefepime monotherapy with meropenem monotherapy.

Statistics

The Fisher X2 exact test and Mann-Whitney U test were used for comparison.

Results

Forty-nine febrile neutopenic episodes were evaluable and these episodes were comparable across the two groups. Of note, the median duration of fever was only 2 days. Bacteremia was present in 12.2% of all episodes. Of those episodes where fever persisted for >7 days, 3/4 had documented bacteremia.

The overall success rate was 77.6%, with 68% in the cefepime and 87.5% in the meropenem arm. This was not statistically significant. The median duration of treatment was 7 days (range 7–18).

Two patients died of febrile neutropenia, one with documented *Candida* sepsis on day 12 and the second on day 13 with no documented culture result. Both patients were not in remission and had received a change of empirical antibiotics on day 4 and addition of empirical amphotericin on day 7.

The solid tumor group had less bacteremia (4/37; 10.8%) versus 2/12 (16.7%; p>0.05) and treatment failure (7/37; 18.95%) versus 4/12 (33.3.%; p>0.05) than the non-Hodgkin lymphoma group.

Conclusions

Both cefepime and meropenem monotherapy were well tolerated and as effective as previously described combination regimens containing aminoglycosides for the empirical treatment of neutropenic children with predominantly low-risk febrile neutropenia with lymphoma and solid tumors.

Study 17

Aksoylar S, Cetingul N, Kantar M. Meropenem plus amikacin versus piperacillin-tazobactam plus netilmicin as empiric therapy for high risk febrile neutropaenia in children. *Pediatr Hematol Oncol* 2004;**21**: 115–23.

Objectives

To evaluate the efficacy and safety of meropenem and amikacin compared with piperacillin-tazobactam plus netilmicin for initial empirical treatment of high-risk febrile neutropenia in children.

Study design

This was a single-center prospective randomized trial. Eligible patients had one of the following criteria: a diagnosis of leukemia (except those in "maintenance") or stage III–IV lymphoma; ANC <100/μL^3 on admission; "uncontrolled" cancer; significant comorbidity at time of admission.

Excluded were those who had received antibiotic therapy in the preceding 72 h. Meropenem (60 mg/kg/day q8h) plus amikacin (15 mg/kg/day q12h) or piperacillin-tazobactam (piperacillin 100 mg/kg, tazobactam 4 mg/kg over 30–60 min q8h) plus netilmicin (7 mg/kg/day) was administered. If fever persisted at 72 h, a glycopepetide was added and if it persisted on the fifth

day, conventional amphotericin B was added. Antibiotics were continued until 48 h without a fever and ANC >500/μL and no identifiable source of infection. Efficacy of response was evaluated at 72 h and again at completion of episode.

Statistics

Statistical analysis utilized the Fisher exact test and the Mann-Whitney U test.

Results

One hundred episodes were evaluated, 50 in each group. The groups were comparable in terms of age, sex, ANC at entry, use of hematological growth factors, classification of infection, and proportion of positive blood cultures.

The duration of neutropenia, duration of treatment, days with fever, and need for modification were similar in both groups. Overall success was achieved in 97/100 episodes. Three patients in induction and not in remission died due to infection.

The incidence of gram-negative bacteria (45%) exceeded the incidence of gram-positive bacteria (37%). There was no significant difference in time to defervescence of fever between the groups, duration of profound neutropenia or duration of antibiotic therapy. No adverse effects were recorded due to antibiotic regimen.

Conclusions

It was concluded that there was no significant difference in the efficacy of the two empirical regimens.

Line infections

Study 18

Snaterse M, Rüger W, Scholte OP, Reimer WJ, Lucas C. Antibiotic-based catheter lock solutions for prevention of catheter-related bloodstream infection: a systematic review of randomized controlled trials. *J Hosp Infect* 2010;**75**:1–11.

Objectives

The main purpose of this review was to determine whether the use of antibiotic-based CVC solutions reduced the rate of CRBSI. A secondary goal was to ascertain the most effective antibiotic lock solution that will prevent or reduce the incidence of CRBSI.

Study design

All relevant publications from MEDLINE (1966–2009) and the Cochrane Central Register of Controlled Trials (CENTRAL) up to 2009 were retrieved and analyzed. Criteria for inclusion were: planned randomized trials, quasi-randomized trials or systematic review/meta-analysis of randomized or quasi-randomized trials, published articles that reviewed the effects of one or more preventative antibiotic-based lock solutions used intermittently in patients with CVCs.

Statistics

Catheter-related bloodstream infection was defined as isolation of the same organism from the catheter segment and peripheral blood or simultaneous quantitative blood cultures with a 5:1 ratio of CVC versus peripheral blood. Bloodstream infection (BSI) was considered as symptoms of infection and at least one positive blood culture. For the dichotomous outcome CRBSI, the overall incidence density ratio (IDR) with a 95% CI and the incidence density difference (IDD) with a 95% CI was calculated by using a review manager (v 4.2.7). The incidence density was calculated by dividing the total number of CRBSIs by the total number of catheter days of follow-up. The number of catheterization days needed to treat was calculated as the inverse of the IDD. Meta-analyses were undertaken using a random effects model for the IDDs or the IDRs to calculate pooled estimates and the 95% CIs. A funnel plot was used as a visual aid to detect publication bias or systematic heterogeneity.

Although the report cited included patients with CVCs undergoing hemodialysis, oncology patients, and high-risk neonates, this review focuses only on the oncology patients.

Results

Six trials were included in the analysis, of which five trials were pediatric studies with tunneled CVCs. The baseline risks for BSI were comparable between trials; mean baseline risk was 1.7 BSIs/1000 catheter days. Most of the trials reported BSI as the main outcome rather than CRBSI. In four of the five pediatric studies, the results were in favor of the antibiotic-based lock solutions but this was statistically significant in only one trial. The pooled results expressed as IDD showed a borderline statistically significant benefit of the antibiotic-based lock solutions (IDD 0.52/1000 catheter-days; 95% CI 1.07–0.02).

There was only one trial that compared antibiotic lock regimens "head to head": vancomycin-heparin versus vancomycin + ciprofloxacin-heparin lock solution. There was no difference in the occurrence of CRBSI between the two regimens (IDD 0.03; 95% CI 0.33–0.27).

Conclusions

It was concluded that routine use of antibiotic-based catheter lock solutions in children with malignant disorders could not be recommended as it only provided a marginal benefit in the prevention of catheter-related bloodstream infections.

Study 19

Ferreira Chacon JM, Hato de Almeida E, de Lourdes Simões R et al. Randomized study of minocycline and edetic acid as a locking solution for central line (Port-A-Cath) in children with cancer. *Chemotherapy* 2011;**57**:285–91.

Objectives

The aim was to evaluate whether minocycline and edetic acid (M-EDTA) used as a lock solution in central venous catheters (CVC) such as Port-A-Cath in children undergoing chemotherapy treatment reduces catheter-associated bloodstream infections (CABSI) when compared with conventional heparin lock solutions.

Study design

This was a single-center prospective randomized study conducted between March 2008 and March 2009. Fifty children were enrolled on the study and were divided into two groups: heparin group (n=26) and M-EDTA group (n=24). All included children were receiving chemotherapy and had an implanted Port-A-Cath CVC. Exclusion criteria were active infections, recent use of antibiotic or allergy to any of the drugs used in the study.

The M-DTA solution contained 30 mg/mL of EDTA and 3 mg/mL of minocycline. The heparin solution concentration was 5000 iu/mL. The catheter-locking solution had the same volume as each catheter's priming solution was introduced after each chemotherapy cycle and remained in the catheter lumen till the start of the next cycle

Prospective blood cultures were obtained at the beginning of the study and at the start of each chemotherapy cycle (weekly or monthly) according to the treatment protocol. A total of 387 blood cultures in the heparin group and 357 in the M-EDTA group were obtained from the catheters after discarding the heparin or M-EDTA lock.

The primary outcome measure was catheter-associated positive blood culture or clinical evidence of bacteremia or sepsis.

Statistics

The Kaplan–Meier method was used to determine the actual survival for each catheter. Other statistical tests included test for comparison of independent proportions, student t test for independent samples, Fisher exact test, log-rank, and Pearson χ^2 test. The level of significance was $p < 0.05$.

Results

Demographic characteristics relating to age, sex, and underlying disease were similar in both randomized groups.

There was a significantly increased incidence of catheter infections in the heparin group compared to the M-EDTA group ($p = 0.001$); the infection rate was 73.1% in the heparin group (19/26 catheters) versus 20.8% in the M-EDTA group (5/24 catheters).

The incidence of infection per catheter/1000 days was 6.3 in the heparin group compared to 1.09 in the M-EDTA group. The mean time free of catheter infection was 4.72 months in the heparin group versus 9.69 months in the M-EDTA group.

Children in the heparin group had a two-fold higher probability of being hospitalized compared to the M-EDTA group (Pearson χ^2 test; $p < 0.05$); the median hospitalization time was 33.5 days (23.5–44) for patients in the heparin group compared to 19.0 days (14.5–25.5) for patients in the M-EDTA group.

There was no difference in antibiotic sensitivity to micro-organisms between the two groups. No side-effects to either M-EDTA or heparin were observed during the study.

Conclusions

It was concluded that M-EDTA was more effective than heparin in preventing catheter infections when used as a locking solution for central venous catheters.

Study 20

Arora RS, Roberts R, Eden TO, Pizer B. Interventions other than anticoagulants and systemic antibiotics for prevention of central venous catheter-related infections in children with cancer. *Cochrane Database Syst Rev* 2010;**12**:CD007785.

Objectives

The main aim was to determine which of the many interventions were effective in preventing CVC-related infections in children with cancer. Secondary aims included effectiveness of each intervention in the following subgroup of patients: implanted versus external catheters, hematological versus nonhematological malignancies, and hemopoietic stem cell transplantation (HSCT) versus no HSCT.

Study design

Only RCTs and quasi-randomized trials in children (<18 years of age) with a malignant disorder who had a long-term tunneled CVC were included in this review.

Electronic searches of MEDLINE (January 1950–January 2009), EMBASE (January 1980–January 2009), CINAHL (January 1982–March 2009) and the COCHRANE Central Register of Controlled Trials (CENTRAL) were performed to extract relevant RCTs. In addition, abstracts of conference proceedings of the American Society of Clinical Oncology (2004–2008), the American Society of Pediatric Hematology/Oncology (2004–2008), the International Society of Pediatric Oncology (2004–2008) and the Multinational Association of Supportive Care in Cancer (2004–2008) were hand searched to extract any relevant information on CVC infections in children. Additionally, ongoing trials from the *meta*Register of Controlled Trials (www.controlled-trials.com/mrct/) and the National Cancer Register (portal.nihr.ac.uk/Pages/NRRArchive.aspx) were also screened.

Data collection was not restricted by language. The results from different databases were merged and duplicate reports of the same study removed. Most disagreements were resolved through discussion.

Statistics

While for dichotomous outcomes, the estimates of effect of an intervention were expressed as a risk ratio with 95% confidence interval (95% CI), for continuous outcomes, weighted mean differences with standard deviations were used to summarize the data for each group with 95% CI. Rare events such as catheter infections were conventionally expressed as per 1000 CVC days with rate ratios (event rate in experimental arm/event rate in the control arm) as a summary statistic. The generic inverse-variance approach in Rev Man was used for meta-analyses of rate ratios with data entered as natural logarithms (log rate ratio and the standard error of the log rate ratio). The significance of any discrepancies in the estimates of treatment from different trials effects was assessed with a random effects model using the I^2 statistic as this method described the percentage of total variation across the studies that was due to heterogeneity rather than to chance (heterogeneity was defined as $I^2 > 50\%$).

Results

Three studies were included in this review; in two of the studies the prophylactic intervention was flushing the CVC with urokinase and in the third study, the prophylactic intervention was a longer interval (15 days) between changing the dressing of the CVC.

Urokinase as prophylactic intervention

The first study enrolled 103 patients between the ages of 1 and 21 years with implanted CVCs. All patients were randomized to monthly catheter flushes – 3 mL of urokinase-heparin (5000 iu/mL of urokinase) versus heparin (300 units of heparin). Only patients who received flushes on six occasions at monthly intervals were included in the analyses.

The second study enrolled 577 patients with both hematological and nonhematological malignancies between the ages of 3 months and 21 years. This study included patients with implanted as well as external catheters. Patients were randomized to two weekly catheter flushes with urokinase (5000 iu/mL) versus heparin (100 units/mL).

Frequency of dressing change

Only one study that enrolled 113 patients between the ages of 1 and 22 years with mainly a hematological malignancy planned for high-dose chemotherapy followed by stem cell transplantation was included in this report. Patients were randomized to catheter dressing every 15 days versus every 4 days. Only those who had external catheters were included in this study.

Effects of interventions

Intervention with prophylactic urokinase
Neither study reported catheter-borne bloodstream infection as an outcome.

One study reported the overall rate of catheter-related infection(CAI) for implanted catheters of 0.4/1000 CVC days in the urokinase-heparin arm versus 0.6/1000 CVC days in the heparin arm, which was not statistically significant.

The second study reported an overall rate of CAI for all types of CVCs of 1.6/1000 CVC days in the urokinase arm versus 2.2/1000 CVC days in the heparin arm (p=0.05). The rate of CAI for external catheters was 2.6/1000 CVC days in the urokinase arm versus 3.9/1000 CVC days in the heparin arm (p=0.04). While the authors commented that there were no significant differences in the rate of CAI for implanted catheters, no actual CAI rates were given.

A meta-analysis of both trials showed a nonsignificant advantage for patients in the urokinase arm (rate ratio 0.72, 95% CI 0.12–4.41). A funnel plot to assess publication bias was not performed due to small patient numbers in the two reported studies.

Neither study reported pocket of infection as an outcome.

While both studies reported premature catheter removal as an outcome, only the second study expressed it with some significance. There were two premature catheter removals in the urokinase arm versus one in the heparin arm. No statistical significance of this result was reported.

Frequency of interval of catheter dressing as an outcome

Catheter-borne bloodstream infection, CAI, exit site infection, and tunnel infection were not reported as outcomes.

There were no premature catheter removals in the intervention arm (catheter dressing every 15 days) or in the control arm (dressing change every 4 days).

Conclusions

The authors concluded that flushing the CVC with urokinase (with or without heparin) compared to heparin alone decreased the rate of catheter-related infections. While catheter dressing change every 15 days did not lead to more premature catheter removals, the authors felt that the data were insufficiently robust to assess whether catheter-related infection rates were also changed.

Index

ABV (doxorubicin–bleomycin–vinblastine), Hodgkin
    lymphoma 107, 111, 115
ABVD (doxorubicin–bleomycin–vinblastine–dacarbazine),
    Hodgkin lymphoma 105, 106, 107, 109, 110, 111,
    112, 114, 115
ACOP (doxorubicin/anthracycline combined with
    cyclophosphamide–vincristine–prednisolone),
    non-Hodgkin lymphoma 95
A-COPP (doxorubicin–cyclophosphamide–vincristine–
    procarbazine–prednisone), Hodgkin
    lymphoma 106, 109
actinomycin D (dactinomycin)
    Ewing sarcoma 34
        and vincristine–ifosfamide 33
    Wilms tumor 34–5, 38, 39
        and vincristine 34
    see also AVA; BCD; IVA; VA; VAC; VACA; VAIA
acute lymphoblastic leukemia see lymphoblastic leukemia
acute myeloid leukemia (AML) 119–45, 223–6
    CNS prophylaxis 123, 144–5
    dexrazoxane as cardioprotectant (with anthracycline
        treatment) in 236–7
    G-CSF 120, 209–10, 214, 216, 223–6
    induction therapy 119–21, 126–34
    maintenance treatment 122–3, 133, 137–9
    postremission therapy 121–3, 126–43
acute myeloid leukemia/myelodysplastic syndrome
    with dexrazoxane 235–7
    with G-CSF 210
ADCOMP (doxorubicin–asparaginase–cyclophosphamide–
    vincristine–methotrexate–prednisone),
    non-Hodgkin lymphoma 95
ADE (cytarabine/ARAC–daunorubicin–etoposide),
    acute myeloid leukemia, (ADE) 119, 120,
    127, 132, 144
adjuvant (postoperative) therapy
    medulloblastoma 71, 74–5, 78–9

osteosarcoma 18
rhabdomyosarcoma 9–10
Wilms tumor 38, 41, 44–5
adolescents, lymphoblastic leukemia 149, 204–6
Adriamycin see doxorubicin
AIE (ARAC–idarubicin–etoposide) 119, 127, 144, 224
AI(E)OP group
    leukemia
        acute myeloid 141, 142
        lymphoblastic 147, 181, 184
    rhabdomyosarcoma 8, 9
Alin C-9/C-11/C-12 studies 170, 170–1
all-trans-retinoic acid (ATRA), acute promyelocytic
    leukemia 120–1, 132–4, 138–9
amifostine
    germ cell tumors 66
    hepatoblastoma 59
amikacin
    ceftriaxone and see ceftriaxone–amikacin
    meropenem and, vs piperacillin/tazobactam
        and netilmicin 263
    piperacillin/tazobactam and 254
        vs carbapenem 260–1
amoxicillin–clavulanate and ofloxacin vs
    ceftriaxone–amikacin 257–8
amphotericin 246, 251, 252, 254, 255, 256, 260,
    262, 263
    liposomal 245, 246, 247–8, 251
anaplastic/undifferentiated tumors
    gliomas 81, 81–2, 82, 85, 86
    large cell lymphomas (ALCL) 88, 89, 91, 95, 100–3
    sarcomas 5, 6, 8, 11, 12, 240, 241
anthracyclines 235–42
    cardiotoxicity see cardiotoxicity
    lymphoblastic leukemia 238–9, 240, 241
        dexrazoxane as cardioprotectant 235–6
        long-term effects 150

Evidence-Based Pediatric Oncology, Third Edition. Edited by Ross Pinkerton, Ananth Shankar and Katherine K. Matthay.
© 2013 John Wiley & Sons, Ltd. Published 2013 by John Wiley & Sons, Ltd.

anthracyclines (*cont'd*)
  non-Hodgkin lymphoma 88, 89, 91, 241
    combined with cyclophosphamide–vincristine–
      prednisolone (ACOP) 95
antibiotics (antibacterials) 243–4, 253–67
  with central venous lines 246, 263–4
antifungals 247–53
  empirical therapy 245–6, 247–8, 250
  prophylactic 245, 248–50
AOPE (doxorubicin–vincristine–etoposide–prednisolone),
    Hodgkin lymphoma 110
AP (doxorubicin–cisplatin), osteosarcoma 15, 16
APO (doxorubicin–prednisone–vincristine), non-Hodgkin
    lymphoma 91, 91–2, 95
ARAC *see* cytarabine
asparaginase
  lymphoblastic leukemia 147–8, 156–7, 160–1, 165–7,
    184, 187, 190, 191, 202–3, 204, 236
    comparisons of different forms 156–7, 165–6,
      190, 202–3
    pegylated 157, 163, 166, 167, 190, 192, 201,
      201, 202–3
    recombinant 164–5
  non-Hodgkin lymphoma 95
  T-cell leukemia/lymphoma 95
astrocytoma 81, 82, 85, 86
AVA (actinomycin D–vincristine–doxorubicin),
    Wilms tumor 39, 40, 41, 45
azacytidine in acute myeloid leukemia 142

B-cell lymphoma 88, 92, 95, 103
  diffuse large (DLBCL) 88, 91, 95, 97, 98, 99, 100
bacterial infections 243, 244
  antibiotics 243–4, 253–67
BCD (cisplatin or bleomycin–cyclophosphamide–
    actinomycin D), osteosarcoma 18, 19, 20
BEP (bleomycin–etoposide–cisplatin), germ cell
    tumors 65, 66, 67
Berlin–Frankfurt–Münster (BFM) group
  acute lymphoblastic leukemia 147, 148, 156, 169, 174,
    175, 176, 181, 182, 186, 187, 189, 192, 197,
    199–200, 217
  acute myeloid leukemia 119, 120, 121, 122, 123, 127, 144,
    209, 210, 224, 226
  G-CSF use 217
  non-Hodgkin lymphoma 88, 90, 92, 95, 96, 101, 102
bevacizumab, glioma 82
BFM group *see* Berlin–Frankfurt–Münster group
bleomycin *see* ABV; ABVD; BCD; BEP; JEB; MOPP-B
blood transfusion requirements, erythropoietin
    reducing 220–1
bloodstream infections and risk with central venous
    catheters 246–7, 263–7
bone marrow suppression *see* myelosuppression
bone marrow transplantation (BMT) 141–3
  acute myeloid leukemia 141–3
  neuroblastoma 47, 50–1, 54, 55

brainstem
  glioma 81, 82, 85, 86
  medulloblastoma 75, 79
Brazilian ALL Study Group trial GBTLI-80 169
Brazilian Childhood Co-operative Group, lymphoblastic
    leukemia 149, 190–1
Brazilian Wilms Tumor Study Group 39
busulphan–melphalan
  Ewing sarcoma 26, 32, 33
  neuroblastoma 48

C5V (cisplatin–5-fluorouracil–vincristine),
    hepatoblastoma 58, 61, 62, 63
CALLCG (Childhood ALL Collaborative Group) 181, 230,
    238–9
Cancer and Leukemia Group B (CALGB)
  Hodgkin lymphoma 109–10
  lymphoblastic leukemia 170, 174
Candida 244, 245, 246, 252–3
carboplatin
  glioma 85
  hepatoblastoma 58–9
    and doxorubicin 59
  medulloblastoma, and lomustine–vincristine 76
  see also CEM; COJEC; JEB
carcinoma
  hepatocellular 61
  papillary thyroid, dexrazoxane-associated risk 237
  renal cell 36
cardiotoxicity (of anthracyclines incl. doxorubicin) 44, 150
  protection from 150, 165, 231, 233–4, 235–8
caspofungin 245, 246, 247–8, 250, 251
catheter-related infections 246–7, 263–7
CCG *see* Children's Cancer Group
CCNU *see* lomustine
CCSG *see* Children's Cancer Study Group
cefepime
  vs meropenem 262–3
  vs piperacillin–tazobactam 262
cefoperazone–sulbactam vs piperacillin–tazobactam 256–7
cefozopran vs piperacillin/tazobactam 253–4
ceftazidime vs meropenem 259–60
ceftriaxone–amikacin 261
  amoxicillin–clavulanate and ofloxacin vs 257–8
  ± ciprofloxacin 261
CEM (carboplatin–etoposide–melphalan),
    neuroblastoma 48
central nervous system
  non-Hodgkin lymphoma 99–100
  prophylaxis (chemotherapy and/or craniospinal/
    neuraxial radiation)
    acute lymphoblastic leukemia 150, 156, 165–6,
      168–78, 182, 200
    acute myeloid leukemia 123, 144–5
    medulloblastoma 70, 71, 74, 76–7, 78–9
    non-Hodgkin lymphoma 89–90, 94
  relapse rate in lymphoblastic leukemia 196

central venous catheter infections 246–7, 263–7
CESS *see* Co-operative Ewing's Sarcoma Study; European Intergroup Cooperative Ewing's Sarcoma Study
chemoradiotherapy
    Ewing sarcoma 27
    glioma 85–6
    Hodgkin lymphoma 106, 107, 109, 110, 111
    medulloblastoma 78
chemotherapy
    acute lymphoblastic leukemia
        continuation/maintenance therapy 149, 180–97
        induction therapy 147–8, 154–67
        long-term effects 150
        new agents 150–1
        postinduction therapy 148, 148–9, 168–97, 204–6
        relapsed patients 198–203
    acute myeloid leukemia 141
        consolidation therapy 121–2, 135–6
        induction 119–21, 126–34
    cardiotoxicity of anthracyclines *see* cardiotoxicity
    Ewing sarcoma 25–32, 240, 241
    germ cell tumors 65–8
    glioma 82–3, 85–6
    hepatoblastoma 58–64, 241
    intrathecal *see* intrathecal therapy
    lymphoma
        Hodgkin 105, 106–8, 109–12, 113–15
        non-Hodgkin 88–104, 241
    medulloblastoma 69–77
    neuroblastoma 50, 51, 53, 54, 55
        induction 47, 50, 51, 53, 54
    osteosarcoma 14–16, 18–20, 22–4
    rhabdomyosarcoma 3, 4–5, 8–10, 240, 241
    veno-occlusive disease caused by *see* hepatic veno-occlusive disease
    Wilms tumor 34–46, 230, 240, 241
    see also myeloablative (chemo)therapy
Childhood ALL Collaborative Group (CALLCG) 181, 230, 238–9
Children's Cancer and Leukemia Study Group, Japanese 182–3
Children's Cancer Group, North American (CCG)
    germ cell tumors 65, 66
    glioma 81–2, 82, 85–6
    hepatoblastoma 58, 61
    leukemia
        acute myeloid 119, 120, 121, 122, 126, 126–7, 127, 129, 137–8, 142
        lymphoblastic 155, 157, 163, 168, 169, 171, 172, 173, 173–4, 181, 181–2, 193–6, 195–6, 204–5, 205–6
    lymphoma
        Hodgkin 107, 110–11
        non-Hodgkin 91, 91–2, 94, 94–5, 97, 99
    medulloblastoma 65, 70, 74, 75–6
    neuroblastoma 51, 53–4, 55
    osteosarcoma 20
Children's Cancer Group, Tokyo, lymphoblastic leukemia 156, 169

Children's Cancer Study Group (UKCCSG)
    G-CSF use 213, 215
    germ cell tumors 65, 66
    hepatoblastoma 58, 64
    leukemia
        acute myeloid 126
        lymphoblastic 171, 171–2, 192
    lymphoma
        Hodgkin 109, 110
        non-Hodgkin 88, 89, 97, 99
    medulloblastoma 74, 76
    osteosarcoma 18–19
    Wilms tumor 34–5, 45–6
Children's Leukemia Cooperative Group of EORTC 172, 187–8
Children's Oncology Group (COG)
    Ewing's sarcoma 25, 26, 29, 31
    germ cell tumours 66, 67
    glioma 81, 82, 83
    hepatoblastoma 63
    leukemia
        acute myeloid 120, 122, 129
        lymphoblastic 147, 148, 162–3, 189, 193–5, 201–2, 204–6
    lymphoma
        Hodgkin 107, 111, 114–15
        non-Hodgkin 90, 91, 91–2
    medulloblastoma 81
    neuroblastoma 47, 48, 53–4, 56
    osteosarcoma 14, 15, 22
    rhabdomyosarcoma 4, 5, 11, 12–13
    Wilms tumor 36
CHOP (cyclophosphamide–doxorubicin–vincristine–prednisone) 05, 88, 89, 91, 94
cilastatin–imipenem vs piperacillin–tazobactam 253–4
ciprofloxacin–ceftriaxone–amikacin 261
cisplatin
    germ cell tumors 65, 66
    hepatoblastoma 59, 63–4
        and doxorubicin 59, 61, 63–4
    medulloblastoma
        with cyclophosphamide–vincristine 71, 79
        with lomustine–vincristine 70, 71, 76, 79
        in vincristine–methylprednisolone–lomustine–hydroxyurea–procarbazine–cisplatin–cyclophosphamide–cytarabine (8 drugs in one day regimen) 70, 74
    neuroblastoma, and teniposide 50
    osteosarcoma
        with doxorubicin 19
        with doxorubicin–methotrexate 20
        intra-arterial 19–20
    see also AP; BCD; BEP; COJEC; doxorubicin–methotrexate–cisplatin; PVB
13-cis-retinoic acid (isotretinoin), neuroblastoma 47, 48, 50, 51, 53, 54, 56, 57
cladribine–cytarabine, acute myeloid leukemia 130–1

clear cell sarcoma of kidney (CCSK) 36, 41
co-amoxiclav (amoxicillin–clavulanate) and ofloxacin vs
  ceftriaxone–amikacin 257–8
COG see Children's Oncology Group
COJEC (cisplatin–vincristine–carboplatin–etoposide–
  cyclophosphamide), neuroblastoma 48, 53, 57, 223
colony-stimulating factors (CSFs) 209–29
  granulocyte see granulocyte-colony stimulating factor
  granulocyte macrophage 219–20
COMP (cyclophosphamide–vincristine–
  methotrexate–prednisone)
  Hodgkin lymphoma 113–14
  non-Hodgkin lymphoma 89, 91, 94, 95, 96
  see also ADCOMP; DCOMP
congestive heart failure with anthracyclines 44, 242
consolidation therapy
  acute myeloid leukemia 121–2, 135–6
  antifungal prophylaxis 252–3
continuation therapy, acute lymphoblastic leukemia 149,
  180–97
Co-operative Ewing's Sarcoma Study (CESS-86) 27
  see also EICESS-92
Co-operative Study Group for Childhood Acute
  Lymphoblastic Leukaemia (COALL) 183, 195–6
COPAD (cyclophosphamide–vincristine–prednisolone–
  doxorubicin), non-Hodgkin lymphoma 89
COPAdM (cyclophosphamide–vincristine–prednisolone–
  doxorubicin–methotrexate), non-Hodgkin
  lymphoma 97, 98, 99, 100
COPP (cyclophosphamide–vincristine–procarbazine–
  prednisolone), Hodgkin lymphoma 107, 111
  see also ACOPP
corticosteroids see steroids and specific types
COSS group (German), osteosarcoma 15, 18, 19
craniospinal radiation, medulloblastoma 70, 71, 74, 76–7,
  78–9
CSFs see colony-stimulating factors
CVPP (cyclophosphamide–vinblastine–procarbazine–
  prednisone), Hodgkin lymphoma 106, 110
cyclophosphamide
  Ewing sarcoma 29–30
  and topotecan 26, 31, 32
  germ cell tumors, added to BEP 66
  medulloblastoma
    with vincristine 74
    with vincristine–cisplatin 71, 79
    with vincristine–methylprednisolone–lomustine–
      hydroxyurea–procarbazine–cisplatin–cytarabine
      (8 drugs in one day regimen) 70, 74
  neuroblastoma
    and doxorubicin 50
    and topotecan 55
  see also ACOP; A-COPP; ADCOMP; BCD; CHOP;
    COMP; COP; COPAD; COPAdM; COPP; CVPP;
    DCOMP; VAC; VACA; VDC; VTC
cyclosporin A to modulate P-glycoprotein in acute myeloid
  leukemia 135–6

cytarabine (ARAC; cytosine arabinoside) 120
  acute lymphoblastic leukemia 197, 204
    high-dose 175–6, 197
    intermediate-dose 197
    intrathecal 163, 171, 173, 173–4, 200
  acute myeloid leukemia 121–2, 126, 127, 128, 130,
    131–2, 133, 134, 135, 137, 138, 141, 142, 144
    with cladribine 130–1
    in CNS prophylaxis 123
    with daunorubicin 119
    with daunorubicin and etoposide (ADE) 119, 120,
      127, 132, 144
    with daunorubicin and thioguanine
      (DAT) 120, 127, 135, 141
    with fludarabine and idarubicin (AIE) 129–30
    with gemtuzumab ozogamicin (GO) 121–2
    with idarubicin and etoposide see idarubicin
    intrathecal 126, 127, 128, 132, 141, 144
    with mitoxantrone (HAM) 121, 127, 137, 144, 224
  medulloblastoma, in 8 drugs in one day regimen
    of vincristine–methylprednisolone–lomustine–
    hydroxyurea–procarbazine–cisplatin–
    cyclophosphamide–cytarabine 70, 74
  non-Hodgkin lymphoma, with etoposide
    (CYVE) 90, 95
cytogenetics
  acute lymphoblastic leukemia 163
    subtypes 146, 149, 151, 161
  acute myeloid leukemia 133, 226
cytokine use, neuroblastoma 47–8, 56–7
cytosine arabinoside see cytarabine
CYVE (cytarabine and etoposide), non-Hodgkin
  lymphoma 90, 99

dactinomycin D see actinomycin D; BCD; IVA; VA; VAC;
  VACA; VAIA
Dana-Farber Cancer Institute (DFCI) ALL
  Consortium 233, 235–6
  protocol 91-01 and 95-01 166–7, 190
  protocol 95-01 165–6
dasatinib 151
DAT (daunorubicin–ARAC-thioguanine) 120, 127,
  135, 141
daunomycin/daunorubicin (DNR)
  acute dexrazoxane 238, 239
  acute myeloid leukemia 126, 127, 128, 133, 134, 138, 141
    with cytarabine (ARAC) 119
    with cytarabine-etoposide 119, 144
    with cytarabine-thioguanine (DAT) 120, 127, 135, 141
    with etoposide 119–20
  non-Hodgkin lymphoma, with COMP (D-COMP) 95
  see also DCTER; IdaDCTER
DCOMP (daunomycin-COMP), non-Hodgkin
  lymphoma 95
DCTER (daunorubicin–cytarabine–etoposide–
  thioguanine–dexamethasone), acute myeloid
  leukemia 119, 121, 126–7

dexamethasone in lymphoblastic leukemia 154–5, 156, 159,
        160, 164, 186, 187, 191, 192
    see also DCTER
dexrazoxane (DXN) 150, 165, 231, 233–4, 235–8
diffuse large B-cell lymphoma (DBLCL) 88, 91, 95, 97, 98,
        99, 100
doxorubicin (Adriamycin)
    acute lymphoblastic leukemia 238, 239
    cardiotoxicity see cardiotoxicity
    hepatoblastoma
        and carboplatin 59
        and cisplatin 59, 61, 63–4
    neuroblastoma, and cyclophosphamide 50
    rhabdomyosarcoma 5
    Wilms tumor 35, 43–4
    see also ABV; ABVD; ACOP; A-COPP; ADCOMP;
        AOPE; AP; APO; AVA; CHOP; COPAD;
        COPAdM; DCOMP; MAP; OPA; VACA;
        VAIA; VDC; VIDE
doxorubicin–methotrexate, osteosarcoma 18, 19, 20
doxorubicin–methotrexate–cisplatin, osteosarcoma 20, 22–4
    and ifosfamide 22–4
dressing changes with central venous lines 266, 267
Dutch Leukaemia Study Group
    ALL VII protocol 167
    ALL VIII protocol 184
    see also Italian–Dutch–Hungarian-ALL-91 trial

Eastern Cooperative Oncology Group (ECOG) trial
        (E1900), acute myeloid leukemia 121–2
ECOG trial (E1900), acute myeloid leukemia 121–2
EDTA (edetic acid) see ethylene diamine tetra-acetic acid
EICESS-92 study 25, 26, 29–30
EICNHL group 89, 91, 100–2
Einhorn regimen (with cisplatin), germ cell tumors 65
epirubicin in lymphoblastic leukemia 160–1
Erwinia asparaginase
    lymphoblastic leukemia 184
        compared with other forms 156–7, 165–6, 190
    T-cell leukemia/lymphoma 160–1
        compared with other forms 95, 165–7, 202–3
erythropoietin (EPO) 211, 220–2
Escherichia coli asparaginase
    lymphoblastic leukemia 183, 184, 190
        compared with other forms 156–7, 165–7, 190, 202–3
    T-cell leukemia/lymphoma, compared with other
        forms 95, 202–3
ethylene diamine tetra-acetic acid (edetic acid; EDTA)
    cyclic derivative (dexrazoxane; DXN) 150, 165, 231,
        233–4, 235–8
    minocycline and, as central line locking solution 246,
        264–5
etoposide (VP-16)
    acute myeloid leukemia 142
        with cytarabine and daunorubicin 119, 120, 127, 132, 144
        with cytarabine and idarubicin see idarubicin
        with mitoxantrone or daunorubicin 119–20

Ewing sarcoma, and ifosfamide 25, 29–30, 31, 32
glioma 85
    see also AOPE; BEP; CEM; CYVE; DCTER; IdaDCTER;
        JEB; PVB; VIDE; VIE
EURAMOS 15, 16
Euro-Ewing-99 25–6
European Intergroup for Childhood NHL (EICNHL) 89,
        91, 100–2
European Intergroup Cooperative Ewing's Sarcoma Study
        (EICESS-92) 25, 26, 29–30
European Neuroblastoma Study Group 51
European Organization for Research into Treatment of
        Cancer (EORTC)
    Children's Leukemia Cooperative Group of 172, 187–8
    lymphoblastic leukemia 156, 172, 175, 177, 183, 187–9
    non-Hodgkin lymphoma 85
    osteosarcoma 15, 18–19
European Osteosarcoma Intergroup (EOI) 15, 19, 24
European Paediatric Soft Tissue Sarcoma Group
        (EpSSG) 4, 5, 6
Ewing sarcoma 25–33
    chemotherapy 25–32, 240–1, 241

FAB/LMB group, non-Hodgkin lymphoma 89–90, 97–100
febrile neutropenia see neutropenia
filgrastim see granulocyte-colony stimulating factor
fluconazole prophylaxis
    in allogeneic stem cell transplantation 249–50
    in remission induction or consolidation
        chemotherapy 252–3
fludarabine–cytarabine–idarubicin, acute myeloid
        leukemia 129–30
5-fluorouracil (in C5V regimen), hepatoblastoma 58, 61,
        62, 63
French Pediatric Oncology Group, germ cell tumors 65
French Society for Paediatric Oncology (SFOP),
        non-Hodgkin lymphoma 88, 89, 91, 95,
        97, 99
fungal infections 244–6, 247–53

G-CSF see granulocyte-colony stimulating factor
GD2, monoclonal antibodies to, neuroblastoma 47–8, 56–7
gefitinib, glioma 83
gemtuzumab ozogamicin (GO), acute myeloid
        leukemia 120, 121, 121–2, 132
germ cell tumors 65–8
German studies
    COSS group, osteosarcoma 15, 18, 19
    GPOH group see GPO(H) group
    HIT group, medulloblastoma 70–1, 76, 79–80
glioblastoma multiforme 81, 82, 85, 86
GM-CSF (granulocyte macrophage colony-stimulating
        factor) 219–20
gonadal germ cell tumours 67
GPO(H) group
    medulloblastoma 76
    Wilms tumor 44–5

granulocyte-colony stimulating factor (G-CSF;
  filgrastim) 213–18, 223–9
  acute lymphoblastic leukemia 213–17
  acute myeloid leukemia 120, 209–10, 214, 216, 223–6
  erythropoietin plus, reducing transfusion
    requirements 220–1
  neuroblastoma 47, 56–7, 57
  non-Hodgkin lymphoma 215, 216, 216
  pegylated 210, 227–8
  receptor isoform IV 120, 210, 226
granulocyte macrophage colony-stimulating factor
  (GM-CSF) 219–20
growth factors, hematopoietic stem cell 209–29

HAM (high-dose cytarabine–mitoxantrone), acute myeloid
  leukemia 121, 127, 137, 144, 224
heart, drug toxicity see cardiotoxicity
hematopoietic stem cell growth factors 209–29
hematopoietic stem cell transplantation
  acute lymphoblastic leukemia 198, 200, 210, 216–17
  acute myeloid leukemia 122–3
    autologous 123, 141–3
  antifungal prophylaxis 248–50
  G-CSF in 216–17
  see also bone marrow transplantation
hepatic veno-occlusive disease (chemotherapy-induced)
  lymphoblastic leukemia patients 149, 193, 193–5, 196
  Wilms tumor patients 45
hepatoblastoma 58–64, 241
hepatocellular carcinoma 61
HIT group, medulloblastoma 70–1, 76, 79–80
Hodgkin lymphoma/disease 105–15, 236–8
hydrocortisone in acute lymphoblastic leukemia,
  intrathecal 173, 174
hydroxyurea, medulloblastoma, in 8 drugs in one day
    regimen of vincristine–methylprednisolone–
    lomustine–hydroxyurea–procarbazine–cisplatin–
    cyclophosphamide–cytarabine 70, 74
hyperfractionated radiotherapy
  lymphoblastic leukemia 172–3
  medulloblastoma 71

IdaDCTER (idarubicin–cytarabine–thioguanine–
    etoposide–daunorubicin), acute myeloid
    leukemia 119, 121, 129–30
idarubicin
  acute myeloid leukemia
    with cytarabine–etoposide (AIE) 119, 127, 144, 224
    with cytarabine–etoposide–thioguanine–daunorubicin
      (IdaDCTER) 119, 121, 129
    with cytarabine–fludarabine 129
  lymphoblastic leukemia 198–9, 238
IDH (Italian–Dutch–Hungarian)-ALL-91 trial 184
ifosfamide
  Ewing sarcoma 29–30
    with etoposide 25, 29–30, 31, 32
    with vincristine–dactinomycin 33

osteosarcoma 15
  with doxorubicin–methotrexate–cisplatin 22–4
  see also IVA; VAIA; VIDE; VIE
imatinib
  glioma 83
  lymphoblastic leukemia 146, 151
imipenem–cilastatin vs piperacillin–tazobactam 253–4
immunosuppression in lymphoblastic leukemia therapy 149
induction (of remission) chemotherapy
  acute lymphoblastic leukemia 146–8, 154–67
  acute myeloid leukemia 119–21, 126–34
  antifungal prophylaxis 252–3
  neuroblastoma 47, 50, 51, 53, 54
  therapy following see postremission/postinduction therapy
infections 243–67
  central venous catheter 246–7, 263–7
  risk stratification/prediction 244, 258–9
intensification therapy, lymphoblastic leukemia 148–9,
    204–6
intergroup studies
  acute lymphoblastic leukemia (IDH ALL 91) 184
  acute myeloid leukemia (INT0129) 132–4
  Ewing sarcoma 31
    INT-0091 25, 26, 27, 29, 31
  hepatoblastoma (P9645) 58, 62
  non-Hodgkin lymphoma, European Intergroup
    (EICNHL) 89, 91, 100–2
  osteosarcoma (INT0133) 16
  rhabdomyosarcoma (IRSG) 3, 4, 5, 8
interleukin-2
  acute myeloid leukemia 122
  neuroblastoma 56
International Society of Paediatric Oncology (SIOP)
  European Neuroblastoma (SIOPEN) 47, 48, 57, 223
  glioma 81
  hepatoblastoma, Childhood Liver Tumour Strategy
    Group (SIOPEL) 58, 59, 60, 63
  medulloblastoma 69, 70, 70–1, 71, 74–5, 75, 76
  rhabdomyosarcoma 3
  Wilms tumor 34, 35, 36, 38, 41, 44–5, 230
intrathecal (IT) therapy (incl. methotrexate)
  acute myeloid leukemia 132, 191
  lymphoblastic leukemia 154, 156, 157, 163, 168–75, 176,
    182, 192, 193, 194, 200, 204
    types and duration 173–4
  medulloblastoma 74
  non-Hodgkin lymphoma 90, 91, 102
iproplatin, glioma 85
irinotecan
  glioma 82
  rhabdomyosarcoma 5
isotretinoin (13-cis-retinoic acid), neuroblastoma 47, 48,
    50, 51, 53, 54, 56, 57
Italian–Dutch–Hungarian (IDH)-ALL-91 trial 184
Italian Sarcoma Group/Scandinavian Sarcoma Group III
    protocol 25, 30
Italian studies see AIEOP group; Rizzoli Institute

itraconazole prophylaxis in autologous stem cell
  transplantation 248–9
IVA/VIA (ifosfamide–vincristine–actinomycin D)
  germ cell tumors 66
  rhabdomyosarcoma 5, 9
  see also VAIA

Japanese Children's Cancer and Leukemia Study Group 182–3
JEB (carboplatin–etoposide–bleomycin), germ cell tumors 65

kidney
  non-Wilms tumors 36
  resection (nephrectomy), Wilms tumor 34, 35, 36, 38,
    39, 40, 41, 45
  Wilms tumors 34–46, 230, 240, 241

large cell lymphoma
  anaplastic (ALCL) 88, 89, 91, 95, 100–3
  diffuse (DBLCL) 88, 91, 95, 97, 98, 99, 100
leukemia 119–206
  acute lymphoblastic *see* lymphoblastic leukemia
  acute myeloid *see* acute myeloid leukemia
liposomal amphotericin 245, 246, 247–8, 251
liposomal muramyl tripeptide phosphatidyl ethanolamine
    (MTP-PE; Mifurtimide) 14, 16, 20, 22–4
liver
  transplantation with hepatoblastoma 59
  tumors 58–64, 241
  see also hepatic veno-occlusive disease
lomustine (CCNU)
  glioma, and prednisolone–vincristine 85–6
  medulloblastoma
    with vincristine 70, 74–5
      and carboplatin 76
      and cisplatin 70, 71, 76, 79
      and methylprednisolone–lomustine–hydroxyurea–
        procarbazine–cisplatin–cyclophosphamide–
        cytarabine (8 drugs in one day regimen) 70, 74
      and prednisolone 74
      and prednisolone–vincristine 74
lumbar puncture, traumatic 148
lymphoblastic leukemia, acute (ALL) 99–100, 146–206,
    240, 241
  anthracyclines in *see* anthracyclines
  CNS prophylaxis 150, 168–78
  erythropoietin 222
  G-CSF in 213–17
  GM-CSF in 219
  long-term effects of therapies 150
  maintenance/continuation therapy 149, 180–97
  postremission/postinduction therapy 148–9, 168–97
    adolescents and young adults 149, 204–6
  relapsed 150, 196, 198–203
    prediction of relapse 162
    prediction of survival in 201–2
  remission induction 146–8, 154–67
lymphoblastic lymphoma 90, 94, 95, 175, 215

lymphoma 88–115
  Hodgkin 105–15, 236–8
  non-Hodgkin *see* non-Hodgkin lymphoma

maintenance therapy
  acute lymphoblastic leukemia (=continuation
    therapy) 149, 180–97
  acute myeloid leukemia 122–3, 133, 137–9
MAP (mitoxantrone–doxorubicin–cisplatin),
    osteosarcoma 15, 16
Mayo clinic, osteosarcoma 14
mechlorethamine (mustine)–vincristine–procarbazine–
    prednisone, Hodgkin lymphoma 113
  see also MOPP; MOPP-B
Medical Research Council (MRC) studies
  acute myeloid leukemia 119–20, 120, 121, 122, 127
  lymphoblastic leukemia *see* UK ALL trials
  osteosarcoma 18–19
Medical Research Council/National Cancer Research Network
    Childhood Leukaemia Working Party 192
medulloblastoma 69–77
melphalan
  Ewing sarcoma, with busulphan 26, 32, 33
  neuroblastoma, with busulphan 48
  rhabdomyosarcoma 5
  see also CEM; VM
Memorial Sloan-Kettering Cancer Center
  lymphoblastic leukemia 155, 169
  osteosarcoma 15, 19
6-mercaptopurine, lymphoblastic leukemia 149, 155, 160,
    183, 186, 187, 190–1, 192–6
  with methotrexate 180, 181–2, 182–3, 183, 186, 187,
    189, 190–1
  6-thioguanine compared with 192–6
meropenem
  amikacin plus, vs piperacillin/tazobactam and
    netilmicin 263
  cefipime vs 262–3
  ceftazidime vs 259–60
methotrexate
  lymphoblastic leukemia 161–4, 182, 189–91, 204
    escalating-dose 162–4
    high-dose 161–2, 174–5, 175, 189–91, 197, 200, 201
    intermediate-dose 174–5, 189–91
    intrathecal 154, 156, 157, 163, 168–75, 182, 192, 193,
      194, 200
    with 6-mercaptopurine 180, 181–2, 182–3, 183, 186,
      187, 189, 190–1
  medulloblastoma, with vincristine 74
  non-Hodgkin lymphoma 88–9, 90, 95–6, 97, 99,
    100–2
  osteosarcoma, with other agents 18, 19, 20
  route and dose 182
  see also ADCOMP; COMP; COPAdM; DCOMP;
    doxorubicin–methotrexate; doxorubicin–
    methotrexate–cisplatin; procarbazine–
    methotrexate–vincristine

methylprednisolone
    lymphoblastic leukemia 154
    medulloblastoma (in 8 drugs in one day regimen
        of vincristine–methylprednisolone–lomustine–
        hydroxyurea–procarbazine–cisplatin–
        cyclophosphamide–cytarabine) 70, 74
Mifurtimide (muramyl tripeptide phosphatidyl
    ethanolamine), liposomal 14, 16, 20, 22–4
minimal residual disease detection in lymphoblastic
    leukemia 149–50
minocycline and edetic acid as central line locking
    solution 246, 264–5
mitoxantrone
    acute myeloid leukemia
      and cytarabine 121, 127, 137, 144, 224
      and etoposide 119–20
    lymphoblastic leukemia 198–9
    osteosarcoma, and doxorubicin–cisplatin (MAP) 15, 16
MMT (malignant mesenchymal tumours) studies 3, 5, 6
monoclonal antibodies
    acute myeloid leukemia 120, 132
    neuroblastoma 47–8, 56–7
    non-Hodgkin's lymphoma 92
MOPP (mustine–vincristine–procarbazine–prednisolone)
    glioma 85
    Hodgkin lymphoma 105, 106, 107, 109, 110, 111
    medulloblastoma 75
MOPP-B (mustine–vincristine–procarbazine–
    prednisolone-bleomycin), Hodgkin
    lymphoma 106, 109
MRC see Medical Research Council
muramyl tripeptide phosphatidyl ethanolamine (MTP-PE),
    liposomal (Mifurtimide) 14, 16, 20, 22–4
mustine (mechlorethamine)–vincristine–procarbazine–
    prednisone, Hodgkin lymphoma 113
    see also MOPP; MOPP-B
myeloablative (chemo)therapy, neuroblastoma 47–8, 50–1,
    53–5
myelodysplastic syndrome and AML see acute myeloid
    leukemia/myelodysplastic syndrome
myeloid leukemia, acute see acute myeloid leukemia
myelosuppression
    CSFs in management of see colony-stimulating factors
    dexrazoxane-induced 231
    in lymphoblastic leukemia therapy 149

National Wilms Tumor Study Group (NWTS;
    NWTSG) 34, 39–41, 43–4
    NWTS-1 39
    NWTS-2 39
    NWTS-3 39–40, 43, 44
    NWTS-4 40, 43, 44
    NWTS-5 35, 41
neoadjuvant (preoperative) therapy
    medulloblastoma 71, 76
    osteosarcoma 18
    Wilms tumor 35, 36, 38, 39, 41, 43–4, 45–6

nephrectomy, Wilms tumor 34, 35, 36, 38, 39, 40, 41, 45
neuraxial radiation see central nervous system
neuroblastoma 47-57m 223–4
neuroectodermal tumor, primitive 31–2, 85
neutropenia, febrile (FBN) 243–63
    G-CSF 215, 216, 217, 218, 223, 225, 228, 229
non-Hodgkin lymphoma 88–104, 187–8, 241
    G-CSF use 215, 216, 216
    lymphoblastic lymphoma 90, 94, 95, 175, 215
nystatin prophylaxis in remission induction or
    consolidation chemotherapy 252–3

ofloxacin and amoxicillin–clavulanate vs
    ceftriaxone–amikacin 257–8
oligodendroglioma, anaplastic 81–2
OPA (vincristine–prednisolone–doxorubicin), Hodgkin
    lymphoma 113–14
OPP (vincristine–procarbazine–prednisolone), glioma 85
osteosarcoma (osteogenic sarcoma) 14–24
    dexrazoxane-associated risk 237

P-glycoprotein modulation with cyclosporin A in acute
    myeloid leukemia 135–6
papillary thyroid carcinoma, dexrazoxane-associated
    risk 237
PCV (prednisolone–lomustine/CCNU–vincristine)
    glioma 85–6
    medulloblastoma 74
    see also MOPP
Pediatric Oncology Group, French (SFOP), germ cell
    tumors 65
Pediatric Oncology Group, North American (POG)
    Ewing tumor 26, 27, 29, 31
    germ cell tumours 65, 67
    glioma 82, 85, 86
    hepatoblastoma 58, 61
    leukemia
      acute lymphoblastic 189
      acute myeloid 120, 121, 122, 135–6, 141
    lymphoma
      Hodgkin 107, 109–10, 114, 236–8
      non-Hodgkin 91, 94, 95
    medulloblastoma 70, 75
    neuroblastoma 50
    osteosarcoma 14, 18, 20
    rhabdomyosarcoma 4, 8, 9
Pediatric Oncology Group, Taiwan, lymphoblastic
    leukemia 160–1
pegylated formulation
    asparaginase, in lymphoblastic leukemia 157, 163, 166,
      167, 190, 192, 201, 202–3
    G-CSF 210, 227–8
pharmacology (pharmacokinetics and
    pharmacodynamics)
    asparaginase 202–3
      recombinant 164–5
    methotrexate 161

Philadelphia chromosome-positive lymphoblastic
        leukemia 146
    older patients 149
piperacillin–tazobactam 254–5
    amikacin plus see amikacin
    cefipime vs 262
    cefoperazone–sulbactam vs 256–7
    cefozopran vs 253–4
    imipenem–cilastatin vs 253–4
    netilmicin plus, vs meropenem–amikacin 263
platinum therapy, intensified, hepatoblastoma 58–9, 62–3
    see also carboplatin; cisplatin; iproplatin
PNET-3 and -4 trials 70, 71, 76
POG see Pediatric Oncology Group
polyglutamates, methotrexate (accumulation in
        leukemia cells) 162
    assessment 161
    relapse prediction 162
postoperative therapy see adjuvant therapy'
postremission/postinduction therapy
    acute lymphoblastic leukemia see lymphoblastic
        leukemia, acute
    acute myeloid leukemia 121–3, 135–43
prednisolone in lymphoblastic leukemia 146–7,
        154–5, 156, 200
    see also ACOP; AOPE; COP; COPAD; COPAdM;
        COPP; MOPP; OPA; PCV
prednisone in lymphoblastic leukemia 159–60
    see also A-COPP; ADCOMP; APO; CHOP; COMP; CVPP;
        DCOMP; mechlorethamine–vincristine–
        procarbazine–prednisone
preoperative therapy see neoadjuvant therapy
PRETEXT criteria 59, 63
primitive neuroectodermal tumor 31–2, 85
procarbazine–methotrexate–vincristine,
        medulloblastoma 70
    see also A-COPP; CVPP; mechlorethamine–vincristine–
        procarbazine–prednisone; MOPP; MOPP-B; OPP
promyelocytic leukemia, acute 120–1, 132–4, 138–9
Pseudomonas 244
purine de novo synthesis, measurement (with high-dose
        methotrexate infusion) 161, 162
PVB (cisplatin–vinblastine–bleomycin), germ
        cell tumors 65

radiation therapy (RT)
    in CNS prophylaxis see central nervous system
    glioma 82, 86
    lymphoma
        Hodgkin 105, 105–6, 109–11
        non-Hodgkin 89–90, 94–5
    medulloblastoma 69, 70–2, 74–6, 78–9
    rhabdomyosarcoma 3, 5–6, 8, 9
    Wilms tumor 34, 35, 36, 38, 39–40
    see also chemoradiotherapy
Radiation Therapy Oncology Group,
        medulloblastoma 69, 70, 74

relapse
    acute lymphoblastic leukemia see lymphoblastic leukemia
    acute myeloid leukemia, G-CSF therapy and G-CSF
        receptor isoform IV and risk of 120, 210, 226
remission
    induction see induction chemotherapy
    therapy after see postremission/postinduction therapy
renal cell carcinoma 36
retinoids
    acute promyelocytic leukemia 120–1, 132–4, 138–9
    neuroblastoma 47, 48, 50, 51, 53, 54, 56, 57
rhabdoid tumor, malignant 36, 40, 43
rhabdomyosarcoma 3–12, 240, 241
Rizzoli Institute, osteosarcoma 15

St Jude group
    acute myeloid leukemia 130, 225
    G-CSF 214, 225
    non-Hodgkin lymphoma 88, 94, 95
sarcoma 240–1, 241
    clear cell, kidney (CCSK)36 41
    erythropoietin use 221, 222
    Ewing 25–33
    GM-CSF use 219, 220
    osteogenic see osteosarcoma
    soft tissue 3–12
    undifferentiated 5, 6, 8, 11, 12, 240, 241
secondary malignant neoplasm (SMN) risk
    with dexrazoxane 231, 235–7
    with G-CSF 210
    with thiopurines 195, 196
SIOP and SIOPEN see International Society of
        Paediatric Oncology
soft tissue sarcoma 3–12
spinal radiation see central nervous system
stem cell, hematopoietic see bone marrow transplantation;
        hematopoietic stem cell growth factors;
        hematopoietic stem cell transplantation
steroids in lymphoblastic leukemia 146–7, 154–6,
        159–60
    pulses 181–2, 186–9
    see also specific types
sulbactam–cefoperazone vs piperacillin–tazobactam 256–7
Summary of previous studies
surgery
    glioma 81–2
    hepatoblastoma 59
    osteosarcoma 18
    Wilms tumor 35, 36
    see also adjuvant (postoperative) therapy;
        neoadjuvant therapy

T-cell acute lymphoblastic leukemia, G-CSF 215
T-cell lymphoma/leukemia 88, 89, 91, 95, 103
    G-CSF 215, 217
Taiwan Pediatric Oncology Group 160–1
    lymphoblastic leukemia 160–1

Tata Memorial Hospital (Mumbai), Hodgkin
    lymphoma 111–12
tazobactam *see* piperacillin–tazobactam
temozolomide, glioma 82
teniposide–cisplatin, neuroblastoma 50
testicular germ cell tumours 67
6-thioguanine (6-TG)
    in acute myeloid leukemia *see* DAT; DCTER; IdaDCTER
    in lymphoblastic leukemia 149, 183, 192–3
        6-mercaptopurine compared with 192–6
thiopurines in lymphoblastic leukemia, comparisons
        between different types 183, 192–6
    see also 6-mercaptopurine; 6-thioguanine
thrombopoietin (TPO) 211
thyroid carcinoma, papillary, dexrazoxane-associated risk 237
tipofarnib, glioma 83
Tokyo Children's Cancer Group, lymphoblastic
    leukemia 156, 169
topotecan
    Ewing sarcoma 31, 32
      and cyclophosphamide 26, 31, 32
    neuroblastoma, and cyclophosphamide 55
    rhabdomyosarcoma 11
    see also VTC
transfusion requirements, erythropoietin reducing 220–1
troponin T levels and dexrazoxane 233
tyrosine kinase inhibitors, lymphoblastic leukemia 146, 151

UK ALL trials 180–1
    97 and 97/99 192, 195–6
    I/II/III 180
    V 180, 183
    VII 168, 169, 182
    VIII 180–1
UK Children's Cancer Study Group *see* Children's Cancer
    Study Group
UKW-3 study 35–6, 45
undifferentiated tumors *see* anaplastic/undifferentiated
    tumors
urokinase with central venous lines 246, 266, 267

VA (vincristine–actinomycin D)
    rhabdomyosarcoma 5
    Wilms tumor 34, 39, 40, 45
VAC (vincristine–actinomycin D–cyclophosphamide)
    Ewing sarcoma 25, 26, 27
    germ cell tumors 65
    rhabdomyosarcoma 4, 5, 8, 9–10
VACA (vincristine–actinomycin D–
        cyclophosphamide–doxorubicin)
    Ewing sarcoma 25, 27, 30
    germ cell tumors 65
VAIA (vincristine–doxorubicin–ifosfamide–dactinomycin),
    Ewing sarcoma 25, 27

VDC (vincristine–doxorubicin–cyclophosphamide), Ewing
    sarcoma 27, 31, 32
veno-occlusive disease *see* hepatic veno-occlusive disease
venous catheter infections, central 246–7, 263–7
VIA *see* IVA
VIDE (vincristine–ifosfamide–doxorubicin–etoposide),
    Ewing sarcoma 26, 33
VIE (ifosfamide–vincristine–etoposide),
    rhabdomyosarcoma 4, 9
vinblastine
    germ cell tumors (in PVB regimen) 65
    non-Hodgkin lymphoma 91–2
      anaplastic large cell lymphoma 102–4
    see also ABV; ABVD; CVPP
vincristine
    Ewing sarcoma, and dactinomycin–ifosfamide 33
    germ cell tumors, and lomustine 79
    glioma, and prednisolone–CCNU 85–6
    lymphoblastic leukemia 160, 163, 170, 172, 174, 181–2,
        186–9, 191, 192, 228
      pulses 16–19, 181–2, 186–9
    medulloblastoma
      with cyclophosphamide 74
      with cyclophosphamide–cisplatin 71, 79
      with lomustine 70, 74–5
      with lomustine–carboplatin 76
      with lomustine–cisplatin 70, 71, 76, 79
      with methotrexate (intrathecal) 74
      with methylprednisolone–lomustine–hydroxyurea–
        procarbazine–cisplatin–cyclophosphamide–
        cytarabine (8 drugs in one day regimen) 70, 74
      with prednisolone–lomustine (CCNU) 74
    Wilms tumor 34, 38, 39, 45
    see also ACOP; A-COPP; ADCOMP; AOPE; APO; AVA;
      C5V; CHOP; COMP; COP; COPAD; COPAdM;
      IVA;mechlorethamine–vincristine–procarbazine–
      prednisone; MOPP; MOPP-B; OPA; OPP;
      procarbazine–methotrexate–vincristine; VA;
      VAC; VACA; VAIA; VIDE; VM
vincristine–methylprednisolone–lomustine–hydroxyurea–
        procarbazine–cisplatin–cyclophosphamide–
        cytarabine (8 drugs in one day),
        medulloblastoma 70, 74
vinorelbine, rhabdomyosarcoma 5
VM, rhabdomyosarcoma 5, 9
voriconazole prophylaxis 245, 246
    allogeneic stem cell transplantation 249–50
VP-16 *see* etoposide
VTC (vincristine–topotecan–cyclophosphamide),
    rhabdomyosarcoma 11–12

Wilms tumor 34–46, 230, 240, 241

young adults, lymphoblastic leukemia 149, 204–6